WITHDRAWN

W700 PAY

D1435016

Simpson's

THE SANDERSON LIBRARY
Learning Resource Centre
Ormskirk & District General Hospital

Forensic Medicine

P009114

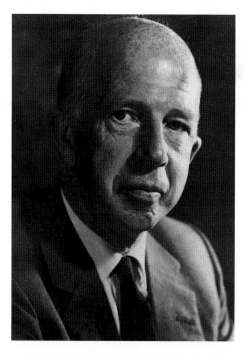

Professor CEDRIC KEITH SIMPSON CBE (1907–85)

MD (Lond), FRCP, FRCPath, MD (Gent), MA (Oxon), LLD (Edin), DMJ

Keith Simpson was the first Professor of Forensic Medicine in the University of London and undoubtedly one of the most eminent forensic pathologists of the twentieth century. He spent all his professional life at Guy's Hospital and he became a household name through his involvement in many notorious murder trials in Britain and overseas. He was made a Commander of the British Empire in 1975.

He was a superb teacher, through both the spoken and the printed word. The first edition of this book appeared in 1947 and in 1958 won the Swiney Prize of the Royal Society of Arts for being the best work on medical jurisprudence to appear in the preceding ten years.

Keith Simpson updated this book for seven further editions. Professor Bernard Knight worked with him on the ninth edition and, after Professor Simpson's death in 1985, updated the text for the tenth and eleventh editions. Richard Shepherd updated *Simpson's Forensic Medicine* for its twelfth edition in 2003.

Simpson's
Forensic Medicine

13th Edition

Jason Payne-James LLM MSc FRCS FFFLM FFSSoc DFM
Consultant Forensic Physician and Honorary Senior Lecturer, Cameron
Forensic Medical Sciences, Barts and The London School of Medicine
and Dentistry, London; Director, Forensic Healthcare Services Ltd, UK

Richard Jones BSc(Hons) MBBS FRCPath MCIEH MFSSoc MFFLM
Home Office Pathologist working at the Wales Institute of Forensic
Medicine, University Hospital of Wales, Cardiff, Wales, UK

Steven B Karch MD FFFLM FFSSoc
Consultant Cardiac Pathologist and Toxicologist, Berkeley, California, USA

John Manlove BA MSc DIC PhD FFSSoc
Manlove Forensics Ltd, Wantage, Oxon, UK

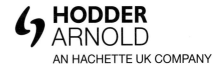
**HODDER
ARNOLD**
AN HACHETTE UK COMPANY

First published in Great Britain in 1947 by Edward Arnold
This thirteenth edition published in 2011 by
Hodder Arnold, an imprint of Hodder Education, a division of Hachette UK
338 Euston Road, London NW1 3BH
http://www.hodderarnold.com

© 2011 Hodder & Stoughton Ltd

All rights reserved. Apart from any use permitted under UK copyright law, this publication may only be reproduced, stored or transmitted, in any form, or by any means with prior permission in writing of the publishers or in the case of reprographic production in accordance with the terms of licences issued by the Copyright Licensing Agency. In the United Kingdom such licences are issued by the Copyright Licensing Agency: Saffron House, 6-10 Kirby Street, London EC1N 8TS.

Whilst the advice and information in this book are believed to be true and accurate at the date of going to press, neither the author[s] nor the publisher can accept any legal responsibility or liability for any errors or omissions that may be made. In particular (but without limiting the generality of the preceding disclaimer) every effort has been made to check drug dosages; however it is still possible that errors have been missed. Furthermore, dosage schedules are constantly being revised and new side-effects recognized. For these reasons the reader is strongly urged to consult the drug companies' printed instructions before administering any of the drugs recommended in this book.

British Library Cataloguing in Publication Data
A catalogue record for this book is available from the British Library

Library of Congress Cataloging-in-Publication Data
A catalog record for this book is available from the Library of Congress

ISBN-13   978 0 340 986 035
ISBN-13 [ISE]   978 0 340 986 042 (International Students' Edition, restricted territorial availability)

In order that we can ensure that students continue to benefit from the availability of our special editions, if you have purchased an ISE copy of this book in an un-authorized country, please email exportenquiries@hodder.co.uk letting us know where, when and from which organization or individual you made the purchase.

1 2 3 4 5 6 7 8 9 10

Commissioning Editor: Caroline Makepeace
Project Editor: Joanna Silman
Production Controller: Kate Harris
Cover Designer: Helen Townson
Indexer: Laurence Errington

Cover image © Ashley Cooper Visuals Unlimited, Science Photo Library

Typeset in 9.5/12 Boton by MPS Limited, a Macmillan Company
Printed and bound in India

What do you think about this book? Or any other Hodder Arnold title?
Please visit our website: www.hodderarnold.com

Contents

About the authors

Jason Payne-James qualified in medicine in 1980 at the London Hospital Medical College. He is a forensic physician and has undertaken additional postgraduate education to higher degree level at Cardiff Law School, the Department of Forensic Medicine and Science at the University of Glasgow and with the University of Ulster, Northern Ireland.

He is external Consultant to the National Policing Improvement Agency and to the National Injuries Database. He is Editor-in-Chief of the Journal of Forensic and Legal Medicine. His forensic medicine clinical and research interests include healthcare of detainees, deaths, harm and near-misses in custody, torture, drugs and alcohol, wound and injury interpretation, sexual assault, neglect, non-accidental injury, restraint and use of force injury, police complaints and age estimation.

He has co-edited, co-authored or contributed to a number of other books including the *Encyclopedia of Forensic & Legal Medicine, Forensic Medicine: Clinical & Pathological Aspects, Symptoms and Signs of Substance Misuse, Artificial Nutrition Support in Clinical Practice, Symptoms and Early Warning Signs, Dr Apple's Symptoms Encyclopaedia, Medico-legal Essentials of Healthcare, Colour Atlas of Forensic Medicine, Age Estimation in the Living – a Practitioner's Guide, Current Practice in Forensic Medicine* and the *Oxford Handbook of Forensic Medicine*.

Richard Jones qualified in Environmental Health in 1994 at the University of Wales (Cardiff Institute of Higher Education), and in medicine in 2002 at Guy's, King's and St Thomas' School of Medicine, London. His postgraduate medical training was in histopathology and forensic pathology and his name appears on the current Home Office Register of Forensic Pathologists. He is the author of *Forensic Medicine for Medical Students*, an educational website (www.forensicmed.co.uk)

Steven B Karch received his undergraduate degree from Brown University, Rhode Island. He attended graduate school in anatomy and cell biology at Stanford. He has an MD from Tulane University and did postgraduate training in neuropathology at the Royal London Hospital and in cardiac pathology at Stanford.

He has published twelve books and is at work on several more, including a novel on Napoleon and his doctors. He was a Forensic Science Editor for Humana Press is now an associate editor for the *Journal of Forensic and Legal Medicine* and the *Journal of Cardiovascular Toxicology*.

John Manlove graduated from Oxford University in 1993 with a degree in biological sciences (1993) from. He has postgraduate qualifications from Imperial College and London (Birkbeck) University. He is one of the Directors of MFL (Manlove Forensics Ltd), an independent forensic provider based in South Oxfordshire providing services across the criminal justice spectrum.

He has been appointed to the position of Honorary Senior Lecturer at Dundee University in the School of Life Sciences and is currently on the council of BAHID (British Association of Human Identification). He is a Fellow of the Forensic Science Society and on the editorial board of *Science and Justice*.

Foreword

The trust placed in forensic practitioners by those administering justice is enormous. Although practitioners provide their evidence at the behest of one party or another in cases where there is not an agreed expert, their duty to the court is clear. They must assist the court, in their reports and in any evidence they give orally, by giving their opinions impartially and honestly to the best of their ability. In all but a tiny handful of cases, this trust is rightly reposed in forensic practitioners. However when it is shown that such trust should not have been reposed or that a practitioner has betrayed the principles adhered to by all but that tiny handful, the effect on the administration of justice and on the integrity of forensic practitioners can be devastating.

I therefore welcome this new edition of *Simpson's Forensic Medicine*. As it claims, it sets out the basics of forensic medicine and related forensic science specialties for those who are commencing careers in forensic medicine or forensic science, or those whose work brings them into contact with situations that require an awareness of the principles.

It is welcome to see that it takes an international perspective. Developments in forensic science and medicine are, of course, worldwide; a development in one country which may contradict the received wisdom in another is these days often seized upon by parties to litigation. Legal developments in one country are being more frequently raised in other countries. These may relate to the manner in which expert evidence is adduced or the weight accorded to it. This internationalisation of forensic practice has enormous benefits, but carries with it acute risks if there is not the strictest adherence to the ethical principles clearly expounded in this work. These days a forensic practitioner must be aware of these changes and the ever greater willingness of lawyers to seek expert opinion from overseas to support their case where none can be found within their own jurisdiction.

In these developments, it is therefore essential that lawyers understand the basic principles of the forensic science and medicine in the cases that come before them and that forensic practitioners and forensic medical practitioners understand the way in which the courts operate and their high duties to the court. This work forms an important bridge between law on the one hand and science and medicine on the other. It is a useful perspective through which to see the need to ensure that developments in the law and developments in forensic practice and forensic medicine move together with ever increasing dialogue.

Lord Justice Thomas
Vice-President of the Queen's Bench Division
and Deputy Head of Criminal Justice

Preface

Since the first edition of *Simpson's Forensic Medicine* was published in 1947 there has been general recognition that the term 'forensic medicine' has expanded considerably to embrace not only forensic pathology but also clinical forensic medicine. In addition, medical practitioners who work within these fields now require knowledge and understanding, not only of medical concepts, but also of both law and forensic science, and how they interact. Indeed, many subjects that may have been considered part of 'forensic medicine', in its old sense, have now developed their own specialties, such as forensic toxicology, forensic science, forensic odontology and forensic anthropology.

The earlier editions of Simpson's were directed predominantly at a purely medical readership. Over 20 years ago Bernard Knight recognized that the readership should and did lie beyond solely a medical readership. There has been a huge increase in the public awareness of forensic techniques and process, led by an expanding media fascination with such subjects. With this has come an increase in the numbers of those wishing to study these areas as undergraduates or subsequently as postgraduates, who may not come from a medical background. What has not changed since Keith Simpson's first edition is that the budding forensic practitioner, or the undergraduate, or the law enforcement officer, or the healthcare professional or the lawyer who wishes to study, or those who by the nature of their work, will at some stage (like it or not) become involved in forensic matters, needs to be aware of and understand the basis of forensic medicine and how it relates to the other specialties.

This, the 13th edition of *Simpson's Forensic Medicine* has been written to assist all those groups, not simply doctors, and to illustrate the basic concept of forensic medicine and related forensic specialties and provide an introduction to the concepts and the principles of practice for those commencing forensic careers, or for those whose daily workload will bring them into contact with situations that require an awareness of these matters. In addition, each chapter provides a range of suggestions for further reading (books, key scientific papers and reviews, web-based sources) about each subject which will provide further in-depth authoritative information. As we all work within multi-professional settings, it is important to have an awareness of the general principles that apply. The perspective provided in this book is generally from that of a doctor. Readers will originate from different countries and different jurisdictions. Examples of relevant regulations, law, codes and practice will generally be derived from the England and Wales jurisdictions. All readers should be aware of those that apply within their professional setting, their own country and their own jurisdiction.

There are considerable changes in content, format and layout from previous editions which we hope will clarify and expand on topics of particular current relevance. Any mistakes or misinterpretations are those of the editors who will happily receive comment and criticism on any aspect of the content. We hope that readers will find that this edition addresses their needs.

Jason Payne-James
London, February 2011

Acknowledgements

A project such as this requires the support and expertise of many, not just the editors or authors.

Jason Payne-James would like to thank colleagues and associates with whom he has collaborated in the last two decades and his family for their support and encouragement. He would also like to thank Philip Shaw, Caroline Makepeace and Joanna Silman in their respective roles at Hodder, Andy Anderson who copy-edited the text and Michèle Clarke who proofread.

Richard Jones would like to thank Mary Hassell, HM Coroner for Cardiff and the Vale of Glamorgan; and Marc Smith, Forensic Medical Photographer, Wales Institute of Forensic Medicine.

John Manlove is grateful for the contribution of Kathy Manlove, James Shackel, Samantha Pickles and Andrew Wade in the preparation of his chapters.

Authors' note

The contents of this book follow the Interpretation Act 1978, so that, unless specifically stated otherwise, words importing the masculine gender include the feminine and words importing the feminine gender include the masculine.

Examples of procedure or functions will be given predominantly from the perspective of a medical practitioner (a doctor), but many of the principles or examples stated will apply also to other professionals. All professionals should be aware of the regulations or codes of conduct that apply to their practice, and of the laws and statutes that apply in their own jurisdiction.

List of picture credits

Figures 3.1 to 3.5 Richard Jones.

Figure 3.6 Reproduced with permission from Saukko P and Knight B. *Knight's Forensic Pathology* 3rd Edition. London: Hodder Arnold, 2004.

Figures 5.9, 5.11 and 5.12 Reproduced with permission from Saukko P and Knight B. *Knight's Forensic Pathology* 3rd Edition. London: Hodder Arnold, 2004.

Figures 6.1-6.7, 6.9b, 6.10, 6.13, 6.15 Richard Jones.

Figure 6.14 Reproduced with permission of Professor E. Lignitz from Saukko P and Knight B. *Knight's Forensic Pathology* 3rd Edition. London: Hodder Arnold, 2004.

Figure 7.2a, 7.3, 7.5, 7.8, 7.12 Reproduced with permission from Saukko P and Knight B. *Knight's Forensic Pathology* 3rd Edition. London: Hodder Arnold, 2004.

Figure 7.4, 7.7, 7.10b, 7.11 Reproduced from Keeling J and Busuttil A. *Paediatric Forensic Medicine and Pathology*. London: Hodder Arnold, 2008.

Figures 8.1-8.18 and 8.20-8.36 Jason Payne-James

Figure 9.3, 9.6-9.8, 9.10, 9.12, 9.14-9.16 Richard Jones

Figure 9.1, 9.2, 9.5, 9.9, 9.11 Reproduced with permission from Saukko P and Knight B. *Knight's Forensic Pathology* 3rd Edition. London: Hodder Arnold, 2004.

Figures 10.6, 10.13 Richard Jones

Figure 10.3, 10.5, 10.7, 10.10 Reproduced with permission from Saukko P and Knight B. *Knight's Forensic Pathology* 3rd Edition. London: Hodder Arnold, 2004.

Figure 10.12 Courtesy of Professor TK Marshall, Queen's University, Belfast

Figures 11.1-11.9 Jason Payne-James

Figures 12 and 12.2 Jason Payne-James

Figures 13.1-13.3 Jason Payne-James

Figure 13.4 Reproduced from Hobbs CJ and Wynne JM. *Physical Signs of Child Abuse: A Color Atlas* 2nd edition. London: WB Saunders, 2001.

Figure 14.4, 14.7 Richard Jones

Figure 15.1, 15.8 Richard Jones

Figure 15.3 and 15.14 Reproduced with permission from Saukko P and Knight B. *Knight's Forensic Pathology* 3rd Edition. London: Hodder Arnold, 2004.

Figure 17.3, 17.4, 17.7, 17.8 Richard Jones

Figure 17.6 Reproduced with permission from Saukko P and Knight B. *Knight's Forensic Pathology* 3rd Edition. London: Hodder Arnold, 2004.

Figures 20.1-20.5, 20.12, 20.13 Jason Payne-James

Figures 20.7, 20.8, 20.11 Steven B Karch

Figures 20.6, 20.9, 20.10, 20.14, 20.15, 20.16, 20.17 Photographs by Dennis J Young, courtesy of the US Drug Enforcement Administration (DEA).

Figure 21.1 Steven B Karch

Figures 23.1-23.9, 23.11-23.15 Manlove Forensics Ltd

Figure 23.10 Image copyright Forensic Science Service (FSS). Reproduced with permission.

Figure 23.16 Image copyright Napier Associates Ltd. Reproduced with permission.

Figure 23.18 Image copyright Board of Trustees of the Armouries

Figure 24.1, 24.2 Manlove Forensics Ltd

Chapter

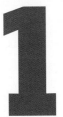

Principles of forensic practice

- Introduction
- Legal systems
- Doctors and the law
- Evidence for courts
- Doctors in court
- Further information sources

■ Introduction

Different countries have different legal systems, which broadly divide into two areas – criminal and civil. The systems have generally evolved over many years or centuries and are influenced by a wide variety of factors including culture, religion and politics. By and large, the rules have been established over many hundreds of years and are generally accepted because they are for the mutual benefit of the population – they are the framework that prevents anarchy. Although there are some common rules (for example concerning murder) that are to be found in every country, there are also considerable variations from country to country in many of the other codes or rules. The laws of a country are usually established by an elected political institution, the population accepts them and they are enforced by the imposition of penalties on those who are found guilty of breaking them.

Members of medical, healthcare and scientific professions are bound by the same general laws as the population as a whole, but they may also be bound by additional laws specific to their area of practice. The training, qualification and registration of doctors, scientists and related professions is of great relevance at the current time, in the light of the recognized need to ensure that evidence, both medical and scientific, that is placed before the court, is established and recognized. Fraudulent professional and 'hired guns' risk undermining their own professions, in addition to causing miscarriages of justice where the innocent may be convicted and the guilty acquitted. It is sometime difficult for medical and scientific professionals to realize that their evidence is only part of a body of evidence, and that unlike in the fictional media, the solving of crimes is generally the result of meticulous painstaking and often tedious effort as part of a multi-professional team.

The great diversity of the legal systems around the world poses a number of problems to the author when giving details of the law in a book such as this. Laws on the same aspect commonly differ widely from country to country, and some medical procedures (e.g. abortion) that are routine practice (subject to appropriate legal controls) in some countries are considered to be a crime in others. Within the United Kingdom, England and Wales has its own legal system, and Scotland and Northern Ireland enjoy their own legal traditions which, although distinct from that of England and Wales, share many traditions. There are also smaller jurisdictions with their own individual variations in the Isle of Man and the Channel Isles. Overarching this is European legislation and with it the possibility of final appeals to the European Court. Other bodies (e.g. the International Criminal Court) may also influence regional issues.

This book will utilize the England and Wales legal system for most examples, making reference to other legal systems when relevant. However, it is crucial that any individual working in, or exposed to, forensic matters is aware of those relevant laws, statutes, codes and regulations that not only apply generally but also specifically to their own area of practice.

■ Legal systems

Laws are rules that govern orderly behaviour in a collective society and the system referred to as 'the Law' is an expression of the formal institutionalization of the promulgation, adjudication and enforcement of rules. There are many national variations but the basic pattern is very similar. The exact structure is frequently developed from and thus determined by the political system, culture and religious attitudes of the country in question. In England and Wales, the principal sources of these laws are Parliament and the decisions of judges in courts of law. Most countries have two main legal systems: criminal courts and civil courts. The first deals predominantly with disputes between the State and individual, the second with disputes between individuals. Most jurisdictions may also have a range of other legal bodies that are part of these systems or part of the overall justice system (e.g. employment tribunals, asylum tribunals, mental health review tribunals and other specialist dispute panels) and such bodies may deal with conflicts that arise between citizens and administrative bodies, or make judgements in other disputes. All such courts, tribunals or bodies may at some stage require input from medical and scientific professionals.

In England and Wales, decisions made by judges in the courts have evolved over time and this body of decisions is referred to as 'common law' or 'case law'. The 'doctrine of precedent' ensures that principles determined in one court will normally be binding on judges in inferior courts. The Supreme Court of the United Kingdom is the highest court in all matters under England and Wales law, Northern Irish law and Scottish civil law. It is the court of last resort and highest appeal court in the United Kingdom; however the High Court of Justiciary remains the supreme court for criminal cases in Scotland. The Supreme Court was established by the Constitutional Reform Act 2005 and started work on 1 October 2009. It assumed the judicial functions of the House of Lords, which were previously undertaken by the Lords of Appeal in Ordinary (commonly called Law Lords). Along with the concept of Parliamentary Sovereignty is that the judiciary are independent of state control, although the courts will still be bound by statutory law. This separation is one that is frequently tested.

Criminal law

Criminal law deals with relationships between the state and the individual and as such is probably the area in which forensic medical expertise is most commonly required. Criminal trials involve offences that are 'against public interest'; these include offences against the person (e.g. murder, assault, grievous bodily harm, rape), property (e.g. burglary, theft, robbery), and public safety and security of the state (terrorism). In these matters the state acts as the voice or the agent of the people. In continental Europe, a form of law derived from the Napoleonic era applies. Napoleonic law is an 'inquisitorial system' and both the prosecution and the defence have to make their cases to the court, which then chooses which is the more credible. Evidence is often taken in written form as depositions, sometimes referred to as 'documentary evidence'. The Anglo-Saxon model applies in England and Wales and in many of the countries that it has influenced in the past. This system is termed the 'adversarial system'. If an act is considered of sufficient importance or gravity, the state 'prosecutes' the individual. Prosecutions for crime in England and Wales are made by the Crown Prosecution Service (CPS), who assess the evidence provided to them by the police. The CPS will make a determination as to whether to proceed with the case and, in general, the following principles are taken into account: prosecutors must be satisfied that there is sufficient evidence to provide a realistic prospect of conviction against each suspect on each charge; they must consider what the defence case may be, and how it is likely to affect the prospects of conviction; a case which does not pass the 'evidential stage' must not proceed, no matter how serious or sensitive it may be. Sir Hartley Shawcross in 1951, who was then Attorney General, stated: '...[this] has never been the rule in this country – I hope it never will be – that suspected criminal offences must automatically be the subject of prosecution'. He added that there should be a prosecution: 'wherever it appears that the offence or the circumstances of its commission is or are of such a character that a prosecution in respect thereof is required in the public interest' (House of Commons Debates). This approach has been endorsed by Attorneys General ever since. Thus, even when there is sufficient evidence to justify a prosecution or to offer an out-of-court disposal, prosecutors must go on to consider whether a prosecution is required in the public interest. The prosecutor must be sure that there are public interest factors tending against prosecution that outweigh those tending in favour, or else the prosecutor is satisfied that the public interest may be properly served, in the first instance, by offering the offender the opportunity to have the matter dealt with by an out-of-court disposal. The more serious the offence or the offender's record of criminal behaviour, the more likely it is that a prosecution will be required in the public interest.

In a criminal trial it is for the prosecution to prove their case to the jury or the magistrates 'beyond reasonable doubt'. If that level cannot be achieved, then the prosecution fails and the individual is acquitted. If the level is achieved then the individual is convicted and a punitive sentence is applied. The defence does not have to prove innocence because any individual is presumed innocent until found guilty. Defence lawyers aim to identify inconsistencies and inaccuracies or weaknesses of the prosecution case and can also present their own evidence.

The penalties that can be imposed in the criminal system commonly include financial (fines) and loss of liberty (imprisonment) and community-based sentences. Some countries allow for corporal punishment (beatings), mutilation (amputation of parts of the body) and capital punishment (execution).

In England and Wales the lowest tier of court (in both civil and criminal cases) is the Magistrates' Court. 'Lay' magistrates sit in the majority of these courts advised by a legally qualified justice's clerk. In some of these courts a district judge will sit alone. Most criminal cases appear in magistrates' courts. The Crown Court sits in a number of centres throughout England and Wales and is the court that deals with more serious offences, and appeals from magistrates' courts. Cases are heard before a judge and a jury of 12 people. Appeals from the Crown Court are made to the Criminal Division of the Court of Appeal. Special courts are utilised for those under 18 years of age.

Civil law

Civil law is concerned with the resolution of disputes between individuals. The aggrieved party undertakes the legal action. Most remedies are financial. All kinds of dispute may be encountered, including those of alleged negligence, contractual failure, debt, and libel or slander. The civil courts can be viewed as a mechanism set up by the state that allows for the fair resolution of disputes in a structured way.

The standard of proof in the civil setting is lower than that in the criminal setting. In civil proceedings, the standard of proof is proof on the balance of probabilities – a fact will be established if it is more likely than not to have happened.

Recently Lord Richards noted in a decision of the Court of Appeal in Re (N) v Mental Health Review Tribunal (2006) QB 468 that English law recognizes only one single standard for the civil standard but went on to explain that the standard was flexible in its application:

> 'Although there is a single standard of proof on the balance of probabilities, it is flexible in its application. In particular, the more serious the allegation or the more serious the consequences if the allegation is proved, the stronger must be the evidence before the court will find the allegation proved on the balance of probabilities. Thus the flexibility of the standard lies not in any adjustment to the degree of probability required for an allegation to be proved (such that a more serious allegation has to be proved to a higher degree of probability), but in the strength or quality of the evidence that will in practice be required for an allegation to be proved on the balance of probabilities.'

If the standard of proof is met, the penalty that can be imposed by these courts is designed to restore the position of the successful claimant to that which they had before the event, and is generally financial compensation (damages). In certain circumstances there may be a punitive element to the judgment.

The Magistrates' Court is used for some cases, but the majority of civil disputes are dealt within the County Court in the presence of a circuit judge. The High Court has unlimited jurisdiction in civil cases and has three divisions:

1 *Chancery* – specializing in matters such as company law;
2 *Family* – specializing in matrimonial issues and child issues; and
3 *Queen's Bench* – dealing with general issues.

In both civil and criminal trials, the person against whom the action is being taken is called the defendant; the accuser in criminal trials is the state and in civil trials it is the plaintiff.

■ Doctors and the law

Doctors and other professionals may become involved with the law in the same way as any other private individual: they may be charged with a criminal offence or they may be sued through the civil court. A doctor may also be witness to a criminal act and may be required to give evidence about it in court.

However, it is hoped that these examples will only apply to the minority of professionals reading this book. For most, the nature of the work may result in that individual providing evidence that may subsequently be tested in court. For doctors are circumstances in which doctors become involved with the law simply because they have professional skills or experience. In these cases, the doctor (or other professional) may have one of two roles in relation to the court, either as a professional or as an expert witness, the delineation of which can sometimes overlap.

Professional witness

A professional witness is one who gives factual evidence. This role is equivalent to a simple witness of an event, but occurs when the doctor is providing factual medical evidence. For example, a casualty doctor may confirm that a leg was broken or that a laceration was present and may report on the treatment given. A primary care physician may confirm that an individual has been diagnosed as having epilepsy or angina. No comment or opinion is generally given and any report or statement deals solely with the relevant medical findings.

Expert witness

An expert witness is one who expresses an opinion about medical facts. An expert will form an opinion, for instance about the cause of the fractured leg or the laceration. An expert will express an opinion about the cause of the epilepsy or the ability of an individual with angina to drive a passenger service vehicle. Before forming an opinion, an expert witness will ensure that the relevant facts

about a case are made available to them and they may also wish to examine the patient. In the United Kingdon the General Medical Council has recently published guidance for doctors acting as expert witnesses (http://www.gmc-uk.org/guidance/ethical_guidance/expert_witness_guidance.asp).

There are often situations of overlap between these professional and expert witness roles. For example a forensic physician may have documented a series of injuries having been asked to assess a victim of crime by the police and then subsequently be asked to express an opinion about causation. A forensic pathologist will produce a report on their post-mortem examination (professional aspect) and then form conclusions and interpretation based upon their findings (expert aspect).

The role of an expert witness should be to give an impartial and unbiased assessment or interpretation of the evidence that they have been asked to consider. The admissibility of expert evidence is in itself a vast area of law. Those practising in the USA will be aware that within US jurisdictions admissibility is based on two tests: the Frye test and the Daubert test. The Frye test (also known as the general acceptance test) was stated (Frye v United States, 293 F. 1013 (D.C.Cir. 1923) as:

> Just when a scientific principle or discovery crosses the line between the experimental and demonstrable stages is difficult to define. Somewhere in the twilight zone the evidential force of the principle must be recognized, and while courts will go a long way in admitting expert testimony deduced from a well-recognized scientific principle or discovery, the thing from which the deduction is made must be sufficiently established to have gained general acceptance in the particular field in which it belongs.

Subsequently in 1975, the Federal Rules of Evidence – Rule 702 provided:

> If scientific, technical, or other specialized knowledge will assist the trier of fact to understand the evidence or to determine a fact in issue, a witness qualified as an expert by knowledge, skill, experience, or training, or education may testify thereto in the form of an opinion or otherwise.

It appeared that Rule 702 superseded Frye and in 1993 this was confirmed in Daubert v Merrell Dow

Pharmaceuticals, Inc. 509 US 579 (1993). This decision held that proof that establishes scientific reliability of expert testimony must be produced before it can be admitted. Factors that judges may consider were:

Whether the proposition is testable
Whether the proposition has been tested
Whether the proposition has been subjected to peer review and publication
Whether the methodology technique has a known or potential error rate
Whether there are standards for using the technique
Whether the methodology is generally accepted.

The question as to whether these principles applied to all experts and not just scientific experts was explored in cases and in 2000 Rule 702 was revised to:

If scientific, technical, or other specialized knowledge will assist the trier of fact to understand the evidence or to determine a fact in issue, a witness qualified as an expert by knowledge, skill, experience, or training, or education may testify thereto in the form of an opinion or otherwise, provided that (1) the testimony is sufficiently based upon reliable facts or data, (2) the testimony is the product of reliable principles and methods, and (3) the witness has applied the principles and methods to the facts of the case.

Committee Notes of the Federal Rules also emphasize that if a witness is relying primarily on experience to reach an opinion, that the witness must explain how that specific experience leads to that particular opinion.

In England and Wales, His Honour Judge Cresswell reviewed the duties of an expert in the Ikarian Reefer case (1993) FSR 563 and identified the following key elements to expert evidence:

1. *Expert evidence presented to the court should be, and should be seen to be, the independent product of the expert uninfluenced as to form or content by the exigencies of litigation.*
2. *An expert witness should provide independent assistance to the Court by way of objective, unbiased opinion in relation to matters within his expertise.*
3. *An expert witness in the High Court should never assume the role of an advocate.*
4. *An expert should state facts or assumptions upon which his opinion is based.*
5. *He should not omit to consider material facts which could detract from his concluded opinion.*
6. *An expert witness should make it clear when a particular question or issue falls outside his area of expertise.*
7. *If an expert's opinion is not properly researched because he considers that insufficient data is available, then this must be stated with an indication that the opinion is no more than a provisional one.*
8. *In cases where an expert witness, who has prepared a report, could not assert that the report contained the truth, the whole truth and nothing but the truth without some qualification, that qualification should be stated in the report.*
9. *If, after exchange of reports, an expert witness changes his views on a material matter having read the other side's report or for any other reason, such change of view should be communicated (through legal representatives) to the other side without delay and when appropriate to the court.*
10. *Where expert evidence refers to photographs, plans, calculations, analyses, measurements, survey reports or other similar documents, these must be provided to the opposite party at the same time as the exchange of reports.*

A more recent case further clarified the role of the expert witness (Toulmin HHJ in Anglo Group plc v Winther Brown & Co. Ltd. 2000)

1. *An expert witness should at all stages in the procedure, on the basis of the evidence as he understands it, provide independent assistance to the court and the parties by way of objective unbiased opinion in relation to matters within his expertise. This applies as much to the initial meetings of experts as to evidence at trial. An expert witness should never assume the role of an advocate.*
2. *The expert's evidence should normally be confined to technical matters on which the court will be assisted by receiving an explanation, or to evidence of common*

5

professional practice. The expert witness should not give evidence or opinions as to what the expert himself would have done in similar circumstances or otherwise seek to usurp the role of the judge.

3. He should cooperate with the expert of the other party or parties in attempting to narrow the technical issues in dispute at the earliest possible stage of the procedure and to eliminate or place in context any peripheral issues. He should cooperate with the other expert(s) in attending without prejudice meetings as necessary and in seeking to find areas of agreement and to define precisely areas of disagreement to be set out in the joint statement of experts ordered by the court.

4. The expert evidence presented to the court should be, and be seen to be, the independent product of the expert uninfluenced as to form or content by the exigencies of the litigation.

5. An expert witness should state the facts or assumptions upon which his opinion is based. He should not omit to consider material facts which could detract from his concluded opinion.

6. An expert witness should make it clear when a particular question or issue falls outside his expertise.

7. Where an expert is of the opinion that his conclusions are based on inadequate factual information he should say so explicitly.

8. An expert should be ready to reconsider his opinion, and if appropriate, to change his mind when he has received new information or has considered the opinion of the other expert. He should do so at the earliest opportunity.

These points remain the essence of the duties of an expert within the England and Wales jurisdiction.

When an expert has been identified it is appropriate that he is aware of relevant court decisions that relate to his role within his own jurisdictions. Extreme scepticism should be used if an individual claiming to be an expert is unaware of the expected roles and duties they should conform to.

Civil court procedure in England and Wales also now allows that, 'where two or more parties wish to submit expert evidence on a particular issue, the court may direct that the evidence on that issue is to be given by a single joint expert, and where the parties who wish to submit the evidence ('the relevant parties') cannot agree who should be the single joint expert, the court may – (a) select the expert from a list prepared or identified by the relevant parties; or (b) direct that the expert be selected in such other manner as the court may direct.'

The aims of these new rules are to enable the court to identify and deal more speedily and fairly with the medical points at issue in a case. Where both parties in both criminal and civil trials appoint experts, courts encourage the experts to meet in advance of court hearings in order to define areas of agreement and disagreement.

The duties of an expert are summarized as being that the expert's duty is to the court and any opinion expressed must not be influenced by the person who requested it, or by whoever is funding it, but must be impartial, taking into account all the evidence, supporting it where possible with established scientific or medical research, and experts should revise the opinion if further or changed evidence becomes available.

This remains an evolving area of law.

▪ Evidence for courts

There are many different courts in England and Wales, including Coroner, Magistrate, Crown, County and the Courts of Appeal. Court structure in other jurisdictions will have similar complexity and, although the exact process doctors and other professionals may experience when attending court will depend to some extent upon which court in which jurisdiction they attend, there are a number of general rules that can be made about giving evidence. In recent years courts have developed better, but not perfect, communication systems, informing witnesses who are required to give evidence in court of their role and the procedures in place, prior to attendance. In England and Wales all courts have witness services that can respond to questions and those who have never been to court before can have the opportunity of being shown the layout and structure of a court.

Statements and reports

A statement in a criminal case is a report that is prepared in a particular form so that it can be used as evidence. There is an initial declaration that ensures that the person preparing the statement is aware that they must not only tell the truth but must also ensure that there is nothing within the report that they know to be false. The effect of this declaration is to render the individual liable for criminal prosecution if they have lied. A statement provided when acting as a professional witness will be based on the contemporaneous notes (notes or records made at the time of examination), and it is important that the statement fairly reflects what was seen or done at the time.

A statement may be accepted by both defence and prosecution, negating the need for court attendance. If, for example, the defence do not accept the findings or facts expressed, the doctor will be called to court to give live evidence and be subject to examination, cross-examination and re-examination.

In civil proceedings a different official style is adopted. In these cases a sworn statement (an affidavit) is made before a lawyer who administers an oath or other formal declaration at the time of signing. This makes the document acceptable to the court.

In many countries, a statement in official form or a sworn affidavit is commonly acceptable alone and personal appearances in court are unusual. However, in the system of law based on Anglo-Saxon principles, personal appearances are common and it is the verbal evidence – tested by the defence – that is important.

If a case comes to trial, any statement made for the prosecution will be made available to all interested parties at the court; at present, the same principle of disclosure does not apply to all reports prepared for the defence in a criminal trial. Thus a defence team may commission a report that is not helpful to the client's defence. This does not have to be disclosed to the prosecution team. The format for reports in civil trial is different. In England and Wales the Ministry of Justice publishes and updates civil, criminal and family procedure rules and practice directions, and these are accessible online. It is important to understand that, although these are published, practice sometime varies from the published rules and directions.

Attending court

If a citizen is asked to appear as a witness for the court, it is the duty of all to comply, and attendance at court is generally presumed without the need to resort to a written order. Courts in England and Wales generally have specific witness liaison units, that liaise with all participants in a case, attempting (often unsuccessfully) to ensure that the dates of any trial are convenient for all witnesses. Court listing offices try to take into account 'dates to avoid' (e.g. clinics or operating sessions, pre-booked holidays or other court commitments), but this is not always successful. When notified that a court case in which you are a witness is going to take place, it is generally possible to agree a specific day on which your attendance is required. However, the court does have total authority and sometimes will compel attendance even when you have other commitments. In this case, a witness summons will be issued. This a court order signed by a judge or other court official that must be obeyed or the individual will be in contempt of court and a fine or imprisonment may result.

Waiting to give evidence involves much time-wasting and frustration, but it is important that witnesses do not delay court proceedings by failure to attend, or being late. Reasons for last-minute changes in the need for court attendance include factors such as a guilty plea being entered on the first day of the trial, or acceptance of a lesser charge.

Giving evidence

When called into court, every witness will, almost invariably, undergo some formality to ensure that they tell the truth. 'Taking the oath' or 'swearing in' requires a religious text (e.g. the New Testament, the Old Testament, the Koran) appropriate to the individual's religious beliefs (if any) or a public declaration can be made in a standard form without the need to touch a religious artefact. This latter process is sometimes referred to as 'affirming'. Regardless of how it is done, the effect of the words is the same: once the oath has been taken, the witness is liable for the penalties of perjury.

Whether called as a witness of fact, a professional witness of fact or an expert witness, the process of giving evidence is the same.

Whoever has 'called' the witness will be the first to examine them under oath; this is called the 'examination in chief' and the witness will be asked to confirm the truth of the facts in their statement(s). This examination may take the form of one catch-all question as to whether the whole of the statement is true, or the truth of individual facts may be dealt with one at a time. If the witness is not an expert, there may be questions to ascertain how the facts were obtained and the results of any examinations or ancillary tests performed. If the witness is an expert, the questioning may be expanded into the opinions that have been expressed and other opinions may be sought.

When this questioning is completed, the other lawyers will have the opportunity to question the witness; this is commonly called 'cross-examination'. This questioning will test the evidence that has been given and will concentrate on those parts of the evidence that are damaging to the lawyer's case. It is likely that both the facts and any opinions given will be tested.

The final part of giving evidence is the 're-examination'. Here, the original lawyer has the opportunity to clarify anything that has been raised in cross-examination but he cannot introduce new topics.

The judge may ask questions at any time if he feels that by doing so it may clarify a point or clear a point of contention, or if he thinks counsel are missing a point. The judge may allow the jury to ask questions. However, most judges will refrain from asking questions until the end of the re-examination.

■ Doctors in court

Any medico-legal report must be prepared and written with care because it will either constitute the medical evidence on that aspect of a case or it will be the basis of any oral evidence that may be given in the future. Any doctor who does not, or cannot, sustain the facts or opinions made in the original report while giving live evidence may, unless there are reasons for the specific alteration in fact or opinion, find themselves embarrassed. Any medical report or statement submitted to courts should always be scrutinized by the author prior to signing and submitting it to avoid factual errors (e.g. identifying the wrong site of an injury or sloppy typographical errors). However, any comments or conclusions within the report are based upon a set of facts that surround that particular case. If other facts or hypotheses are suggested by the lawyers in court during their examination, a doctor should reconsider the medical evidence in the light of these new facts or hypotheses and, if

necessary, should accept that, in view of the different basis, his conclusions may be different. If the doctor does not know the answer to the question he should say so, and if necessary ask the judge for guidance in the face of particularly persistent counsel. Similarly, if a question is outwith the area of expertise of the witness, it is right and appropriate to say so and to decline to answer the question.

Anyone appearing before any court in either role should ensure that their dress and demeanour are compatible with the role of an authoritative professional. It is imperative that doctors retain a professional demeanour and give their evidence in a clear, balanced and dispassionate manner.

The oath or affirmation should be taken in a clear voice. Most court proceedings are tape-recorded and microphones are often placed for that purpose, not for amplifying speech. In some courts, witnesses will be invited to sit, whereas in others they will be required to stand. Many expert witnesses prefer to stand as they feel that it adds to their professionalism, but this decision must be matter of personal preference. Whether standing or sitting, the doctor should remain alert to the proceedings and should not lounge or slouch. The doctor should look at the person asking the questions and, if there is one, at the jury when giving their answers; they should remain business-like and polite at all times.

Evidence should also be given in a clear voice that is loud enough to reach across the court room. Take time in responding and be aware that judges (and lawyers) will be writing down or typing responses. Most witnesses will at some time have been requested to 'Pause, please' as the legal profession attempt to keep up with complex medical or scientific points.

When replying to questions, it is important to keep the answers to the point of the question and as short as possible: an over-talkative witness who loses the facts in a welter of words is as bad as a monosyllabic witness. Questions should be answered fully and then the witness should stop and wait for the next question. On no account should a witness try to fill the silence with an explanation or expansion of the answer. If the lawyers want an explanation or expansion of any answer, they will, no doubt, ask for it. Clear, concise and complete should be the watchwords when answering questions.

Becoming hostile, angry or rude as a witness while giving evidence does not help in conveying credibility of the witness to a court. Part of the role

1 Principles of forensic practice

of the lawyers questioning is to try and elicit such responses, which invariably are viewed badly by juries – expect to have qualifications and experienced and opinions challenged. It is important to remember that it is the lawyers who are in control in the courtroom and they will very quickly take advantage of any witness who shows such emotions. No matter how you behave as a witness, you will remain giving evidence until the court says that you are released; it is not possible to bluff, boast or bombast a way out of this situation – and every witness must remember that they are under oath. A judge will normally intervene if he feels that the questioning is unreasonable or unfair.

A witness must be alert to attempts by lawyers unreasonably to circumscribe answers: 'yes' or 'no' may be adequate for simple questions but they are simply not sufficient for most questions and, if told to answer a complex question 'with a simple "yes" or "no" doctor', he should decline to do so and, if necessary, explain to the judge that it is not possible to answer such a complex question in that way.

The old forensic adage of 'dress up, stand up, speak up and shut up' is still entirely applicable and it is unwise to ignore such simple and practical advice.

Preparation of medical reports

The diversity of uses of a report is reflected in the individuals or groups that may request one: a report may be requested by the police, prosecutors, Coroners, judges, medical administrators, government departments, city authorities or lawyers of all types. The most important question that doctors must ask themselves before agreeing to write a report is whether they (1) have the expertise to write such a report and (2) have the authority to write such a report. A good rule of thumb is to ensure that, when medical records will need to be reviewed, written permission to access and use those records has been given, either by the individual themselves, or by an individual or body with the power to give that consent. If consent has not been sought, advice should be sought from the relevant court or body for permission to proceed. The fact of a request, even from a court, does not mean that a doctor can necessarily ignore the rules of medical confidentiality; however, a direct order from a court is a different matter and should, if valid, be obeyed. Any concerns about such matters should be raised with the appropriate medical defence organization.

Medical confidentiality is dealt with in greater detail in Chapter 2, but in general terms the consent of a living patient is required and, if at all possible, this should be given in writing to the doctor. There are exceptions, particularly where serious crime is involved. In some countries or jurisdictions both doctor and patient may be subject to different rules that allow reports to be written without consent. If no consent was provided, this should be stated in the report, as should the basis on which the report was written. Any practitioners should make themselves aware of the relevant laws and codes of conduct applicable to them within their current jurisdiction.

In general, in most countries it is considered inappropriate for non-judicial state agencies to order a doctor to provide confidential information against the wishes of the patient, although where a serious crime has been committed the doctor may have a public duty to assist the law-enforcement system. It is usual for the complainant of an assault to be entirely happy to give permission for the release of medical facts so that the perpetrator can be brought to justice. However, consent cannot be assumed, especially if the alleged perpetrator is the husband, wife or other member of the family. It is also important to remember that consent to disclose the effects of an alleged assault does not imply consent to disclose all the medical details of the victim, and a doctor must limit his report to relevant details only.

Mandatory reporting of medical issues may be relevant in some countries; often these relate to terrorism, child abuse, use of a weapon and other violent crime.

Structure of a statement or report

The basis of most reports and statements lies in the contemporaneous notes made at the time of an examination and it is essential to remember that copies of these notes will be required in court if you are called to give live evidence.

Many court or tribunal settings have specific protocols for written report production but in general most will include the information and details referred to below. When instructed to prepare an expert report always clarify whether or not a specific structure is required and if so, follow it assiduously.

A simple professional witness statement (one that simply reports facts found at examination) will be headed by specific legal wording. Included may be the doctor's professional address and qualifications should follow. The date of the report is essential and the time(s), date(s) and place(s) of any examination(s) should be listed, as should the details of any other person who was present during the examination(s). Indicate who requested the statement, and when. Confirm your understanding of your role at the time (e.g. 'I was called by the police to examine an alleged victim of assault to document his injuries'). Confirm that the patient has given consent for the release of the medical information (if no consent is available it must be sought). By referral to contemporaneous notes outline the history that you were aware of (... 'Mr X told me that...'). In simple terms summarize your medical findings. If information other than observation during a physical examination (e.g. medical records, X-rays) forms part of the basis of the report, it too must be recorded.

Clarity and simplicity of expression make the whole process simpler. Statements can be constructed along the same lines as the clinical notes – they should structured, detailed (but not over-elaborate – no one needs to be impressed with complex medical and scientific terms) and accurate. Do not include every single aspect of a medical history unless it is relevant and consent has been given for its disclosure. A court does not need to know every detail, but it does need to know every relevant detail, and a good report will give the relevant facts clearly, concisely and completely, and in a way that an intelligent person without medical training can understand.

Medical abbreviations should be used with care and highly technical terms, especially those relating to complex pieces of equipment or techniques, should be explained in simple, but not condescending, terms. Abbreviations in common usage such as ECG can generally be used without explanation although occasionally further explanation is required.

It is preferable not to submit handwritten or proforma type statements unless absolutely unavoidable. A clear, concise and complete report or statement may prevent the need for court attendance at all, and if you do have to give evidence, it is much easier to do so from a report that is legible. The contemporaneous clinical notes may be required to support the statement and it is wise to ensure that all handwriting within such notes has been reviewed (and interpreted) prior to entering the witness box.

Autopsy reports are a specialist type of report and may be commissioned by the Coroner, the police or any other legally competent person or body. Again, as with expert reports, there may be standardized protocols or proforma. The authority to perform the examination will replace the consent given by a live patient, and is equally important. The history and background to the death will be obtained by the police or the Coroner's officer, but the doctor should seek any additional details that appear to be relevant, including speaking to any clinicians involved in the care of the deceased and reviewing the hospital notes. A visit to the scene of death in non-suspicious deaths, especially if there are any unusual or unexplained aspects, is to be encouraged.

An autopsy report is confidential and should only be disclosed to the legal authority who commissioned the examination. Disclosure to others, who must be interested parties, may only be made with the specific permission of the commissioning authority and, in general terms, it would be sensible to allow that authority to deal with any requests for copies of the report.

Doctors must resist any attempt to change or delete any parts of their report by lawyers who may feel those parts are detrimental to their case; any requests to rewrite and resubmit a report with alterations for these reasons should be refused. Lawyers may sometimes need to be reminded of the role of the doctor and their duties, both as doctors and as experts. Pressure from lawyers to revise or manipulate a report inappropriately warrants referral to their professional body, and the court should be informed. The doctor should always seek the advice of the judge of matters arising that may result in potential breaches of these important duties.

■ Further information sources

Anglo Group plc v Winther Brown & Co Ltd and others (2000) All ER (D) 294.

Boccaccini MT, Brodsky SL. Believability of expert and lay witnesses: implications for trial consultation. *Professional Psychology: Research and Practice* 2002; **33:** 384–8.

Burton JL, Rutty GN (eds). *The Hospital Autopsy: A Manual of Fundamental Autopsy Practice*, 3rd edn. London: Hodder Arnold, 2010.

1 Principles of forensic practice

Cooper J, Neuhaus IM. The 'hired gun' effect: assessing the effect of pay, frequency of testifying and credentials on the perception of expert testimony. *Law and Human Behavior* 2000; **24**: 149–71.

Court of Appeal in Re (N) v Mental Health Review Tribunal (2006) QB 468.

Crown Prosecution Service. Code for Crown Prosecutors. http://www.cps.gov.uk/publications/code_for_crown_prosecutors/ (accessed 11 February 2011).

Daubert v Merrell Dow Pharmaceuticals, Inc. 509 US 579 (1993). http://www.law.cornell.edu/supct/html/92-102.ZS.html (accessed 23 November 2010).

Federal Rules of Evidence Article I. General provisions, Rule 702. http://www.law.cornell.edu/rules/fre/rules.htm#Rule702 (accessed 23 November 2010).

Freckelton I. A Guide to the Provision of Forensic Medical Evidence. In: Gall J, Payne-James JJ (eds) *Current Practice in Forensic Medicine*. London: Wiley, 2011.

Freckelton I, Selby H. *Expert Evidence: Law, Practice, Procedure and Advocacy*, 4th edn. Sydney: Thomson Reuters, 2009.

Frye v United States, 293 F. 1013 (D.C.Cir. 1923). http://www.law.ufl.edu/faculty/little/topic8.pdf (accessed 23 November 2010).

General Medical Council. Guidance for doctors acting as expert witnesses. http://www.gmc-uk.org/guidance/ethical_guidance/expert_witness_guidance.asp (accessed 23 November 2010).

House of Commons Debates, Volume 483, 29 January 1951 (quote of Hartley Shawcross).

Ikarian Reefer 1993 2 LILR 68, 81–82.

Lynch J. *Clinical Responsibility*. Oxford: Radcliffe Publishing, 2009.

Ministry of Justice (England and Wales). Civil Procedure Rules. http://www.justice.gov.uk/civil/procrules_fin/ (accessed 23 November 2010).

Ministry of Justice (England and Wales). Criminal Procedure Rules http://www.justice.gov.uk/criminal/procrules_fin/index.htm (accessed 23 November 2010).

Ministry of Justice (England and Wales). Family Procedure Rules. http://www.justice.gov.uk/family/procrules/index.htm (accessed 23 November 2010).

Ministry of Justice (England and Wales). Procedure rules: http://www.justice.gov.uk/procedure.htm (accessed 23 November 2010).

Payne-James JJ, Dean P, Wall I. *Medicolegal Essentials in Healthcare*, 2nd edn. London: Greenwich Medical Media, 2004.

Re (N) v Mental Health Review Tribunal 2006, QB468.

Stark MM. *Clinical Forensic Medicine: a Physician's Guide*, 3rd edn. New York: Humana Press, 2011.

Toulmin HHJ in Anglo Group plc v Winther Brown & Co. Ltd. 2000. http://www.hrothgar.co.uk/YAWS/frmreps/anglo.htm (accessed 23 November 2010).

Chapter

2

The ethics of medical practice

■ Introduction

Medical practice has many forms and can embrace many backgrounds and discipline. Examples include the predominantly science-based 'Western medicine', traditional Chinese medicine, Ayurvedic medicine in India, and the many native systems from Africa and Asia. It is not unusual for more than one system to work together such as Chinese and Western medicine in parts of China. There are other alternative and complementary forms of medicine with varying degrees of evidence and science on which they are based. These alternative forms of medicine may have their own traditions, conventions and variably active codes of conduct. The focus of this chapter will relate to the relatively easily defined science-based 'Western medicine', although to describe modern, science-based medicine as 'Western medicine' is historically inaccurate because its origins can be traced through ancient Greece to a synthesis of Asian, North African and European medicine.

■ Duties, promises and pledges

The Greek tradition of medical practice was epitomized by the Hippocratic School on the island of Kos around 400 BC. It was there that the foundations of both modern medicine and the ethical facets of the practice of that medicine were laid. A form of words universally known as the Hippocratic Oath was developed at and for those times, but the fact that it remains the basis of ethical medical behaviour, even though some of the detail is now obsolete, is a testament to its simple common sense and universal acceptance. A generally accepted translation is as follows:

I swear by Apollo the physician and Aesculapius and Health and All-heal and all the gods and goddesses, that according to my ability and judgement, I will keep this Oath and this stipulation – to hold him who taught me this art, equally dear to me as my own parents, to make him partner in my livelihood: when he is in need of money, to share mine with him; to consider his family as my own brothers and to teach them this art, if they want to learn it, without fee or indenture. To impart precept, oral instruction and all other instruction to my own sons, the sons of my teacher and to those who have taken the disciple's oath, but to no-one else. I will use treatment to help the sick according to my ability and judgement, but never with a view to injury or wrong-doing. Neither will I administer a poison to anybody when asked to do so nor will I suggest such a course. Similarly, I will not give a woman a pessary to produce abortion. But I will keep pure and holy both my life and my art. I will not use the knife, not even sufferers with the stone, but leave this to be done by men who are practitioners of this work. Into whatsoever houses I enter, I will go into them for the benefit of the sick and will abstain from every voluntary act of mischief or corruption: and further, from the seduction of females or males, of freeman or slaves. And whatever I shall see or hear in the course of my profession or not in connection with it, which ought not to be spoken of abroad, I will not divulge, reckoning that all such should be kept secret. While I carry out this oath, and not break it, may it be granted to me to enjoy life and the practice of the art, respected by all men: but if I should transgress it, may the reverse be my lot.

It is commonly believed that all medical practitioners (in the United Kingdom defined as a medical practitioner registered by the General Medical Council) have taken the Hippocratic Oath. This is in fact not the case but the key principles espoused form the basis of what is broadly called 'medical ethics'. The principles of medical ethics have developed over several thousand years and continue to evolve and change, influenced by society, the legal profession and the medical profession itself. Virtually every day a news story will run in the media which may have its basis in the interpretation of aspects of medical ethics, such as euthanasia and abortion. The laws governing the practice of medicine vary from country to country, but the broad principles of medical ethics are universal and are formulated not only by national medical associations, but by international

organizations such as the World Medical Association (WMA).

■ International codes of medical ethics

Assorted bodies explore and attempt to define matters of medical ethics. The WMA was founded in 1947, and a central objective of the WMA has been to establish and promote the highest possible standards of ethical behaviour and care by physicians. In pursuit of this goal, the WMA has adopted global policy statements on a range of ethical issues related to medical professionalism, patient care, research on human subjects and public health. The WMA Council and its standing committees regularly review and update existing policies and continually develop new policy on emerging ethical issues. As a result of the horrific violations of medical ethics during the 1939–45 war, the international medical community restated the Hippocratic Oath in a modern form in the Declaration of Geneva in 1948 most recently amended and revised in 2006 to state:

> *At the time of being admitted as a member of the medical profession:*
> *I solemnly pledge to consecrate my life to the service of humanity;*
> *I will give to my teachers the respect and gratitude that is their due;*
> *I will practise my profession with conscience and dignity;*
> *The health of my patient will be my first consideration;*
> *I will respect the secrets that are confided in me, even after the patient has died;*
> *I will maintain by all the means in my power, the honour and the noble traditions of the medical profession;*
> *My colleagues will be my sisters and brothers;*
> *I will not permit considerations of age, disease or disability, creed, ethnic origin, gender, nationality, political affiliation, race, sexual orientation, social standing or any other factor to intervene between my duty and my patient;*
> *I will maintain the utmost respect for human life;*
> *I will not use my medical knowledge to violate human rights and civil liberties, even under threat;*
> *I make these promises solemnly, freely and upon my honour.*

Box 2.1 Duties of a physician as defined by the World Medical Association

Duties of a physician in general

A physician shall:

- Always exercise his/her independent professional judgment and maintain the highest standards of professional conduct
- Respect a competent patient's right to accept or refuse treatment
- Not allow his/her judgment to be influenced by personal profit or unfair discrimination
- Be dedicated to providing competent medical service in full professional and moral independence, with compassion and respect for human dignity
- Deal honestly with patients and colleagues, and report to the appropriate authorities those physicians who practise unethically or incompetently or who engage in fraud or deception
- Not receive any financial benefits or other incentives solely for referring patients or prescribing specific products
- Respect the rights and preferences of patients, colleagues, and other health professionals
- Recognize his/her important role in educating the public but use due caution in divulging discoveries or new techniques or treatment through non-professional channels
- Certify only that which he/she has personally verified
- Strive to use health care resources in the best way to benefit patients and their community
- Seek appropriate care and attention if he/she suffers from mental or physical illness
- Respect the local and national codes of ethics

Duties of physicians to patients

A physician shall:

- Always bear in mind the obligation to respect human life
- Act in the patient's best interest when providing medical care
- Owe his/her patients complete loyalty and all the scientific resources available to him/her. Whenever an examination or treatment is beyond the physician's capacity, he/she should consult with or refer to another physician who has the necessary ability
- Respect a patient's right to confidentiality. It is ethical to disclose confidential information when the patient consents to it or when there is a real and imminent threat of harm to the patient or to others and this threat can be only removed by a breach of confidentiality
- Give emergency care as a humanitarian duty unless he/she is assured that others are willing and able to give such care
- In situations when he/she is acting for a third party, ensure that the patient has full knowledge of that situation
- Not enter into a sexual relationship with his/her current patient or into any other abusive or exploitative relationship

Duties of physicians to colleagues

A physician shall:

- Behave towards colleagues as he/she would have them behave towards him/her
- Not undermine the patient–physician relationship of colleagues in order to attract patients
- When medically necessary, communicate with colleagues who are involved in the care of the same patient. This communication should respect patient confidentiality and be confined to necessary information

WMA International code of Medical Ethics. Latest amendment: WMA General Assembly, Pilanesberg, South Africa, October 2006. Copyright World Medical Association. All rights reserved.

Table 2.1 Example Declarations of the World Medical Association (many are revised and amended in different years)

Year	Declaration	Key topic
1948	The Declaration of Geneva	Humanitarian goals of medicine
1964	The Declaration of Helsinki	Human experimentation and clinical trials
1970	The Declaration of Oslo	Therapeutic abortion
1973	The Declaration of Munich	Racial, political discrimination in medicine
1975	The Declaration of Tokyo	Torture and other cruel and degrading treatment or punishment
1981	The Declaration of Lisbon	Rights of the patient
1983	The Declaration of Venice	Terminal illness
1983	The Declaration of Oslo	Therapeutic abortion
1984	The Declaration of San Paolo	Pollution
1987	The Declaration of Madrid	Professional autonomy and self-regulation
2006	The Declaration of Ottawa	Child health
2009	The Declaration of Delhi	Health and climate change

The WMA has also amended the 'Duties of a Physician in General' on a number of occasions – most recently in 2006. Box 2.1 shows these duties of physicians, in general, to patients and to colleagues.

The principles espoused by these duties and the pledges are embraced in one form or another by most medical bodies representing medical practitioners around the world. Table 2.1 identifies some of the WMA Declarations in recent years, and shows the breadth of subject matter that requires consideration. Often these amend or revise previous declarations (the Declaration of Geneva of 1948 being most recently amended in 2006).

■ Duties of doctors – UK perspective

Increasingly, regulatory bodies are defining in relatively unambiguous terms how professionals should work. The General Medical Council in the UK has published a document on how a registered medical practitioner (a doctor) should undertake good medical practice. *Good Medical Practice*, published by the General Medical Council, advises doctors on their duties. Extracts from *Good Medical Practice* are provided in Box 2.2.

The General Medical Council publishes advice and guidance for doctors in the UK in a number of specific areas, for example concerning the use of

---

Box 2.2 Duties of a doctor (from *Good Medical Practice*)

In 'Good Medical Practice' the terms 'you must' and 'you should' are used in the following ways: 'You must' is used for an overriding duty or principle; 'You should' is used when we are providing an explanation of how you will meet the overriding duty; 'You should' is also used where the duty or principle will not apply in all situations or circumstances, or where there are factors outside your control that affect whether or how you can comply with the guidance. Serious or persistent failure to follow this guidance will put your registration at risk.

The duties of a doctor registered with the General Medical Council

Patients must be able to trust doctors with their lives and health. To justify that trust you must show respect for human life and you must:

- Make the care of your patient your first concern
- Protect and promote the health of patients and the public
- Provide a good standard of practice and care
- Keep your professional knowledge and skills up to date
- Recognize and work within the limits of your competence
- Work with colleagues in the ways that best serve patients' interests
- Treat patients as individuals and respect their dignity
- Treat patients politely and considerately
- Respect patients' right to confidentiality
- Work in partnership with patients
- Listen to patients and respond to their concerns and preferences
- Give patients the information they want or need in a way they can understand
- Respect patients' right to reach decisions with you about their treatment and care
- Support patients in caring for themselves to improve and maintain their health
- Be honest and open and act with integrity
- Act without delay if you have good reason to believe that you or a colleague may be putting patients at risk
- Never discriminate unfairly against patients or colleagues
- Never abuse your patients' trust in you or the public's trust in the profession.
- You are personally accountable for your professional practice and must always be prepared to justify your decisions and actions.

Good doctors - paragraph 1

1. Patients need good doctors. Good doctors make the care of their patients their first concern: they are competent, keep their knowledge

and skills up to date, establish and maintain good relationships with patients and colleagues (those a doctor works with, whether or not they are also doctors), are honest and trustworthy, and act with integrity.

Good clinical care – paragraphs 2 and 3

Providing good clinical care.

2. Good clinical care must include:
   a. adequately assessing the patient's conditions, taking account of the history (including the symptoms, and psychological and social factors), the patient's views, and where necessary examining the patient
   b. providing or arranging advice, investigations or treatment where necessary
   c. referring a patient to another practitioner, when this is in the patient's best interests.

3. In providing care you must:
   a. recognize and work within the limits of your competence
   b. prescribe drugs or treatment, including repeat prescriptions, only when you have adequate knowledge of the patient's health, and are satisfied that the drugs or treatment serve the patient's needs
   c. provide effective treatments based on the best available evidence
   d. take steps to alleviate pain and distress whether or not a cure may be possible
   e. respect the patient's right to seek a second opinion
   f. keep clear, accurate and legible records, reporting the relevant clinical findings, the decisions made, the information given to patients and any drugs prescribed or other investigation or treatment
   g. make records at the same time as the events you are recording or as soon as possible afterwards
   h. be readily accessible when you are on duty
   i. consult and take advice from colleagues, where appropriate
   j. make good use of the resources available to you.

Good Medical Practice published by the General Medical Council in 2006 and available online at: http://www.gmc-uk.org/guidance/good_medical_practice/index.asp

chaperones when undertaking intimate examinations. Box 2.3 shows the following advice given by the GMC on this subject in November 2006.

Box 2.3 Guidelines for intimate examinations

The GMC regularly receives complaints from patients who feel that doctors have behaved inappropriately during an intimate examination. Intimate examinations, that is examinations of the breasts, genitalia or rectum, can be stressful and embarrassing for patients. When conducting intimate examinations you should:

- Explain to the patient why an examination is necessary and give the patient an opportunity to ask questions
- Explain what the examination will involve, in a way the patient can understand, so that the patient has a clear idea of what to expect, including any potential pain or discomfort (paragraph 13 of our booklet *Seeking patients' consent* gives further guidance on presenting information to patients)
- Obtain the patient's permission before the examination and be prepared to discontinue the examination if the patient asks you to. You should record that permission has been obtained
- Keep discussion relevant and avoid unnecessary personal comments
- Offer a chaperone or invite the patient (in advance if possible) to have a relative or friend present. If the patient does not want a chaperone, you should record that the offer was made and declined. If a chaperone is present, you should record that fact and make a note of the chaperone's identity. If for justifiable practical reasons you cannot offer a chaperone, you should explain that to the patient and, if possible, offer to delay the examination to a later date. You should record the discussion and its outcome
- Give the patient privacy to undress and dress and use drapes to maintain the patient's dignity. Do not assist the patient in removing clothing unless you have clarified with them that your assistance is required.

From *Maintaining boundaries–guidance for doctors*. General Medical Council, 2006.

It is up to the medical practitioner to determine for each patient seen, in whatever clinical setting (including custodial and penal facilities) that they are following such guidance. Clearly, however, irrespective of the cause for the examination, based on the General Medical Council (GMC) guidelines, visual assessment or physical examination that involves touching, by hand, of an intimate area will constitute an intimate examination and it is appropriate for the relevant principles described in Box 2.3 to be put into practice. It is advisable to record all such information within contemporaneous medical records, including if a patient declines to have a chaperone present. A medical practitioner should always be mindful of how any actions might be perceived at a later date by anyone reviewing their conduct, and to ensure they can justify whatever action they took.

Other healthcare professionals may nowadays have expanded roles in healthcare and for example in England and Wales nurses and paramedics may assess detainees in police custody. Sexual Assault Nurse Examiners are in practice increasingly around the world. All will have their own professional standards and accountability, and the duties that they have to their patients may be very explicit (similar to GMC guidelines) or more generalized. The Nursing and Midwifery Council (NMC) in the UK which is the professional body for nurses has a Code of Professional Conduct with principles much the same as those for doctors. Box 2.4 gives a summary of the NMC code of professional conduct: standards for conduct, performance and ethics, and each of these components is expanded in further detail in the full code.

Box 2.4 Summary of professional conduct standards for nurses

The people in your care must be able to trust you with their health and well-being

To justify that trust, you must:

- make the care of people your first concern, treating them as individuals and respecting their dignity
- work with others to protect and promote the health and well-being of those in your care, their families and carers, and the wider community
- provide a high standard of practice and care at all times
- be open and honest, act with integrity and uphold the reputation of your profession.

As a professional, you are personally accountable for actions and omissions in your practice, and must always be able to justify your decisions.

You must always act lawfully, whether those laws relate to your professional practice or personal life.

Failure to comply with this code may bring your fitness to practise into question and endanger your registration.

From *The code standards for conduct, performance and ethics for nurses and midwives*. Nursing and Midwifery Council, 2008.

The Health Professions Council (HPC) is a body created by statute in England and Wales, which regulates healthcare professionals (e.g. arts therapists, biomedical scientists, chiropodists/podiatrists, clinical scientists, dietitians, hearing aid dispensers, occupational therapists, operating department practitioners, orthoptists, paramedics, physiotherapists, practitioner psychologists, prosthetists/orthotists, radiographers, and speech and language therapists). The HPC was set up to protect the public and keeps a register of health professionals who meet its standards for training, professional skills, behaviour and health. All of these professions have at least one professional title that is protected by law, including those shown above. This means, for example, that anyone using the titles 'physiotherapist' or 'dietitian' must be registered with the HPC.

It is a criminal offence for someone to claim that they are registered with the HPC when they are not, or to use a protected title they are not entitled to use.

Medical ethics in practice

The formal role of ethics in contemporary medicine has expanded dramatically in recent years and is reflected in many issues, such as the use of research and ethics committees for the consideration of research on humans, and the increasing role of clinical ethicists who may work closely with other professional such as geneticists and transplant centres. Medical ethics is incorporated into medical school curricula as the need for knowledge of such matters becomes increasingly important with high-technology medicine creating clinical scenarios that were unthinkable even three decades ago.

Examples of the type of subject that may be embraced in discussions on medical ethics may include:

- patient autonomy and their right to refuse or choose treatment
- non-maleficence – do no harm
- beneficence – acting in the patient's best interests
- dignity
- honesty – providing informed consent
- justice – how healthcare is apportioned when health and financial resources may be limited.

It is important for doctors and other healthcare professionals to be aware of these issues, even if they do not provide immediate answers to clinical dilemmas. Sometimes these factors conflict – for example, a Jehovah's witness declining a blood transfusion even though the doctor knows that death will ensue.

There are few medical or healthcare activities that do not have some ethical considerations, varying from research on patients to medical confidentiality, from informed consent to doctor–doctor relationships. Often, law develops as a result of public and political debate on such issues. Breaches of such ethics may result in disciplinary processes and the sanctions that can be applied by professional bodies against the doctor found guilty of unethical practices.

Although the spectrum of unethical conduct is wide, certain universally relevant subjects are

recognized. The seriousness with which each is viewed may vary considerably in different parts of the world.

Confidentiality

The two main elements of medical duties that raise most concern and question are those of confidentiality and consent. Many publications deliberate on these points. Within the United Kingdom the GMC has published guidance on both confidentiality and consent, which gives explicit background and practical guidance to UK medical practitioners. Many other countries will provide similar information orientated to the local jurisdiction and statute. Readers should be aware of the guidance within their own locality.

The UK guidance emphasizes that patients have a right to expect that information about them will be held in confidence by their doctors. Confidentiality is a primary, but not an absolute duty. Doctors must use their own judgement to apply the principles of confidentiality and be prepared to later explain and justify any decisions or actions taken when they have apparently breached that confidentiality.

The key to a doctor–patient relationship is trust. If patients are not assured about confidentiality then they may be put off seeking medical attention or providing doctors with the right information to ensure they get optimal care. There is, however, a balance to be struck in providing appropriate information to others to ensure safe, effective care for the patients themselves and the wider community. The emphasis is on communication to the patient of relevant information so that they are aware that relevant medical information may be disclosed to other healthcare professionals. In the course of this disclosure non-medical healthcare professionals may also have access to personal information.

There are, however, a number of permissible situations when confidentiality may not apply. Box 2.5 identifies those circumstances where confidential information may be allowably disclosed by medical practitioners. In England and Wales there is a system by which a senior personnel member within the National Health Service (NHS) acts as a 'Caldicott Guardian' and is responsible for protecting the confidentiality of patient and service-user information and enabling appropriate information-sharing. Each NHS organization is required to have a Caldicott

Guardian. The mandate covers all organizations that have access to patient records, so it includes acute trusts, ambulance trusts, mental health trusts, primary care trusts, strategic health authorities and special health authorities such as NHS Direct. Caldicott Guardians were also introduced into social care in 2002.

Box 2.5 When confidentiality may not apply

- If required by law
- If the patient consents – implicitly or expressly
- If justified in the public interest (examples identified below)
- Reporting concerns about driving capabilities
- Reporting gunshot and knife wounds
- Reporting serious communicable diseases
- Reporting in relation to insurance or employment purposes

If a doctor holds personal information about patients, the UK health departments provide guidance on how that data must be held, for what period of time and how it must be disposed of. Protection of computers, including passwords, and paper-based records is expected. Sanctions have been taken against doctors who have allowed medical records to be left where the public or other unauthorized personnel have access to them.

Disclosures required by law

Disclosure may be required because of statute, for example notification of known or suspected types of communicable disease. Certain government agencies or bodies may have statutory power to access patient's records. Patients' medical records and related personal information may be required by regulatory bodies if there has been a complaint against a healthcare professional. In all cases it is essential that every opportunity is taken to seek the patient's express consent before disclosure. If disclosure is not consented to, then legal advice and advice from a medical defence organization should be sought before disclosure is made.

The determination of whether or not disclosure is in the public interest may not be one that can be made alone. Information must be disclosed at the order of a judge or a presiding officer of a court. It is appropriate if the request appears immaterial to the case in hand to raise objections, clearly stating the reasons for these objections. Again, in such a situation it may be appropriate to seek the advice of a medical defence organization or a Caldicott

Guardian. Disclosure to others (e.g. police officers) should not be done without consent, unless reasons for disclosure apply. In Scotland, with its own jurisdiction, limited medical information may be disclosed without consent before a criminal trial.

Disclosing information with consent

Certain patients may wish to withhold particular aspects of personal information, and unless other reasons for disclosure apply this wish must be respected. If such a request might influence aspects of medical care, it should be ensured that the patient is fully aware that withholding information may compromise that care. Those who are provided with such information must be reminded of their own duty of confidence. Clinical situations such as medical emergencies may mean that information is passed without consent, and an explanation should later be given to the patient advising them of the reasons for that disclosure. Disclosure may also be permitted for audit if the patient is aware of that possibility and they have not objected to it.

Disclosure requiring express consent

Doctors must always seek specific consent to disclose personal information for any reason beyond clinical care and audit. Typical requests may apply to benefit claims or insurance claims. The patient must always be made aware of the nature and extent of information being disclosed. The information disclosed must be unbiased, relevant and limited to the needs expressed. The patient should generally be offered the opportunity to see any report or disclosure prior to it being disclosed, unless potentially non-disclosable confidential information about another person is contained within it.

Disclosure in the public interest

The principle of confidentially is key to a doctor–patient relationship and the protection conferred enables patients, who might otherwise not disclose relevant medical issues, to have the confidence to discuss such matters with their doctor. However, there are situations where, in the public interest (for example to protect specific individuals or society in general from risks of serious harm) disclosure of otherwise confidential information may be required. In some settings, therefore, if the patient has not given consent, or expressly withheld it, disclosure may be permissible. Decisions to disclose must weigh the interests of the patient, other individuals, or society in general, the risks of harm to all and the risks to the doctor–patient relationship, and come to a balanced decision that can be justified both at the time and later. In addition to risks of harm, there are more general areas where disclosure may be permissible in the public interest and these can relate to areas such as research, education and public health. The opportunity to anonymize such information should always be taken if appropriate, although in many settings it may be possible to obtain consent. A decision to disclose must also take into account the practicalities of getting consent in relation to the need for disclosure.

Disclosures to protect the patient or others

Some patients require disclosure of information for their own protection, but if competent, a refusal to consent to disclosure should be respected, while ensuring that they are fully aware of the reasons why a disclosure is considered in their interests. In the criminal setting, issues of domestic violence are examples of where disclosure may be appropriate but refused by the patient. Disclosure without consent may be justified when others are at risk of serious harm or death that may be reduced by such disclosure. Some circumstances, which often may relate to serious crime (e.g. murder, rape and child abuse) require the prompt disclosure of information to appropriate bodies (e.g. police). Such an approach may also be appropriate if there is a belief that the patient (adult or child) is a victim of neglect or physical, sexual or emotional abuse. If appropriate, the patient should be informed of a decision to disclose before doing so.

Disclosure concerning patients without the capacity to consent

A number of factors may be relevant in the setting where a patient lacks the capacity to consent. Is the lack of capacity temporary or permanent? If

temporary, is there any immediate necessity for disclosure, and can disclosure be deferred until the patient regains capacity to consent? If the patient has someone who has a lawful role in making decisions for them, they should be consulted. In all settings it is expected that the doctor is seen to act in the patient's best interests, and this should take into account views of others, including family and other healthcare professionals.

Disclosure after death

The duty of confidentiality persists after death. Careful consideration must be given, and reasons must be appropriate, for disclosure. Disclosure may be required by Coroners, or others responsible for the investigation of deaths and on statutory forms such as death certificates.

■ Consent

In order to give consent to a treatment, an investigation or a process, an individual must have sufficient capacity, they must possess sufficient understanding or knowledge of the proposed intervention and their agreement to undergo the proposed treatment, investigation or process must be voluntary – that is, it must be freely given and not tainted by any degree of coercion or undue influence from others.

Patients with capacity to make decisions

Consent is a key concept of healthcare and it is expected that all decisions about treatment and healthcare come about as a result of collaboration between doctors and patients. Consent should be based on trust, openness and good communication. In the UK doctors are expected to work in partnership with their patients in order to optimize care. Doctors must listen to patients and respect their views about health. They should discuss the diagnosis, prognosis, treatment and care, and share appropriate information with their patients so that the patients can make informed decisions. They must then allow patients to make decisions themselves and respect those decisions once made. The path by which the decision have been taken should be documented contemporaneously in the clinical record. Consent may given orally or in writing – this is express or explicit consent. Consent may also be given implicitly, for example by allowing blood pressure to be taken by removing clothing to give access to the arm. It is generally accepted that for higher risk or more complex procedures, if there is a risk to life or lifestyle, for research or in the criminal setting (e.g. the taking of intimate samples) that written consent is appropriate. In some settings written consent is mandatory.

Assuming that the patient has capacity to make their own decisions the following four stages should be followed when considering treatment:

1 Both doctor and patient make an assessment taking into account the patient's medical history, views, experience and knowledge.
2 The doctor identifies relevant investigations and treatment to benefit the patient and explains the options with their respective potential risks, burdens and side-effects (including having no treatment or investigation) – the doctor may recommend a particular option, but the decision remains the patient's.
3 The patient weighs up the potential benefits, risks and burdens and any related issues and makes a decision as to how to proceed – the patient may sometimes make a decision that appears irrational to the doctor.
4 The patient may request a treatment that the doctor considers of no overall benefit – the doctor does not have to provide that treatment but must explain their reasons to the patient.

The responsibility for seeking consent is that of the doctor undertaking the investigation or treatment. Such a duty can be delegated if the person to whom it is delegated is appropriately trained and has appropriate knowledge of the treatment or investigation proposed .

Any discussion about risks of a treatment or type of management (including no treatment) must identify and, where possible, quantify side-effects, complications (both major and minor) and their potential consequences (e.g. disability or death). In Chester v Afshar (2004) Lord Bingham stated 'a surgeon owes a general duty to a patient to warn him or her in general terms of possible serious risks involved in the procedure. The only qualification is that there may be wholly exceptional cases where objectively in the best interests of the patient the surgeon may be excused from giving a warning... in modern law medical paternalism no longer rules and a patient has a *prima facie* right to be informed by a surgeon of a small, but well-established, risk of serious injury as a result of surgery.'

Young people, children and consent

Age is not a rigid factor in ability to consent, although it is generally accepted that those aged 16 years and older have the capacity to make decisions about treatment or care. Many children aged under 16 years may also have the capacity to understand and consider options. In the UK the GMC publishes guidance on making decisions in those aged under 18 years and how capacity and best interests may be assessed. The capacity of children below the age of 16 years to consent to medical treatment depends on whether the child has achieved a sufficient understanding and intelligence to appreciate the purpose, nature, consequences and risks of a particular treatment (including no treatment) and has the ability to appraise the medical advice. This concept in England and Wales is known as 'Gillick Competence' and is dependent on the child's chronological age, mental age, and emotional maturity while recognizing a child's increasing autonomy with age.

Patients without capacity to make decisions

If patients are unable to make decisions for themselves, the doctor must engage with those who are close to the patient and with colleagues involved in the healthcare. In England and Wales decisions about those who lack capacity is governed by the Mental Capacity Act 2005. If the patient expresses an opinion with regard to treatment this must be taken into account and follow the specific relevant law. Doctors should make the assumption that every adult has capacity and capacity is only seen to be lacking once it is established (using all means available) that the individual cannot, understand, retain, use or weigh up the information needed either to make the decision, or make clear their wishes. The Mental Capacity Act 2005 Codes give specific advice on assessing capacity.

If a patient lacks capacity and a decision is made on their behalf, the doctor must:

- make the care of the patient the primary concern;
- ensure that the patient is treated as an individual and with dignity;
- support and encourage the patient to be involved in decisions about treatment and care within the limits of their abilities;
- treat the patient with respect and without discrimination. This must be taken into account with all other factors that might otherwise affect consent.

■ Regulation of doctors and other professionals

The General Medical Council

Regulation of the work of healthcare professionals is governed in many countries around the world by regulatory bodies that may have powers to assess the individual's performance and work. In the United Kingdom the regulatory body for registered medical practitioners (doctors) is the GMC, which was established by statute and to whom complaints may be made if they cannot be resolved locally (e.g. in hospital or community settings) or if they are of a certain degree of seriousness. Although the ethical precept of informed consent has attracted attention in a variety of legal jurisdictions it was not until the twenty-first century that the GMC acknowledged this concept when advising medical practitioners on the issue of consent. This evolution occurred with a developing respect for autonomy or 'self-rule' and 'self-determination'.

The GMC registers doctors to practise medicine in the UK. Its purpose is to protect, promote and maintain the health and safety of the public by ensuring proper standards in the practice of medicine. The law gives the GMC four main functions under the Medical Act 1983:

- keeping up-to-date registers of qualified doctors
- fostering good medical practice
- promoting high standards of medical education and training
- dealing firmly and fairly with doctors whose fitness to practise is in doubt.

The GMC fulfils its role by controlling entry to the medical register and setting the standards for medical schools and postgraduate education and training. The GMC has legal powers designed to maintain the standards the public have a right to expect of doctors. If a doctor fails to meet those standards, the GMC acts to protect patients from harm – if necessary, by removing the doctor from the register and removing their right to practise medicine.

The GMC was originally established by the Medical Act of 1858. It has a governing body, the Council, which has 24 members of which 12 are doctors and 12 are lay members. Before the GMC can stop or limit a doctor's right to practise medicine, it needs evidence of impaired fitness to practise. Examples of such evidence includes doctors who have not kept their medical knowledge and skills up to date and are not competent, have taken advantage of their role as a doctor or have done something wrong, are too ill, or have not adequately managed a health problem to enable them to work safely. The GMC can also issue a warning to a doctor where the doctor's fitness to practise is not impaired but there has been a significant departure from the principles set out in the GMC's guidance for doctors, *Good Medical Practice*. A warning will be disclosed to a doctor's employer and to any other enquirer during a 5-year period. A warning will not be appropriate where the concerns relate exclusively to a doctor's physical or mental health.

Legal framework for GMC fitness to practise procedures

The legal framework for the Fitness to Practise procedures is set out in Medical Act 1983 and the Fitness to Practise Rules 2004. These are frequently amended and revised (at the time of writing, most recently in 2009) and reference should be made to the GMC to be aware of the current process. The Medical Act gives the GMC powers and responsibilities for taking action when questions arise about doctors' fitness to practise. The detailed arrangements for how these matters are investigated and adjudicated upon are set out in rules which have the force of law.

Procedures are divided into two separate stages: 'Investigation' and 'Adjudication'. The investigation stages investigate cases to assess whether there is a need to refer them for adjudication. The adjudication stage consists of a hearing of those cases that have been referred to a Fitness to Practise Panel.

Where the complaint raises questions about the doctor's fitness to practise, an investigation will commence and the complaint will be disclosed to the doctor and his/her employer/sponsoring body. This is intended to ensure that there is a complete overview of the doctor's practice and makes the information available to those responsible for local clinical governance. Further information may be sought from the complainant, whose consent will be needed to disclose the complaint to the doctor.

The doctor is given an opportunity to comment on the complaint. An investigation may need further documentary evidence from employers, the complainant or other parties, witness statements, expert reports on clinical matters, an assessment of the doctor's performance and an assessment of the doctor's health.

At the end of the investigation of allegations against a doctor, the case will be considered by two senior GMC staff known as case examiners (one medical and one non-medical) who can conclude the case with no further action, issue a warning, refer the case to a the Panel or agree undertakings. Cases can only be concluded or referred to a Fitness to Practise Panel with the agreement of both a medical and non-medical case examiner. If they fail to agree, the matter will be considered by the Investigation Committee, a statutory committee of the GMC. A warning will be appropriate where the concerns indicate a significant departure from the standards set out in the GMC's guidance for doctors, *Good Medical Practice*, or if there is a significant cause for concern following assessment.

At any stage of the investigation a doctor may be referred to an Interim Orders Panel (IOP), which can suspend or restrict a doctor's practice while the investigation continues. Cases referred to the IOP are those where the doctor faces allegations of such a nature that it may be necessary for the protection of members of the public, or it may be in the public interest or in the interests of the doctor for the doctor's registration to be restricted whilst the allegations are resolved. An IOP may make an order suspending a doctor's registration or imposing conditions upon a doctor's registration for a maximum period of 18 months. An IOP must review the order within 6 months of the order being imposed, and thereafter, at intervals of no more than 6 months. If an IOP wishes to extend an order beyond the period initially set, the GMC will apply to the High Court for permission to do so.

The Fitness to Practise Panel hears evidence and decides whether a doctor's fitness to practise is impaired. Fitness to Practise hearings are the final stage of procedures following a complaint about a doctor.

A Fitness to Practise Panel is composed of medical and non-medical persons and normally comprises three to five panelists. In addition to the chairman, who may be medical or non-medical, there must be at least one medical and one non-medical panelist on each panel. A legal assessor sits with each panel and advises on points of law and of mixed law and fact, including the procedure and powers of the panel. One or more specialist advisers may also be present to provide advice to the panel in relation to medical issues regarding a doctor's health or performance. The GMC is normally represented at the hearing by a barrister. The doctor is invited to attend and is usually present and legally represented. Both parties may call witnesses to give evidence and if they do so the witness may be cross-examined by the other party. The panel may also put questions to the witnesses. The panels meet in public, except where they are considering confidential information concerning the doctor's health or they are considering making an interim order.

Once the panel has heard the evidence, it must decide whether the facts alleged have been found proved and whether, on the basis of the facts found proved, the doctor's fitness to practise is impaired and, if so, whether any action should be taken against the doctor's registration. If the panel concludes that the doctor's fitness to practise is impaired, the following sanctions are available: to take no action; to accept undertakings offered by the doctor provided that the panel is satisfied that such undertakings protect patients and the wider public interest; to place conditions on the doctor's registration; to suspend the doctor's registration; or to erase the doctor's name from the Medical Register, so that they can no longer practise.

Doctors have a right of appeal to the High Court (Court of Session in Scotland) against any decision by a panel to restrict or remove their registration. The Council for Healthcare Regulatory Excellence (which oversees and scrutinizes nine healthcare regulatory bodies in the UK) may also appeal against certain decisions if they consider the decision was too lenient. Any doctor whose name was erased from the Medical Register ('the Register') by a Fitness to Practise Panel can apply for their name to be restored to the Register. Doctors cannot apply to have their name restored to the Register until after a period of 5 years has elapsed since the date their name was erased.

Regulatory bodies for other healthcare professionals in the UK follow a general style similar to that of the GMC when assessing the performance of practitioners.

■ Further information sources

Biggs H. *Healthcare Research Ethics and Law: Regulation, Review and Responsibility.* London: Routledge Cavendish, 2010.

Caldicott Guardian Manual 2010. http://www.dh.gov.uk/prod_consum_dh/groups/dh_digitalassets/@dh/@en/@ps/documents/digitalasset/dh_114506.pdf (accessed 23 November 2010).

Chester (Respondent) v Afshar (Appellant) (2004) UKHL 41 Pt 2. http://www.publications.parliament.uk/pa/ld200304/ldjudgmt/jd041014/cheste-1.htm (accessed 23 November 2010).

Council for Healthcare Regulatory Excellence. http://www.chre.org.uk/.

Fitness to Practice Rules 2004. http://www.gmc-uk.org/consolidated_version_of_FTP_Rules.pdf.26875225.pdf (accessed 23 November 2010).

General Medical Council. http://www.gmc-uk.org/.

General Medical Council. *Good Medical Practice.* Manchester: General Medical Council, 2006; http://www.gmc-uk.org/guidance/good_medical_practice/index.asp

General Medical Council *Confidentiality. Guidance for Doctors.* Manchester: GMC, 2009; http://www.gmc-uk.org/static/documents/content/Confidentiality_core_2009.pdf

General Medical Council *Consent: Patients and Doctors Making Decisions Together. Guidance for Doctors.* Manchester: GMC, 2008; http://www.gmc-uk.org/Consent_0510.pdf_32611803.pdf

Gillick v West Norfolk and Wisbech AHA [1986] AC 112. http://www.hrcr.org/safrica/childrens_rights/Gillick_WestNorfolk.htm (accessed 23 November 2010).

Health Professions Council. http://www.hpc-uk.org.

Lynch J. *Health Records in Court.* Oxford: Radcliffe Publishing, 2009.

Lynch J. *Clinical Responsibility.* Oxford: Radcliffe Publishing, 2009.

McLean S. *Autonomy, Consent and the Law.* London: Routledge Cavendish, 2010.

McLean S, Mason JK. *Legal and Ethical Aspects of Healthcare.* London: Greenwich Medical Media, 2003.

Medical Act 1858. http://www.legislation.gov.uk/ukpga/1858/90/pdfs/ukpga_18580090_en.pdf (accessed 23 November 2010).

Medical Act 1983. http://www.opsi.gov.uk/si/si2006/draft/20064681.htm (accessed 23 November 2010).

Mental Capacity Act 2005. http://www.legislation.gov.uk/ukpga/2005/9/contents (accessed 23 November 2010).

Nursing and Midwifery Council. http://www.nmc-uk.org.

Pattinson SD. *Medical Law and Ethics*, 2nd edn. London: Sweet & Maxwell, 2009.

Payne-James JJ, Dean P, Wall I. *Medicolegal Essentials in Healthcare*, 2nd edn. London: Greenwich Medical Media, 2004.

World Medical Association. http://www.wma.net/.

World Medical Association. *WMA International Code of Medical Ethics.* http://www.wma.net/en/30publications/10policies/c8/index.html (accessed 23 November 2010).

Chapter

3

The medical aspects of death

■ Introduction

All doctors encounter death, and the dying, at some time in their medical career, and must have an understanding of the medical and legal aspects of these phenomena.

■ Definition of death

Only organisms that have experienced life can die, as death represents the cessation of life in a previously living organism. Medically and scientifically, death is not an event; it is a process in which cellular metabolic processes in different tissues and organs cease to function at different rates.

This differential rate of cellular death has resulted in much debate – ethical, religious and moral – as to when 'death' actually occurs. The practical solution to this argument is to consider the death of a single cell (cellular death) and the cessation of the integrated functioning of an individual (somatic death) as two separate aspects.

Cellular death

Cellular death means the cessation of respiration (the utilization of oxygen) and the normal metabolic activity in the body tissues and cells. Cessation of respiration is soon followed by autolysis and decay, which, if it affects the whole body, is indisputable evidence of true death. The differences in cellular metabolism determine the rate at which cells die and this can be very variable – except, perhaps, in the synchronous death of all of the cells following, for example, a nearby nuclear explosion.

Skin and bone will remain metabolically active and thus 'alive' for many hours and these cells can be successfully cultured days after somatic death. White blood cells are capable of movement for up to 12 hours after cardiac arrest – a fact that makes the concept of microscopic identification of a 'vital reaction' to injury of doubtful reliability. The cortical neuron, on the other hand, will die after only 3–7 minutes of complete oxygen deprivation. A body dies cell by cell and the complete process may take many hours.

Somatic death and resuscitation

Somatic death means that the individual will never again communicate or deliberately interact with the environment. The individual is irreversibly unconscious and unaware of both the world and their own existence. The key word in this definition is 'irreversible', as lack of communication and interaction with the environment may occur in a variety of settings such as deep sleep, under anaesthesia, under the influence of drugs or alcohol or as a result of a temporary coma.

There is no statutory definition of death in the United Kingdom but, following proposed 'brain death criteria' by the Conference of Medical Royal Colleges in 1976, the courts in England and Northern Ireland have adopted these criteria as part of the law for the diagnosis of death.

The Academy of Medical Royal Colleges has published a code of practice for the diagnosis of death, stating that 'death entails the irreversible loss of those essential characteristics which are necessary to the existence of a living human person and, thus, the definition of death should be regarded as the irreversible loss of the capacity to breathe.'

Criteria for the diagnosis and confirmation of death are specified following cardiorespiratory arrest, in a primary care setting and in hospital, and following irreversible cessation of brain-stem function, where specified conditions have been fulfilled (see Boxes 3.1–3.3).

Advances in resuscitation techniques in ventilation and in the support of the unconscious patient have resulted in the survival of patients that would otherwise have died as a result of direct cerebral trauma or of cerebral hypoxia from whatever cause.

Previously, brain-stem death would lead inexorably to respiratory arrest and this would cause myocardial hypoxia and cardiac arrest. Artificial ventilation breaks that chain and while ventilation is continued, myocardial hypoxia and cardiac arrest are prevented.

There is a spectrum of survival: some will recover both spontaneous respiration and consciousness, others will never regain consciousness but will regain the ability to breathe on their own and some will regain neither consciousness nor the ability to breathe and will require permanent artificial ventilation to remain 'alive'.

Box 3.1 Criteria for the diagnosis and confirmation of death following cardiorespiratory arrest

- Simultaneous and irreversible onset of apnoea and unconsciousness in the absence of the circulation, following 'full and extensive attempts' at reversal of any contributing causes of cardiorespiratory arrest
- One of the following applies:
  - criteria for not attempting cardiopulmonary resuscitation (CPR) are fulfilled, or
  - CPR attempts have failed, or
  - life-sustaining treatment has been withdrawn, where a decision has been made that such treatment is not in the patient's best interest, or where there is an 'advance decision' from the patient to refuse such treatment
- The person responsible for confirming death observes the individual for a minimum of 5 minutes, ensuring an absence of a central pulse on palpation and an absence of heart sounds on auscultation
- In a hospital setting, supplementary 'evidence' of death may be provided in the form of asystole on a continuous electrocardiogram (ECG) display, absence of contractile activity using echocardiography or absence of pulsatile flow using direct intra-arterial pressure monitoring
- Confirmation of the absence of pupillary responses to light, of the corneal reflexes and any motor response to supra-orbital pressure
- The time of death is recorded when these criteria have been fulfilled

Adapted from Academy of Medical Royal Colleges (2008) *A Code of Practice for the Diagnosis and Confirmation of Death. Report of a Working Party*, London.

Box 3.2 Criteria for the diagnosis of death following irreversible cessation of brain-stem function (adults and children over the age of 2 months)

- Absence of brain-stem reflexes:
  - pupils are fixed and do not respond to changes in light intensity
  - corneal reflex is absent
  - oculovestibular reflexes are absent when ice-cold water is introduced into the ear canals
  - no motor responses within the cranial nerve distribution can be elicited by stimulation of any somatic area
  - no cough reflex response to bronchial stimulation by a suction catheter placed in the trachea down to the carina
  - no gag response to stimulation of the posterior pharynx with a spatula
  - no spontaneous respiratory response following disconnection from the ventilator ('apnoea test'), where arterial blood gas sampling confirms an increase in $PaCO_2$ by more than 0.5 kPa above the starting level
- Brain-stem testing should be made by at least two medical practitioners, registered for more than 5 years, and who are competent in the interpretation of such tests; at least one of these individuals must be a consultant
- Ancillary investigations – cerebral angiography, perfusion and neurophysiological – may be appropriate in some circumstances; brain-stem tests cannot be performed, for example, where there are extensive maxillofacial injuries

Adapted from Academy of Medical Royal Colleges (2008) *A Code of Practice for the Diagnosis and Confirmation of Death. Report of a Working Party*, London.

Box 3.3 Conditions necessary for the diagnosis and confirmation of death following irreversible cessation of brain-stem function

- Irreversible brain damage resulting from damage of known aetiology or, following continuing clinical observation and investigation, there is no possibility of a reversible or treatable underlying cause being present
- Potentially reversible causes of coma have been excluded
- There is no evidence that the state is caused by depressant drugs, for example narcotics, hypnotics or tranquillizers; specific antagonists may need to be used
- Hypothermia as the cause of unconsciousness has been excluded
- Potentially reversible circulatory, metabolic and endocrine disturbances have been excluded as the cause of the continuation of unconsciousness, including hyperglycaemia or hypoglycaemia
- Potentially reversible causes of apnoea have been excluded, for example the effects of neuromuscular blocking agents

Adapted from Academy of Medical Royal Colleges (2008) *A Code of Practice for the Diagnosis and Confirmation of Death. Report of a Working Party*, London.

Vegetative state

In some individuals, resuscitation is successful in that brain-stem function is retained in the absence of cortical function, resulting in a so-called 'vegetative state (VS)' – wakefulness without awareness – from which they may recover, or alternatively may enter a 'minimally conscious state' (MCS). If the VS persists for 12 months following traumatic brain injury or 6 months after another cause, the VS is judged to be 'permanent' under Royal College of Physicians guidelines (2003). In such circumstances, the withdrawal of hydration and assisted nutrition can be considered in the 'best interests' of the patient.

The first, and most significant, case regarding the legality of such withdrawal of 'life sustaining' treatment concerned Tony Bland, in 'persistent vegetative state' following an accident at a football ground (Airedale NHS Trust v Bland). Since that case, in which permission to remove assisted feeding was granted, additional cases have sought to clarify the position following the enactment of the Human Rights Act 1998, the 'right to life' and the right not to be subjected to inhuman and degrading treatment.

Research into functional magnetic resonance imaging (MRI) has identified individuals thought to be in VS with brain activity more in keeping with a diagnosis of MCS. While none of these individuals

has recovered beyond that state, the law and practice relating to the withdrawal of 'life sustaining' treatment in the VS may be subject to change in the future.

Tissue and organ transplantation

The laws relating to tissue and organ donation and transplantation are dependent upon the religious and ethical views of the country in which they apply. The laws vary in both extent and detail around the world, but there are very few countries where transplantation is expressly forbidden and few religions that forbid it – Jehovah's Witnesses are one such group; they also reject transfusion of donated blood.

The organs and tissues to be transplanted may come from one of several sources, which are outlined below.

Homologous transplantation

Tissue is moved between sites on the same body. For example, skin grafts may be taken from the thigh to place on a burn site or bone chips from the pelvis may be taken to assist in the healing of a fracture of a long bone. Homologous blood transfusion can be used where there is a religious objection to the use of anonymously donated blood.

Live donation

In this process, tissue is taken from a living donor whose tissues have been matched to, or are compatible with, those of the recipient. The most common example is blood transfusion but marrow transplantation is now also very common. Other live donations usually involve the kidneys as these are paired organs and donors can, if the remaining kidney is healthy, maintain their electrolyte and water balance with only one kidney.

Most kidneys for transplant are derived from cadaveric donation, but live donation is also possible and this, associated with a high demand for kidneys, especially in Western countries, has resulted in a few surgeons seeking donors (in particular poor people from developing countries) who would be willing to sell one of their kidneys.

This practice is illegal in many countries and, if not specifically illegal, it is certainly unethical.

With increasing surgical skill, the transplantation of a part of a single organ with large physiological reserve (such as the liver) has been more widespread.

Cadaveric donation

In many countries, cadaveric donation is the major source of all tissues for transplantation. The surgical techniques to harvest the organs are improving, as are the storage and transportation techniques, but the best results are still obtained if the organs are obtained while circulation is present or immediately after cessation of the circulation. The aim is to minimize the 'warm ischaemic time'. Some organs (e.g. kidneys) are more resilient to anoxia than others and can survive up to 30 minutes after cessation of cardiac activity.

Cadaveric donation is now so well established that most developed countries have sophisticated laws to regulate it. However, these laws vary greatly: some countries allow the removal of organs regardless of the wishes of the relatives, whereas other countries allow for an 'opting-out' process in which organs can be taken for transplantation unless there is an objection from relatives. The converse of that system is the one practised in the UK, which requires 'opting in'. In this system, the transplant team must ensure that the donor either gave active permission during life or at least did not object and that no close relative objects after death.

The statutory framework governing organ donation from the living and the dead for transplantation is now to be found in the Human Tissue Act 2004 in England, Wales and Northern Ireland – with a similar framework in Scotland – and the Human Tissue Authority has produced a Code of Practice to be followed in such circumstances. Consent for transplantation forms the underlying requirement, and the Act identifies the relevant 'qualifying relationships' regarding who may give such consent.

If an autopsy will be required by law for any reason, the permission of the Coroner, Procurator Fiscal or other legal officer investigating the death must be obtained before harvesting of tissue or organs is undertaken. In general, there is seldom any reason for the legal officer investigating the death to object to organ or tissue donation because it is self-evident that injured, diseased or damaged organs are unlikely to be harvested and certainly will not be transplanted and so will be available for examination.

Description of intraoperative findings by transplant surgeons will suffice in many cases, although it may sometimes be desirable for the pathologist who will subsequently perform the autopsy to be present at the organ retrieval procedure in order to see the extent of external and internal trauma 'first-hand'. In what is almost always a tragic unexpected death, the donation of organs may be the one positive feature and can often be of great assistance to the relatives in knowing that the death of a loved one has resulted in a good outcome for someone.

Xenografts

Grafting of animal tissue into humans has always seemed tempting and clinical trials have been performed with limited success. There is considerable difficulty with cross-matching the tissues and considerable concern about the possibility of transfer of animal viruses to an immunocompromised human host. Strains of donor animals, usually pigs, are being bred in clinically clean conditions to prevent viral contamination, but there is still no guarantee of a close or ideal tissue match. Also, the complexity of their breeding and rearing means that these animals are expensive.

Cloning

A potentially cheaper solution involves the cloning of animals for use as transplant donors. This research took a step forward with the successful cloning of Dolly the sheep in 1996. However, other advances have been slow to appear and although cloning remains a theoretical course of action, much research is still to be done, with its attendant moral and ethical considerations.

■ Cause of death determination and certification

When deciding on what to ascribe an individual's death to, the doctor is making a judgement about causation, which may be relatively straightforward in an individual who has a documented history of ischaemic heart disease and who experiences a cardiac arrest in hospital while on a cardiac monitor. Difficulties arise, for example, where an individual suffers a traumatic event, but has severe underlying natural disease, or where there are many potentially fatal conditions, each capable of providing an explanation for death at that time.

The degree of certainty with which the doctor is required to decide the cause of death may vary between jurisdictions, and it may be more 'intellectually honest' to provide the cause of death determination in a more 'narrative' style, such as is increasingly seen in Coroners' verdicts at inquests in England and Wales.

The law relating to causation is complex, varies between jurisdictions and is a subject outside the scope of this book. However, common themes in this area of law are that 'the cause' is something that is 'substantial and significant' (i.e. it is sufficient to have caused death), and that the outcome would not have occurred 'but for' the occurrence of the illness, disease or alleged action/omission of another person (i.e. it was necessary for such illness or other factor to have occurred for the outcome to be fatal).

In general, if a doctor knows the cause of death, and that cause of death is 'natural' (without any suspicious or unusual features), they may issue a certificate of the medical cause of death (commonly called a 'death certificate'). Which doctor may do this varies: in some countries the doctor must have seen and treated the patient before death, whereas in other countries any doctor who has seen the body after death may issue a certificate.

The format for certifying the cause of death is now defined by the World Health Organization (WHO) and is an international standard that is used in most countries. The system divides the cause of death into two parts: the first part (Part I) describes the condition(s) that led directly to death; Part II is for other conditions, not related to those listed in Part I, that have also contributed to death.

Part I is divided into subsections and generally three – (a), (b) and (c) – are printed on the certificate. These subsections are for disease processes that have led directly to death and that are causally related to one another, (a) being caused by or is a consequence of (b), which in turn is caused by or is a consequence of (c), etc. It is important to realize that, in this system of death certification, it is the disease lowest in the Part I list that is the most important, as it is the primary pathological condition in the 'chain of events' leading to death. It is this disease that is most important statistically and which is used to compile national and international mortality statistics.

Doctors should not record the mode of death (e.g. coma, heart failure) in isolation on the death certificate but, if a mode is specified, it should be qualified by indicating the underlying pathological abnormality leading to that mode of death. For example:

Ia Cardiac failure
Ib Hypertrophic cardiomyopathy
or
Ia Coma
Ib Subarachnoid haemorrhage
Ic Ruptured congenital aneurysm.

Some jurisdictions will allow specific causes of death that would not be acceptable elsewhere. In the UK it is acceptable in certain situations, i.e. if the patient is over 80 years of age, to record 'Ia: Old age'.

At the other end of the age range, the diagnosis of sudden infant death syndrome (SIDS) is now well established; unfortunately, the diagnostic criteria are seldom as well known and even less frequently are they applied to the letter.

The utility of the second part of the death certificate is perhaps questionable, and has a tendency to be used as something of a 'dustbin' to record all, many or some of the diseases afflicting the patient at the time of death, regardless of their causative role in that death. Guidance for doctors completing medical certificates of the cause of death has been produced by the Office for National Statistics.

The reliability of the information contained within the death certificate depends wholly on the integrity and competency of the certifying doctor. Concerns regarding the utility of the death certificate in the UK, prompted in part by the investigation into the homicidal activities of an English doctor, Harold Shipman, which came to light in the late 1990s, have led to proposals for legislative reform in England and Wales. It is anticipated that all death certificates will be scrutinized by a 'medical examiner' who will form a new link between the local health authority and Coroner, identifying cases for further investigation and trends in the local population.

International classifications of disease are now well established and the WHO produced a book, *International Statistical Classification of Diseases and Related Health Problems* (ICD), which can be

BIRTHS AND DEATHS REGISTRATION ACT 1953

(Form prescribed by the Registration of Births, Death and Marriages (Amendment) Regulations 1968)

MEDICAL CERTIFICATE OF CAUSE OF DEATH

For use only by a Registered Medical Practitioner WHO HAS BEEN IN ATTENDANCE during the deceased's last illness, and to be delivered by him forthwith to the Registrar of Births and Deaths

Registrar to enter No of Death Entry

Name of deceased ....

Date of death as stated to me .... day of .... 19....

Place of death ....

Age as stated to me ....

Last seen alive by me .... day of ....

1 The certified cause of death takes account of information obtained from post-mortem.

2 Information from post-mortem may be available later.

3 Post-mortem not being held.

4 I have reported this death to the Coroner for further action.

[See overleaf]

Please ring appropriate digit/s and letter

a Seen after death by me.

b Seen after death by another medical practitioner.

c Not seen after death by a medical practitioner.

CAUSE OF DEATH

The condition thought to be the 'Underlying Cause of Death' should appear in the lowest completed line of Part I

These particulars not to be entered in death register

Approximate interval between onset and death

I(a) Disease or condition directly leading to death† ....

(b) Other disease or condition, if any, leading to I(a) ....

(c) Other disease or condition, if any, leading to I(b) ....

II Other significant conditions CONTRIBUTING TO THE DEATH but not related to the disease or condition causing it. ....

†This does not mean the mode of dying, such as heart failure, asphyxia, asthenia, etc; it means the disease, injury, or complication which caused death.

The death might have been due to or contributed to by the employment followed at some time by the deceased. □ Please tick where applicable

I hereby certify that I was in medical attendance during the above named deceased's last illness, and that the particulars and cause of death above written are true to the best of my knowledge and belief.

Signature ....

Qualifications as registered by General Medical Council

Residence.................... Date ....

For deaths in hospital: Please give the name of the consultant responsible for the above-named as a patient. ....

(Form prescribed by the Registration of Births, Deaths and Marriages Regulations 1968)

NOTICE TO INFORMANT

I hereby give notice that I have this day signed a medical certificate of cause of death of

....

Signature

Date

This notice is to be delivered by the informant to the registrar of births and deaths for the sub-district in which the death occurred.

The certifying medical practitioner must give this notice to the person who is qualified and liable to act as informant for the registration of death (see list overleaf).

DUTIES OF INFORMANT

Failure to deliver this notice to the registrar renders the informant liable to prosecution. The death cannot be registered until the medical certificate has reached the registrar.

When the death is registered the informant must be prepared to give to the registrar the following particulars relating to the deceased:

1. The date and place of death.

2. The full name and surname (and the maiden surname if the deceased was a woman who had married).

3. The date and place of birth.

4. The occupation (and if the deceased was a married woman or a widow the name and occupation of her husband).

5. The usual address.

6. Whether the deceased was in receipt of a pension or allowance from public funds.

7. If the deceased was married, the date of birth of the surviving widow or widower.

THE DECEASED'S MEDICAL CARD SHOULD BE DELIVERED TO THE REGISTRAR

Figure 3.1 Reproduction of death certificate (doctor's counterfoil omitted).

used for both clinical diagnoses and death certificates. In this classification, each condition is given a four-digit ICD code, which simplifies both data recording and data analysis and allows information from many national and international sources to be compared.

In some countries, doctors also have to record the manner of death (e.g. homicide, suicide) on the death certificate, as advocated by the WHO; however, in most Western countries with an efficient medico-legal investigative system, the conclusion about the manner of death is delegated to a legal officer, for example the Coroner in England and Wales, the Procurator Fiscal in Scotland or the Medical Examiner in some of the states of the USA (Figure 3.1)

■ Medico-legal investigation of death

If a death is natural and a doctor can sign a death certificate, this allows the relatives to continue with the process of disposal of the body, whether by burial or cremation. If the death is not natural or if no doctor can complete a death certificate, some other method of investigating and certifying the death must be in place. In England and Wales there are approximately 500 000 deaths each year, of which over half are certified by doctors without referral to Coroners. In 2009, just under 230 000 deaths were reported to Coroners, of which approximately 106 000 required a post-mortem examination to determine the cause of death.

The types of deaths that cannot be certified by a doctor are examined by a variety of legal officers in other countries: Coroners, procurators fiscal, medical examiners, magistrates, judges and even police officers. The exact systems of referral, responsibility and investigation differ widely, but the general framework is much the same. The systems are arranged to identify and investigate deaths that are, or might be, unnatural, overtly criminal, suspicious, traumatic or caused by poisoning, or that might simply be deaths that are unexpected or unexplained (Figure 3.2).

There is currently no common-law duty for a doctor to report an unnatural death to the Coroner, but legislative changes are imminent in England and Wales, and will place a statutory duty on all doctors

to report certain categories of death to the Coroner. The Registrar of Deaths already has such a duty to inform the Coroner about any death that appears to be unnatural or where the rules about completion of the death certificate have not been complied with.

Following the death of a person who has not been receiving medical supervision, and where no doctor was in attendance, the fact of death can be confirmed by nurses, paramedics and other healthcare professionals as well as by doctors. The police will usually investigate the scene and the circumstances of the death and report their findings to the Coroner or other legal authority. The Coroner, through his officers, will attempt to find a family practitioner to obtain medical details. That family practitioner, if found, may be able to complete the death certificate if he is aware of sufficient natural disease and if the scene and circumstances of the death are not suspicious.

If no family practitioner can be found, or if the practitioner is unwilling to issue a death certificate, the Coroner will usually exercise his or her right to require an autopsy, but in Scotland the ability to perform only an external examination of the body on cases such as this – the so-called 'view and grant'– is well established.

This all-embracing coronial power to order autopsies is not found in other countries, where autopsies are often much more restricted. It is not surprising, therefore, that the autopsy rate varies widely from jurisdiction to jurisdiction; in some cases it is nearly

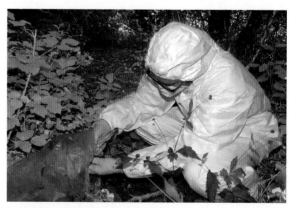

Figure 3.2 Examination of skeletal remains at a wooded 'scene'. The forensic pathologist wears appropriate protective equipment in order to prevent contamination of the remains. The attendance at a 'scene' follows discussion with the crime scene manager regarding the health and safety implications of the 'scene', the approach to the body/remains and a forensic strategy for the recovery of 'trace evidence', including swabs and 'tape lifts' from sites such as exposed skin surfaces and body orifices.

100 per cent but it may fall as low as 5–10 per cent. Some jurisdictions with low autopsy rates insist on the external examination of the body by a doctor with medico-legal training. Autopsy examinations are not the complete and final answer to every death, but without an internal examination it can be impossible to be certain about the cause and the mechanism of death. At least one-third of the causes of death given by doctors have been shown to be incorrect by a subsequent autopsy.

In England and Wales, Coroners' jurisdiction begins when they are informed that a body of a person is lying within their district, and there is reasonable cause to suspect that the deceased died a violent or unnatural death, has died a sudden death of unknown cause, or has died in custody or prison (Coroners Act 1988, Section 8). Deaths are usually referred to the Coroner by doctors, police and members of the public. The circumstances in which the Registrar of Deaths currently must refer a death to the Coroner are contained in the Registration of Births and Deaths Regulations 1987:

- the deceased was not attended in his last illness by the doctor completing the certificate;
- the deceased had not been seen by a doctor either after death or within 14 days prior to death;
- where the cause of death is unknown;
- where death appears to be due to poisoning or to industrial disease;
- where death may have been unnatural or where it may have been caused by violence or neglect or abortion or where it is associated with suspicious circumstances;
- where death occurred during a surgical operation or before recovery from an anaesthetic.

Once a death is reported, the Coroner, if satisfied that it is from natural causes, can decide not to pursue any further enquiries and to ask the doctor to issue a death certificate. Alternatively, and more commonly, he may order an autopsy and, if this reveals that death was from natural causes, may issue a certificate to allow for disposal of the body. If the autopsy cannot establish that death was from natural causes, or if there is a public interest in the death, the Coroner may hold an inquest (a public inquiry into the death). The modern inquest is severely restricted in its functions and the verdicts it may return. An inquest seeks to answer four questions: who the person is, when and where they died and how they died (Coroners Rules 1984). The 'who', 'when' and 'where' questions seldom pose a problem; it is the answer to the fourth question – the 'how' – that is often the most difficult.

The Coroner can sit with or without a jury, except in some specific cases (e.g. deaths on a rail-track or in a prison) when they must sit with a jury. The Coroner's court cannot form any view about either criminal or civil blame for the death.

A Coroner or the jury has a prescribed list of possible verdicts and, although riders or comments may be attached to these verdicts, they must not indicate or imply blame. The commonly used verdicts include:

- unlawful killing (which includes murder, manslaughter, infanticide, death by dangerous driving);
- lawful killing (legal use of lethal force by a police officer);
- accident (misadventure);
- killed himself/herself (suicide);
- natural causes;
- industrial disease;
- abuse of drugs (dependent or non-dependent);
- open verdict (where the evidence is insufficient to reach any other verdict).

There is an increasing trend, however, for the Coroner to deliver a 'narrative verdict' which is a factual record of how, and in what circumstances, the death occurred, and this is often used in those cases in which the cause of death does not fit easily into any of the 'short-form' verdicts. Within the narrative verdict the Coroner may request an inquest jury (if the inquest is held before a jury) to address specific questions perceived to be of concern.

■ The autopsy

The words autopsy, necropsy and post-mortem examination are synonymous, although postmortem examination can have a broader meaning encompassing any examination made after death, including a simple external examination. In general terms, autopsies can be performed for two reasons: clinical interest and medico-legal purposes.

The clinical autopsy is performed in a hospital mortuary after consent for the examination has been sought from, and granted by, the relatives of the deceased. The doctors treating the patient should know why their patient has died and be able to complete a death certificate even in the absence of an autopsy. These examinations have been used in the past for the teaching of medical students and others, and for research, but have been in decline worldwide for several decades.

The medico-legal autopsy is performed on behalf of the state. The aims of these examinations are much broader than those of the clinical autopsy; they aim to:

- identify the body;
- estimate the time of death;
- identify and document the nature and number of injuries;
- interpret the significance and effect of the injuries;
- identify the presence of any natural disease;
- interpret the significance and effect of the natural disease present;
- identify the presence of poisons; and
- interpret the effect of any medical or surgical treatment.

Autopsies can, in theory, be performed by any doctor, but ideally they should be performed by a properly trained pathologist. Medico-legal autopsies are a specialized version of the standard autopsy and should be performed by pathologists who have had the necessary training and experience in forensic pathology. The autopsy should be performed in a mortuary with adequate facilities (Figure 3.3). Guidelines for an autopsy are contained in Appendix 1 (p.240).

However, where there are no trained staff or no adequate facilities – which can occur not only in some developing countries but also in some so-called developed countries that do not adequately fund their medico-legal systems – non-specialist doctors may occasionally have to perform autopsies and histopathologists may have to perform medico-legal autopsies. A poorly performed autopsy may be considerably worse than no autopsy at all; it is certainly worse than an autopsy delayed for a short while to await the arrival of a specialist.

The first crucial part of any autopsy is observation and documentation and these skills should lie within the competence of almost every doctor. All documentation should be in writing, and diagrams, drawings and annotations must be signed and dated at the end of the examination. Photographs are extremely useful in all medico-legal autopsies, but

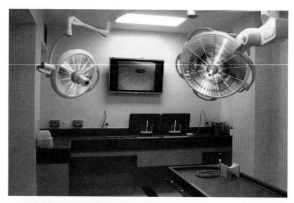

Figure 3.3 Modern forensic autopsy facilities, including directional overhead lighting – with inbuilt video projection and recording capability – to facilitate optimal forensic pathological examinations.

are essential in suspicious deaths. Photographic documentation of injuries should include a scale and some anatomical reference point for ease of review.

Many autopsies will require ancillary investigations, such as radiological, toxicological, biochemical and microscopic analyses. (Figure 3.4, Figure 3.5) These will all have financial implications. Such matters and unwillingness of some individuals to allow autopsy on relatives have been active drivers in exploring other means of undertaking appropriate examinations to establish cause of death. There is substantial interest in many countries into the utility of more modern radiological modalities, such as computed tomography (CT) and MRI, in a post-mortem setting, and results of studies suggest that there is potential for virtual autopsy ('virtopsy') techniques playing a significant role, where such facilities are available, in reducing the requirement for a full

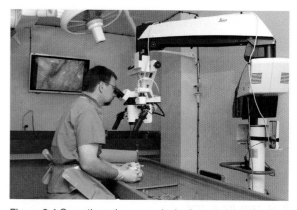

Figure 3.4 Operating microscopy in the forensic autopsy suite facilitates detailed examination and documentation of pathological findings.

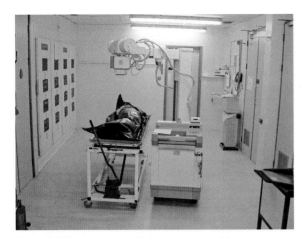

Figure 3.5 Post-mortem radiology is important in many cases in forensic pathology. Note the body is enclosed in a body bag to prevent contamination of the body and loss of 'trace evidence' from the surface of the body, prior to autopsy. Hands (and usually feet) are similarly protected by paper or plastic bags before recovery of a body from a scene.

autopsy examination. The use of imaging techniques in forensic medicine also has potential for wider application in the clinical setting for survivors of, for example, manual strangulation or stabbing, where injury characteristics can be better defined.

◼ The Minnesota protocol

A model autopsy protocol has been produced by the United Nations within the context of the investigation of human rights abuses – the Minnesota Protocol (the United Nations Manual on the Effective Presentation and Investigation of Extra-legal, Arbitrary and Summary Executions) – but which can be used for dealing with 'difficult or sensitive' or controversial cases. The protocol, which covers all stages of the pathological death investigation process, from scene examination to ancillary tests, recognizes the need for such cases to be dealt with by objective, experienced, well-equipped and well-trained pathologists, and much of the detail contained within the protocol codifies the standards already followed by forensic pathologists when performing suspicious death autopsies in many countries.

◼ Exhumation

It is rare for a body to be removed from its grave for further examination; the most common reasons for exhumation are personal, for example if a family chooses to move the body or if a cemetery is to be closed or altered. Various legal formalities must be observed before permission to exhume a body can be given, but these lie outside the scope of this book. Once legal permission has been given, the correct site of the grave must be determined from plans and records of the cemetery, as well as inscriptions on headstones.

In some countries with a low autopsy rate, for example Belgium, exhumations are more common, as legal arguments about an accident or an insurance claim, etc., require an examination of the body to establish the medical facts.

The mechanics of removal of a coffin require some thought and the practice of actually lifting the coffin before dawn owes more to Hollywood than to practical needs. As the body may need to be examined as quickly as possible because of decomposition, the mortuary, the pathologist, the police and everyone else with a legitimate interest must be aware of the time arranged.

An examination of a body after exhumation is seldom as good as the examination of a fresh body, but it is surprising how well-preserved a body may remain and how useful such an examination often is. It is almost impossible to predict how well preserved a body might be, as there are so many confounding factors (Figure 3.6). The autopsy that follows an exhumation should be the same as that performed at any other time, and should be performed by a skilled and experienced forensic pathologist.

If there is a possibility that poisoning may have played a part in the death, samples of soil should

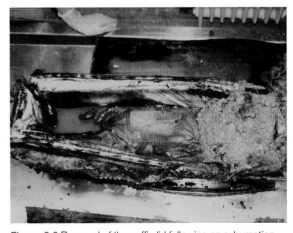

Figure 3.6 Removal of the coffin lid following an exhumation. Liquid mud covers the upper body following leakage of the coffin lid.

be taken from above, below and to the sides of the coffin and submitted for toxicological examination. A control sample should also be taken from a distant part of the cemetery. Additional samples should be taken of any fluid or solid material within the coffin; these control samples may prove useful if any suggestion of contamination is raised at a later date.

■ Further reading

Academy of Medical Royal Colleges. http://www.aomrc.org.uk

Academy of Medical Royal Colleges. 2008. *A Code of Practice for the Diagnosis and Confirmation of Death. Report of a Working Party.* London: Academy of Medical Royal Colleges (http://www.aomrc.org.uk/).

Airedale NHS Trust v Bland (1993) AC789 at 898. http://www.bailii.org/uk/cases/UKHL/1992/5.html (accessed 22 November 2010).

BBC. 1997. Dolly the sheep is cloned: http://news.bbc.co.uk/onthisday/hi/dates/stories/february/22/newsid_4245000/4245877.stm (accessed 22 November 2010).

Bolliger SA, Thali MJ, Ross S, Buck U, Naether S, Vock P. Virtual autopsy using imaging: bridging radiologic and forensic sciences. A review of the Virtopsy and similar projects. *European Radiology* 2008; **18**: 273–82.

Bolliger SA, Filograna L, Spendlove D, Thali MJ, Dirnhofer S, Ross S. Postmortem imaging-guided biopsy as an adjuvant to minimally invasive autopsy with CT and postmortem angiography: a feasibility study. *AJR American Journal of Roentgenology* 2010; **195**: 1051–6.

Burton JL, Rutty GN (eds). *The Hospital Autopsy: A Manual of Fundamental Autopsy Practice,* 3rd edn. London: Hodder Arnold, 2010.

Coroners Rules (as amended) 1984 SI No. 552.

Coroners Act 1988. http://www.legislation.gov.uk/ukpga/1988/13/contents (accessed 22 November 2010).

Dolly the sheep: http://news.bbc.co.uk/1/hi/sci/tech/2764039.stm

Human Rights Act 1998. http://www.legislation.gov.uk/ukpga/1998/42/contents (accessed 22 November 2010).

Human Tissue Act 2004 C.30. http://www.legislation.gov.uk/ukpga/2004/30 (accessed 22 November 2010).

Human Tissue Authority. *Code of Practice 2. Donation of Solid Organs for Transplantation.* London: Human Tissue Authority, 2009 (http://www.hta.gov.uk/).

McLean SA. Permanent vegetative state: the legal position. *Neuropsychological Rehabilitation* 2005; **15**: 237–250.

Office for National Statistics. 2008. *Guidance for doctors completing Medical Certificates of Cause of Death in England and Wales. F66 Guidance.* London: Office for National Statistics.

Pattinson SD. *Medical Law and Ethics*, 2nd edn. London: Sweet & Maxwell, 2009.

Registration of Births and Deaths Regulations 1987 No. 2088. http://www.legislation.gov.uk/uksi/1987/2088/contents/made (accessed 22 November 2010).

Royal College of Physicians. *The Vegetative State: Guidelines on Diagnosis and Management. Report of a Working Party.* London: Royal College of Physicians, 2003; http://www.rcplondon.ac.uk/pubs/contents/47a262a7-350a-490a-b88d-6f58bbf076a3.pdf

Shipman Enquiry: http://www.the-shipman-inquiry.org.uk/reports.asp (accessed 22 November 2010).

Skene L, Wilkinson D, Kahane G, Savulescu J. Neuroimaging and the withdrawal of life-sustaining treatment from patients in vegetative state. *Medical Law Review* 2009; **17**: 245–261.

United Nations. *Manual on the Effective Prevention and Investigation of Extra-Legal, Arbitrary and Summary Executions.* www.umn.edu/humanrts/instree/executioninvestigation-91.html (accessed 9 February 2011).

http://whqlibdoc.who.int/publications/9241560622.pdf (accessed 9 February 2011).

World Health Organization (WHO). *International Statistical Classification of Diseases and Related Health Problems.* ICB-10 (10th revision of volume 2) (2nd edn) (available at http://www.who.int/classifications/icd-10_2nd_ed_volume2.pdf) (accessed 12 January 2011) and (accessed 22 November 2010).

WHO Online ICD-10 Training Tool. http://apps.who.int/classifications/apps/icd/ICD10Training/ICD-10%20Death%20Certificate/html/index.html (accessed 12 January 2011).

3 The medical aspects of death

Chapter 4

Identification of the living and the dead

- Introduction
- Methods of identification
- Identity of decomposed or skeletalized remains
- Mass disasters
- Age estimation in the living
- Further information sources

Introduction

Loss of identity, either deliberate (e.g. because someone does not wish their identity to be known, or wishes to conceal the identity of another) or unintentional (e.g. in mass disasters, or loss of confirmatory papers), is a frequent problem for individuals and authorities in cases of both the living and the deceased.

Proper identification of a body is one of the key questions to be answered when a body is found and in the investigation of any death and forms the first part of a Coroner's inquest (see Chapter 3, p. 31). If decomposition or post-mortem changes are advanced then visual identification may not be possible and other techniques may be required to confirm identify. If there is substantial injury (e.g. in aircraft crashes or bombings) or deliberate mutilation other techniques will be required to establish identity.

Governments should have systems in place for the rapid implementation of mass disaster responses in situations of multiple deaths so that casualties and deceased can be identified as expeditiously as possible, for both legal process and reassurance and comfort of relatives.

The detailed assessment of the dead for evidence of identity is a specialized task for a multi-professional team that includes the forensic pathologist, forensic odontologist, anthropologist, radiologist, and other experts, but every doctor should have some idea of the features that can be used to establish the identity of a person, dead or alive.

The same practitioners may also be required to establish the age of an individual whose identity may be known, but whose age is not. Criminal cases and asylum applications are common settings where age may influence how that person is dealt with and age estimation of the living is an increasingly frequent requirement at the request of courts and tribunals.

A number of means of identification (e.g. fingerprints, DNA) are assisted in some countries by well-established databases, such as the National DNA Database in the UK (see p. 222). Presence on these databases is often related to some form of previous criminal involvement, and thus the person or body with no previous criminal record may prove to be more difficult to identify than those with such a record.

■ Methods of identification

Identification criteria

Identification criteria may be termed primary or secondary, with a third group assisting in identification. Primary identification criteria are fingerprints, DNA, dental and unique medical characteristics. Secondary criteria include features such as deformity, marks and scars, X-rays, personal effects and distinctive clothing. Features that may provide some assistance in identification include clothing, photographs and location. Additional techniques such as gait analysis from CCTV can be useful when other features cannot be used.

DNA profiling

The specificity of DNA profiles is so great in statistical terms that it can be reliably specific to any individual (see p. 219).

The molecule of DNA has two strands of sugar and phosphate molecules that are linked by combinations of four bases – adenine, thymine, cytosine and guanine – forming a double helix structure. Only about 10 per cent of the molecule is used for genetic coding (the active genes), the remainder being 'silent'. In these silent zones, there are between 200 and 14 000 repeats of identical sequences of the four bases. Jeffreys found that adjacent sequences were constant for a given individual and that they were transmitted, like blood groups, from the DNA of each parent. Only uni-ovular twins have the same sequences, and the chances of two unrelated individuals sharing the same sequence is one in a billion, or higher. The statistical analysis of DNA identification is extremely complex and it is important that any calculations are based upon the DNA characteristics of a relevant population and not upon the characteristics of a 'standard' population somewhere else in the world.

There is now no need to match blood with blood and semen with semen, as all the DNA in one individual's body must of necessity be identical. A perpetrator leaving any of his or her cells or biological fluids at a scene is leaving proof of their presence at the scene.

Comparison of DNA profiles with assumed or known family members or against known databases can ensure a person's identity is established. If these comparisons cannot be done, other tests must be used.

As the forensic scientists become more and more proficient at extracting and amplifying smaller and smaller amounts of genetic material, so the risks of contamination increase. Scene examination must now be approached with great care and with sufficient protective clothing to prevent the investigators obscuring any relevant DNA by their own material being inadvertently shed from exposed skin, or by sneezing. There is now a need for investigators to provide exclusion DNA samples in the same way as exclusion fingerprints were once provided.

Examination of dental structures

Forensic odontology (see p. 238) techniques are widely used in the establishing or confirmation of identity when bodies are found, or after mass disaster. Pre-existing dental records and charts and radiographic images can be compared with examination of teeth of the deceased. The odontologist may also be asked to make dental charts of bodies whose identity remains unknown or unconfirmed despite a police investigation, so that, should dental information become available at a later date, the two sets of records may be then be compared. Neither a living individual nor a body can be identified simply by taking a dental chart – that chart has to be compared with, and found to match, a chart whose origins are known (Figure 4.1).

The forensic odontologist is of prime importance in mass disasters where trauma is likely to make visual identification impossible. The great advantage of dental identification is that the teeth are the hardest and most resistant tissues in the body and can survive total decomposition and even severe fire, short of actual cremation (Figure 4.2).

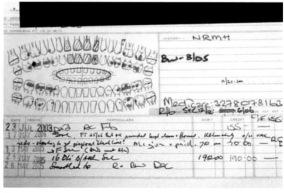

Figure 4.1 Dental chart.

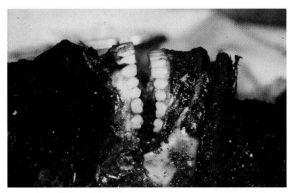

Figure 4.2 Retained dentition after fire.

Where no previous records are available, examination of the mouth and the teeth can still give some general information on age, sex, diet and ethnic origin.

Fingerprints

The recovery of the fingerprints from decomposing and damaged bodies requires the use of specialized techniques which are the province of the fingerprint expert (see also p. 227). Prints may often be obtained from desquamated skin or from the underlying epidermis after shedding of the stratum corneum following prolonged submersion.

Morphological characteristics

Identity cannot be established by the simple measurement of a set of parameters of an individual or a body. It can only be established by matching the parameters that can be measured or seen on an individual with the same parameters that were known to apply to, or to be present on, a named individual. Identification is established by matching a range of general observations made about the body to a range of general information known to be true about that particular individual. The finding of a unique medical feature, or a combination of specific features, that is known to be possessed by that individual alone will add considerable weight to the conclusions.

In both the living and dead, the height, weight and general physique need to be recorded and compared. Hair colour and length, including bleaching or dyeing, the presence of a beard or moustache and the amount and distribution of other body hair, including sites that are commonly shaved, all need to be established. Skin pigmentation, racial and ethnic facial appearances, such as flared nostrils and epicanthic folds are also obvious features that need to be recorded in a standard fashion. All clothing, jewellery and other ornaments on the person must be recorded and photographed as they may provide useful information about the sex, race and even occupation and social status of the body, even if they are not sufficient for identification. Tattoos, surgical scars, old injuries, congenital deformities, striae from childbirth, tribal scars or markings, circumcision, moles, warts and other skin blemishes, etc., must be carefully recorded and, if unusual, photographed because a relative, friend or doctor may be able to confirm an identity from these features.

In a living person or an intact body, the facial appearance is all important, both from ethnic and racial aspects and from individual appearances. Frontal and profile photographs should be taken for comparison.

Tattoos and body piercings

The main use of tattoos and piercings in forensic medicine is in the identification of the bodies of unknown persons. Once again, the simple presence of a tattoo does not constitute identification and there has to be a comparison with the tattoos of a known individual. Ante-mortem images can be very helpful when compared with images of the deceased, which can be used if a visual identification is not possible or so that they can be circulated when the identity is not known.

There is a huge diversity of skin tattoos in Western society, some of which may have specific meaning or significance within certain subgroups of society. However, there is also much folklore about the significance of tattoos, a large amount of which may have been relevant in the past. Now that designs originating from throughout the world are used as body decoration internationally, little assistance is provided by assessing the tattoo design. Names and dates of birth within tattoos may be useful. Decomposing bodies should be examined carefully for tattoos, which may be rendered more visible when the superficial desquamated stratum corneum is removed.

Body piercing is widespread, and the site and type of piercing should be noted and piercings can be used as part of visual identification or can be recovered for identification by relatives if visual identification is not possible.

Identity of decomposed or skeletalized remains

When presumed skeletal remains are discovered, the investigators will want to know the answers to a number of questions. The answers to these questions may require the expertise of pathologists, anthropologists, odontologists, radiologists and scientists. Questions include:

- Are the remains actually bones? Sometimes stones or even pieces of wood are mistaken by the public or police for bones: the anatomical shape, character and texture should be obvious to a doctor.
- Are the remains human? Most doctor should be able to identify most intact long bones. A forensic pathologist will be able to identify almost all of the human skeleton, although phalanges, carpal and tarsal bones can be extremely difficult to positively identify as human because some animals, such as the bear, have paw bones almost identical to the human hand. It may be extremely difficult to identify fragmented bones, and the greater skills and experience of an experienced anthropologist or anatomist are invaluable. Cremated bones pose particular difficulties and these should only be examined by specialists.
- Am I dealing with one or more bodies (is there co-mingling of body parts)? This question can be answered very simply if there are two skulls or two left femurs. However, if there are no obvious duplications, it is important to examine each bone carefully to assess whether the sizes and appearances match. It can be extremely difficult to exclude the possibility of co-mingling of skeletal remains, and expert anthropological advice should be sought if there is any doubt.
- What sex are the bones? The skull and the pelvis offer the best information on sexing; although the femur and sternum can provide assistance, they are of less direct value. It is important to attempt to determine the sex of each of these bones and not to rely on the assessment of just one. Examination by an anthropologist or anatomist is vital.
- What is the age of the person? This will require a multi-professional approach utilizing the skills of the pathologist, anthropologist, odontologist and radiologist, each contributing to the overall picture.
- What is the height (stature) of the person? The head to heel measurement of even a completely fresh dead body is seldom the same as the person's standing height in life, owing to a combination of factors, including muscle relaxation and shrinkage of intervertebral discs. If a whole skeleton is present, an approximate height can be obtained by direct measurement but, because of variable joint spaces, articular cartilage, etc., this can only be, at best, an approximation. If only some bones are available, calculations can be made from established tables
- What is the race or ethnic origin? This is very much the field of trained anthropologists and should not be attempted without their assistance.
- Can a personal identity be discovered? The previous criteria can allot bones to various groups of age and sex but putting a name to the individual depends, as does all identification, upon having reliable ante-mortem data. Occasionally, foreign bodies such as bullets or other metallic fragments may be found embedded in the skeleton; these may either relate to the cause of death or may simply be an incidental finding. Most body implants (e.g. pacemakers, joint replacement) bear a unique reference number which identify the maker – these and other unique medical data are often useful in establishing identity.

Where pre-mortem clinical radiographs are available, the comparison of these with the post-mortem films may give a definite identity. If a skull X-ray is available, comparison of the frontal sinus patterns is incontrovertible as no two people have the same frontal sinus outline. Expert comparisons of the lateral skull X-ray and radiographs of the upper ribs, humeri and femurs can provide useful information based partly, in the limbs, on the pattern of the cancellous bone.

Mass disasters

A mass disaster requires appropriate collection of forensic samples; continuity and integrity of the sample trail; and once analysed the application of appropriate evidential standards. At the time it may not be known whether an event has happened by accident, natural disaster or as a crime. Ante-mortem data from potential decedents, including dental, fingerprint and DNA samples should be sought at the earliest opportunity for later comparison. Fingerprints can be obtained from personal items, in the home or workplace or crime databases. DNA samples can be obtained from similar items but also families. Dental practitioners should be approached to provide dental records, radiographs and casts where available. Matching of the ante-mortem data with the post-mortem samples may be done manually or using specialized software systems so that identities can be confirmed.

If multiple deaths are caused by some form of disaster the process of Disaster Victim Identification (DVI) should be established. In England and Wales a formal process called an Identification Commission and chaired by the Coroner will consider each identification to ensure that an accurate identification is made. Body recovery teams will identify where the deceased are. They will then be photographed before they are moved to assist any criminal investigation and to assist the Coroner in establishing cause of death. At the mortuary any personal items will be retrieved. These will be used as indicators of the potential identity of the person. Investigators will then go with a family liaison officer to recover items that could assist the identification, such as personal items from the deceased's home that may yield fingerprints or DNA, or their dental records from their dentist. Once identification evidence has been collected this will be presented to the Identification Commission who will decide if it meets the standards required to confirm identity. Further evidence may need to be collected. If identity reaches the standard of proof required then the evidence will then be used for an inquest in the death to be opened.

■ Age estimation in the living

Many doctors will be asked to estimate or evaluate the age of an individual but few will have the knowledge or skills of assessing age or be aware of the limitations, even when undertaken correctly. A small number will have the necessary skill to undertake an age estimation and provide responses appropriate to the respective degrees of certainty required in criminal or civil proceedings.

For the deceased, investigation of identity and age is generally undertaken by order of, and with the consent of, authorities – the Coroner in England & Wales.

In the living, other constraints apply. The essential element of any age estimation procedure is to ensure that it complies with, and fulfils, all local and/or national legal and ethical requirements. All practitioners, clinical or forensic, must take full responsibility for their actions in relation to the human rights of the subject undergoing investigation. It is essential that the practitioner, clinical or forensic, undertaking the estimation is ex-perienced in the interpretation and presentation of data emanating from the investigation. They must have a current and extensive understanding of the limitations of their investigation both in relation to the physical technology available to them and to the nature of the database to which they will refer, for comparison purposes. This also requires that the practitioner have a realistic understanding of the variation expressed by the human form and the extrinsic and intrinsic factors that may affect any age-estimation process.

Four main means of age estimation are available (see below), and the more of these that are used the more likely it is that the result of the examination will correlate well with the chronological age of the individual. Underestimation of age is unlikely to raise any issue in relation to an infringement of human rights (as younger persons tend to be treated better in law) but an over-estimation of age can have adverse effects. It is essential that the final estimation is robust and conveys a realistic range within which the chronological age is most likely to occur. Any element of doubt must result in an increased range of possibilities. It is not possible in any circumstance to ascertain with certainty whether an individual is 20 or 21 years of age. An assessment of 20 years ranges from a specific calendar date (birthday) to a date that is 364 days beyond that date and only one day short of the assessment of an age of 21 years. The means of assessment that should be used now to estimate age in the living are:

■ social and psychological evaluation – this requires evaluation by a highly trained clinician or social work practitioner;
■ external estimation of age – this evaluation must be undertaken by a qualified clinician (a forensic physician, or a paediatrician for the child

Stage	G = genitals (boys)		B = breasts (girls)		P = pubic hair (girls)	
1	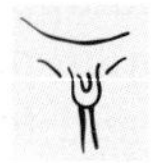	Pre-adolescent	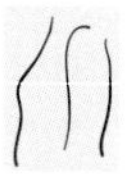	Pre-adoloscent	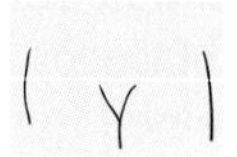	No hair
2	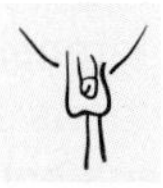	Scrotum pink and texture change, slight enlargement of the penis	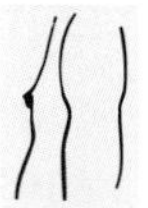	Breast bud	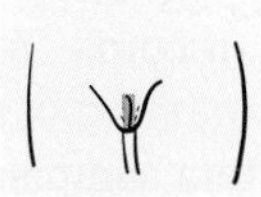	Few fine hairs
3	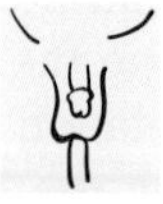	Longer penis larger testes	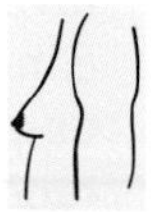	Larger, but no nipple contour separation	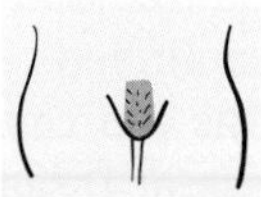	Darkens, coarsens, starts to curl
4	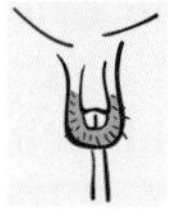	Penis increases in breadth, dark scrotum	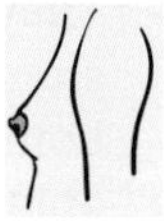	Areola and pailla from secondary mound. Menarche usually commeneces at this stage	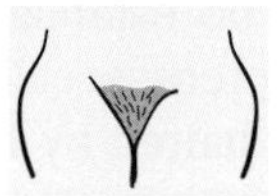	Adult type, smaller area
5	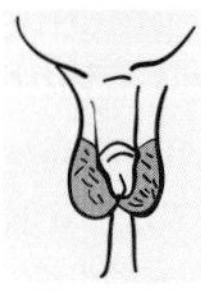	Adult size	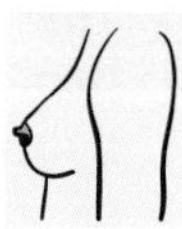	Mature (pailla projects, areola follows breast contour)	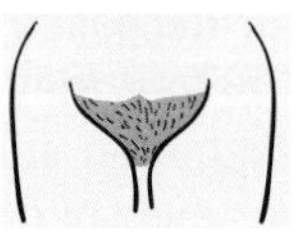	Adult type

Figure 4.3 Tanner staging.

and geriatrician for the elderly – examination by more than one practitioner may be appropriate);

■ skeletal estimation of age – this investigation cannot be undertaken visually and therefore relies on technology to assist the process (exposure to much of the relevant technology has risk from ionizing radiation and can only be undertaken with informed consent)

■ dental estimation of age.

Certain aspects of each of these means of assessment are well recognized. External estimation of age should use Tanner staging to assess child maturity (Figure 4.3). Skeletal estimation will assess hand/wrist radiographs in the first instance, which are compared against standards previously published. A visual intraoral inspection will inform the practitioner as to the stage of emergence and loss of the dentition and is particularly useful for age evaluation in the pre-pubertal years. Pubertal and post-pubertal individuals will, however, require a radiographic investigation.

■ Further information sources

A v. London Borough of Croydon and Secretary of State for the Home Department; WK v. Secretary of State for the Home Department and Kent County Council, [2009] EWHC 939 (Admin), UK: High Court (England and Wales), 8 May 2009. http://www.unhcr.org/refworld/docid/4a251daf2.html (accessed 22 November 2010).

A by his litigation friend Mejzninin vs. Croydon London, Borough Council [2008] EWHC 2921 (Admin). http://www.childrenslegalcentre.com/OneStopCMS/Core/CrawlerResourceServer.aspx?resource=76D78C51-B4F2-4F9F-9904-51A50ADC8634&mode=link&guid=fc8af87a1ce544dea1dd05eb961e2882 (accessed 22 November 2003).

Benson J, Williams J. Age determination in refugee children. *Australian Family Physician* 2008; **37**: 821–824.

Black S, Aggrawal A, Payne-James JJ. *Age Estimation in the Living*. Wiley, London 2010.

Bowers CM. *Forensic Dental Evidence: An Investigator's Handbook*, 2nd edn. Academic Press, Amsterdam 2011.

Crawley H. *When Is a Child Not a Child? Asylum, Age Disputes and the Process of Age Assessment*. London Immigration Law Practitioners' Association (ILPA), 2007.

Crossner CG, Mansfeld L. Determination of dental age in adopted non-European children. *Swedish Dental Journal* 1983; **7:** 1–10.

Dalitz GD. Age determination of adult human remains by teeth examination. *Journal of the Forensic Science Society* 1962; **3:** 11–21.

Dvorak J, George J, Junge A, Hodler J. Age determination by magnetic resonance imaging of the wrist in adolescent male football players. *British Journal of Sports Medicine* 2007; **41,** 45–52.

Euling SY, Herman-Giddens ME, Lee PA *et al.* Examination of US puberty timing data from 1940 to 1994 for secular trends: panel findings. *Pediatrics* 2009; **121**(Suppl 3): S172–S191.

Flecker H. Roentgenographic observations of the times of appearance of epiphyses and their fusion with the diaphyses. *Journal of Anatomy* 1933; **67:** 118–64.

Gilsanz V, Ratib, O. *Hand Bone Age. A Digital Atlas of Skeletal Maturity*. Berlin: Springer, 2005.

Gleiser I, Hunt EE Jr. The permanent mandibular first molar; its calcification, eruption and decay. *American Journal of Physical Anthropology* 1955; **13:** 253–84.

Greulich WW, Pyle SI. *Radiographic Atlas of Skeletal Development of the Hand and Wrist*. Stanford, CA: Stanford University Press 1959.

Jeffrys AJ, Wilson V, Thein SL. Hypervariable minisatellite regions in human DNA. *Nature* 1985; **314:** 67–73.

Kaplowitz PB, Oberfield SE. Reexamination of the age limit for defining when puberty is precocious in girls in the United States: implications for evaluation and treatment. Drug and Therapeutics and Executive Committees of the Lawson Wilkins Pediatric Endocrine Society. *Pediatrics* 1999; **104:** 936–41.

Kvaal SI, Kolltveit KM, Thompsen IO, Solheim T. Age determination of adults from radiographs. *Forensic Science International* 1995; **74,** 175–85.

Lindstrom N. Regional sex trafficking in the Balkans: transnational networks in an enlarged Europe. *Problems of Post-Communism* 2004; **51:** 45–52.

Liversidge HM, Molleson TI. Developing permanent tooth length as an estimate of age. *Journal of Forensic Sciences* 1999 44: 917–20.

Liverpool City Council (R, on the application of) vs. London Borough of Hillingdon [2008] EWHC 1702 (Admin).

Marshall WA. Growth and sexual maturation in normal puberty. *Clinics in Endocrinology and Metabolism* 1975; **4:** 3–25.

Marshall WA, Tanner JM. Variations in pattern of pubertal changes in girls. *Archives of Diseases in Childhood* 1969; **44,** 291–303.

Marshall WA, Tanner JM. Variations in the pattern of pubertal changes in boys. *Archives of Diseases in Childhood* 1970; **45:** 13–23.

Martrille L, Baccino E. Age estimation in the living. In: Payne-James JJ, Corey T, Henderson C, Byard R. (eds) *Encyclopedia of Forensic and Legal Medicine*. Oxford: Elsevier, 2005.

Pyle SI, Waterhouse AM, Greulich WW. *A Radiographic Standard of Reference for the Growing Hand and Wrist*.

Cleveland, OH: The Press of Case Western Reserve University. 1971.

Ritz S, Schütz HW, Peper C. (1993) Postmortem estimation of age at death based on aspartic acid racemization in dentin: its applicability for root dentin. *International Journal of Legal Medicine* 1993; **105:** 289–293.

Royal College of Paediatrics and Child Health. *The Health Of Refugee Children: Guidelines For Paediatricians*. London: Royal College of Paediatrics and Child Health, 1999.

Saunders E. *The Teeth, a Test of Age, Considered with Reference to the Factory Children, Addressed to the Members of Both Houses of Parliament*. London: Renshaw,1837; 1–2.

Schaefer M, Black SM, Scheuer L. *Juvenile Osteology: A Laboratory and Field Manual*. London: Elsevier, 2009.

Scheuer JL, Black SM. *The Juvenile Skeleton*. London: Academic Press, 2004.

Schmeling A, Olze A, Reisinger W, Geserick G. Age estimation of living people undergoing criminal proceedings. *Lancet* 2001; **358:** 89–90.

Schmeling A, Grundmann C, Fuhrmann A. *et al.* Criteria for age estimation in living individuals. *International Journal of Legal Medicine* 2008; **122,** 457–60.

Schmidt S, Mühler M, Schmeling A, Reisinger W, Schulz R. Magnetic resonance imaging of the clavicular ossification. *International Journal of Legal Medicine* 2007; **121:** 321–4.

Solheim T. A new method for dental age estimation in adults. *Forensic Science International* 1993; **59:** 137–47.

Tanner JM. *Foetus into Man: Physical Growth from Conception to Maturity*. London: Open Books, 1978.

Tanner JM, Whitehouse RH. Clinical longitudinal standards for height, weight, height velocity, weight velocity and stages of puberty. *Archives of Diseases in Childhood* 1976; **51,** 170–9.

Tanner JM, Whitehouse RH, Healy MJR. *A New System for Estimating Skeletal Maturity from the Hand and Wrist, with Standards Derived from a Study of 2,600 Healthy British Children*. Paris: Centre International de l'Enfance, 1962.

Tanner JM, Whitehouse RH, Marshall WA, Healy, MJR, Goldstein H. *Assessment of Skeletal Maturity and Prediction of Adult Height (TW2 Method)*, 2nd edn. London: Academic Press, 1975.

Tanner JM, Healy MJR, Goldstein H, Cameron N. *Assessment of Skeletal Maturity and Prediction of Adult Height (TW3 Method)*. London: W.B. Saunders, 2001.

Todd TW. *Atlas of Skeletal Maturation*. St Louis, MO: C.V. Mosby, 1937.

Ubelaker DH. *Human Skeletal Remains: Excavation, Analysis and Interpretation*. Washington, DC: Smithsonian Institute Press, 1978.

van der Linden FPGM, Duterloo HS. *The Development of the Human Dentition: An Atlas*. Hagerstown, MD: Harper and Row, 1976.

Wheeler MD. Physical changes of puberty. *Endocrinology and Metabolism Clinics of North America* 1991; **20:** 1–14.

Wittwer-Backofen U, Gampe J, Vaupel JW. Tooth cementum annulation for age estimation: results from a large known-age validation study. *American Journal of Physical Anthropology* 2004; **123,** 119–29.

Chapter 5

The appearance of the body after death

Introduction

It is accepted that, if irreversible cardiac arrest has occurred, the individual has died and eventually all of the cells of the body will cease their normal metabolic functions and the changes of decomposition will begin.

Initially, these changes can only be detected biochemically as the metabolism in the cells alters to autolytic pathways. Eventually the changes become visible and these visible changes are important for two reasons: first, because a doctor needs to know the normal progress of decomposition so that he does not misinterpret these normal changes for signs of an unnatural death and, second, because they may be used in estimating how long the individual has been dead (i.e. the post-mortem interval, or PMI).

The appearance of the body after death reflects PMI-dependent changes, but the reliability and accuracy of traditional 'markers' of the PMI has become increasingly doubtful, given their dependence on incompletely understood biological and environmental factors.

The early post-mortem interval

Rapid changes after death

When the heart stops and breathing ceases, there is an immediate fall in blood pressure and the supply of oxygen to the cells of the body ceases. Initially, the cells that can use anoxic pathways will do so until their metabolic reserves are exhausted, and then their metabolism will begin to fail. With loss of neuronal activity, all nervous activity ceases, the reflexes are lost and breathing stops. In the eye the corneal reflex ceases and the pupils stop reacting to light. The retinal vessels, viewed with an ophthalmoscope, show the break-up or fragmentation of the columns of blood, which is called 'trucking' or 'shunting' as the appearance has suggested the movement of railway carriages. The eyes themselves lose their intraocular tension.

The muscles rapidly become flaccid (primary flaccidity), with complete loss of tone, but they may retain their reactivity and may respond to touch or taps and other forms of stimulation for some hours after cardiac arrest. Discharges of the dying motor neurons may stimulate small groups of muscle cells and lead to focal twitching, although these decrease with time.

The fall in blood pressure and cessation of circulation of the blood usually render the skin, conjunctivae and mucous membranes pale. The skin of the face and the lips may remain red or blue in colour in hypoxic/congestive deaths. The hair follicles die at the same time as the rest of the skin and there is no truth in the belief that hair continues to grow after death, although the beard may appear more prominent against a pale skin.

Loss of muscle tone may result in voiding of urine; this is such a common finding that no relationship with deaths from epilepsy or asphyxia can be established. Emission of semen is also found in some deaths, therefore, the presence of semen cannot be used as an indicator of sexual activity shortly before death.

Regurgitation of gastric contents is a very common feature of terminal collapse and it is a common complication of resuscitation. Gastric contents are identified in the mouth or airways in a significant proportion of all autopsies. The presence of such material cannot be used to indicate that gastric content aspiration was the cause of death unless it is supported by eyewitness accounts or by microscopic identification of food debris in peripheral airways in association with an inflammatory response.

Rigor mortis

Rigor mortis is, at its simplest, a temperature-dependent physicochemical change that occurs within muscle cells as a result of lack of oxygen. The lack of oxygen means that energy cannot be obtained from glycogen via glucose using oxidative phosphorylation and so adenosine triphosphate (ATP) production from this process ceases and the secondary anoxic process takes over for a short time but, as lactic acid is a by-product of anoxic respiration, the cell cytoplasm becomes increasingly acidic. In the face of low ATP and high acidity, the actin and myosin fibres bind together and form a gel. The outward result of these complex cellular metabolic changes is that the muscles become stiff. However, they do not shorten unless they are under tension.

It is clear from the short discussion above that if muscle glycogen levels are low, or if the muscle cells are acidic at the time of death as a result of exercise,

the process of rigor will develop faster. Electrocution is also associated with rapidly developing rigor and this may be caused by the repeated stimulation of the muscles. Conversely, in the young, the old or the emaciated, rigor may be extremely hard to detect because of the low muscle bulk.

Rigor develops uniformly throughout the body but it is generally first detectable in the smaller muscle groups such as those around the eyes and mouth, the jaw and the fingers. It appears to advance down the body from the head to the legs as larger and larger muscle groups become stiffened. The only use of assessing the presence or absence of rigor lies in the estimation of the time of death, and the key word here is 'estimation', as rigor is such a variable process that it can never provide an accurate assessment of the time of death. Extreme caution should be exercised in trying to assign a time of death based on the very subjective assessment of the degree and extent of rigor. Charts or tables that assign times since death based on the assessment of rigor should be viewed with great scepticism. On its own, rigor mortis has very little utility as a marker of the PMI because of the large number of factors that influence it.

The chemical processes that result in the stiffening of the muscles, in common with all chemical processes, are affected by temperature: the colder the temperature the slower the reactions and vice versa. In a cold body, the onset of rigor will be delayed and the length of time that its effects on the muscles can be detected will be prolonged, whereas in a body lying in a warm environment, the onset of rigor and its duration will be short.

It is also important to be aware of the microenvironment around the body when assessing rigor: a body lying in front of a fire or in a bath of hot water will develop rigor more rapidly than if it were lying outside in winter. When the post-mortem cooling of a body is extreme, the stiffening of the body may result from the physical effects of cooling or freezing rather than rigor. This will become apparent when the body is moved to a warmer environment (usually the mortuary) and the stiffening caused by cold is seen to disappear as the body warms. Continued observation may reveal that true rigor then develops as the cellular chemical processes recommence.

In temperate conditions rigor can commonly be detected in the face between approximately 1 hour and 4 hours and in the limbs between approximately 3 hours and 6 hours after death, with the strength of rigor increasing to a maximum by approximately 18 hours after death. Once established, rigor will remain for up to approximately 50 hours after death until autolysis and decomposition of muscle cells intervenes and muscles become flaccid again. These times are only guidelines and can never be absolute.

It is best to test for rigor across a joint using very gentle pressure from one or two fingers only; the aim is to detect the presence and extent of the stiffness, not to 'break' it. If rigor is broken by applying too much force, those muscle groups cannot reliably be tested again.

Cadaveric rigidity

'Cadaveric rigidity' is said to be the stiffness of muscles that has its onset immediately at death, and the basis for this concept is the finding of items gripped firmly in the hand of the deceased before the onset of normal rigor. Most cases are said to be related to individuals who are at high levels of emotional or physical stress immediately before death and many reports relate to battlefield casualties, but there are many reports of individuals recovered from rivers with weeds or twigs grasped firmly in their hand or the finger of a suicidal shooting found tightly gripping the trigger. It is suggested that the mechanism for this phenomenon is possibly neurogenic, but no scientifically satisfactory explanation has been given. It is clearly not the same chemical process as true rigor and it is better that the term 'instantaneous rigor' is no longer used as it implies an equivalence with a process for which there is a scientific explanation (Figure 5.1).

Post-mortem hypostasis

Cessation of the circulation and the relaxation of the muscular tone of the vascular bed allow simple fluid movement to occur within the blood vessels. Post-mortem hypostasis or post-mortem lividity are the terms used to describe the visual manifestation of this phenomenon. Theoretically, currents will occur between warmer and colder areas of the body and this may be of importance in the redistribution of drugs and chemicals after death. There is also filling of the dependent blood vessels.

The passive settling of red blood cells under the influence of gravity to blood vessels in the lowest areas of the body is of forensic interest. This results

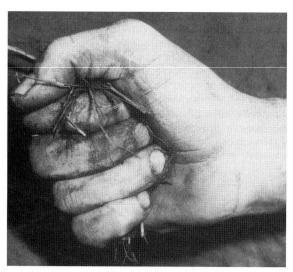

Figure 5.1 Cadaveric rigidity – a rare post-mortem finding that may be seen in bodies recovered from water, where vegetation is found tightly 'gripped' in the hand.

in a pink or bluish colour to these lowest areas and it is this colour change that is called post-mortem hypostasis or lividity. Hypostasis is not always seen in a body and it may be absent in the young, the old and the clinically anaemic or in those who have died from severe blood loss. It may be masked by dark skin colours, by jaundice or by some dermatological conditions.

Post-mortem hypostasis occurs where superficial blood vessels can be distended by blood. Compression of skin in contact with a firm surface, for example, prevents such distension, and results in areas of relative or complete pallor within hypostasis. Relative pallor within hypostasis may also be caused by pressure of clothing or by contact of one area of the body with another, in which case 'mirror image' pallor may be seen (Figure 5.2).

The site and distribution of the hypostasis must be considered in the light of the position of the body after death. A body left suspended after hanging will develop deep hypostasis of the lower legs and arms, with none visible on the torso (Figure 5.3), whereas a body that has partially fallen head first out of bed will have the most prominent hypostatic changes of the head and upper chest.

If a body has laid face downwards, or with the head in a position lower than the rest of the body, hypostasis can cause significant problems for interpretation. Hypostasis in the relatively lax soft tissues of the face can lead to intense congestion and the formation of petechial haemorrhages in the skin of

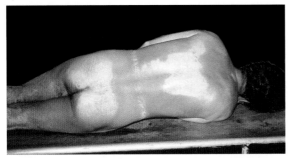

Figure 5.2 Post-mortem hypostasis in a posterior distribution. Areas of pallor can be seen as a result of pressure of the body on a firm surface, whereas parts of the body not in direct contact with that surface are purple/ pink because of the 'settling of blood under gravity'. This body has been lying on its back since death.

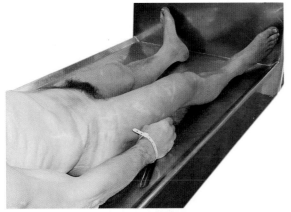

Figure 5.3 Post-mortem hypostasis distribution following hanging. Note the skin discoloration is in the legs and hands because of the vertical body position after death and the green discoloration in the right iliac fossa region.

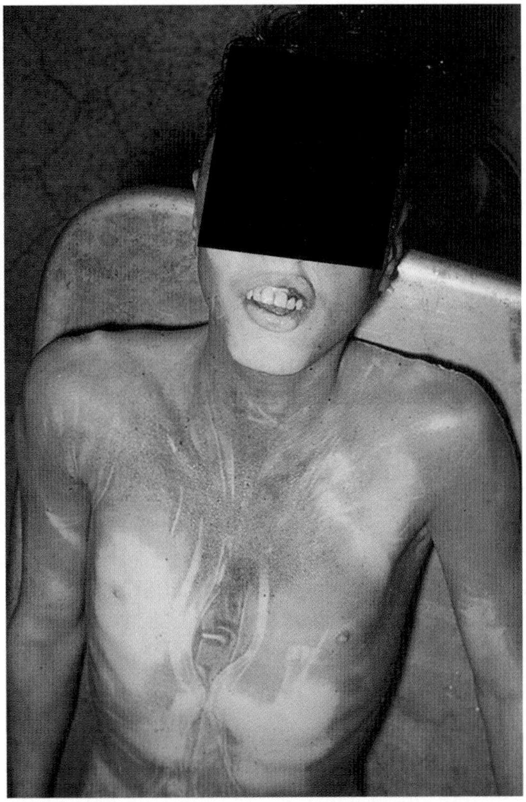

Figure 5.4 Post-mortem hypostasis pattern on the front of a body found face down on a bed. The linear marks are formed by pressure from creases in a blanket. Pallor around the mouth and nose are caused by pressure against the bed and do not necessarily indicate marks of suffocation.

the face, and in the conjunctivae, raising concerns about the possibility of pressure having been applied to the neck. Areas of pallor around the mouth and nose may also add to the impression of pressure having been applied to those areas implying 'suffocation' (Figure 5.4). In such circumstances, the pathologist must attempt to exclude pressure to the mouth, nose and neck as having a role in the death by careful examination and dissection of those structures following removal of the brain and heart, and looking for bruising and skeletal injury.

The colour of hypostasis is variable and may extend from pink to dark pink to deep purple and, in some congestive hypoxic states, to blue. In general, no attempt should be made to form any conclusions about the cause of death from these variations of colour, but there are, however, a few colour changes that may act as indicators of possible causes of death: the cherry pink colour of carbon monoxide poisoning, the dark red or brick red colour associated with cyanide poisoning and infection by *Clostridium perfringens*, which is said to result in bronze hypostasis.

Bodies stored in refrigerators frequently have pink hypostasis, and while pink hypostasis is also seen in hypothermia victims, they may also have prominent pink/red staining over large joints, the precise cause of which is uncertain, but this may represent haemolytic staining.

The time taken for hypostasis to appear is so variable that it has no reliable role in determining the time of death. Movement of a body will have an effect on hypostasis, as the red blood cells continue to move under the influence of gravity. Even after the normal post-mortem coagulation of the blood has occurred, movement of the red blood cells, although severely reduced, still continues. This continued ability of the red blood cells to move is important because changes in the position of a body after the initial development of hypostasis will result in redistribution of the hypostasis and examination of the body may reveal two overlapping patterns.

Cooling of the body after death

The cooling of the body after death can be viewed as a simple physical property of a warm object in a cooler environment. Newton's Law of Cooling states that heat will pass from the warmer body to the cooler environment and the temperature of the body will fall. However, a body is not a uniform structure: its temperature will not fall evenly and, because each body will lie in its own unique environment, each body will cool at a different speed, depending upon the many factors surrounding it (Figure 5.5).

In order to use body temperature as an indicator of the time of death the following three basic forensic assumptions must be made:

1 The first assumption is that the body temperature was 37°C at the time of death. However, many factors affect body temperature in life, including variation throughout any 24-hour period (i.e. diurnal variation), exercise, infection and the menstrual cycle.

2 The second assumption is that it is possible to take one, or perhaps a few, post-mortem body temperature readings and, using mathematical formulae, to extrapolate that data and generate a reliable estimate of the time taken by that body to cool to that measured temperature.

3 The third assumption is that the body has lain in a thermally static environment; this is generally not the case and even bodies lying in a confined domestic environment may be subject to the daily variations of the central heating system, while the variations imposed on a body lying outside are potentially so great that no sensible 'average' can be achieved.

Many other variables and factors also affect the rate of cooling of a body (Box 5.1) and together they show why the sensible forensic pathologist will be reluctant to make any pronouncement on the time of death based on the body temperature alone.

Box 5.1 Examples of factors affecting the rate of cooling of a body

- Mass of the body
- Mass/surface area
- Body temperature at the time of death
- Site of reading of body temperature(s)
- Posture of the body – extended or curled into a fetal position
- Clothing – type of material, position on the body – or lack of it
- Obesity – fat is a good insulator
- Emaciation – lack of muscle bulk allows a body to cool faster
- Environmental temperature
- Winds, draughts, rain, humidity

■ Other post-mortem changes

As the post-mortem interval increases, the body undergoes additional changes that reflect tissue 'breakdown', autolysis and progressive decomposition/ putrefaction.

Decomposition/putrefaction

In the cycle of life, dead bodies are usually returned, through reduction into their various components, to the chemical pool that is the earth. Some components will do this by entering the food chain at almost any level – from ant to tiger – whereas others will be reduced to simple chemicals by autolytic enzymatic processes built into the lysosomes of each cell.

The early changes of decomposition are important because they may be confused by the police or members of the public with the signs of violence or trauma.

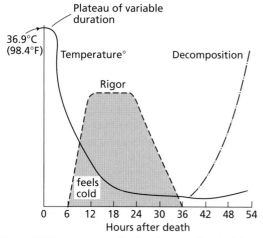

Figure 5.5 The sequence of major changes after death in a temperate environment. Note that the core body temperature does not show a fall for the first hour or so.

Decomposition results in liquefaction of the soft tissues over a period of time, the appearance of which, and the rate of progress of which, is a function of the ambient temperature: the warmer the temperature, the earlier the process starts and the faster it progresses. In temperate climates the process is usually first visible to the naked eye at about 3–4 days as an area of green discoloration of the right iliac fossa of the anterior abdominal wall. This 'greening' is the result of the extension of the commensal gut bacteria through the bowel wall and into the skin, where they decompose haemoglobin, resulting in the green colour. The right iliac fossa is the usual origin as the caecum lies close to the abdominal wall at this site. This green colour is but an external marker of the profound changes that are occurring in the body as the gut bacteria find their way out of the bowel lumen into the abdominal cavity and the blood vessels.

The blood vessels provide an excellent channel through which the bacteria can spread with some ease throughout the body. Their passage is marked by the decomposition of haemoglobin which, when present in the superficial vessels, results in linear branching patterns of variable discoloration of the skin that is called 'marbling' (Figure 5.6). Over time, generalized skin discoloration occurs and, as the superficial layers of the skin lose cohesion, blisters containing red or brown fluid form in many areas. When the blisters burst, the skin sloughs off.

Considerable gas formation in soft tissues and body cavities is common and the body begins to swell, with bloating of the face, abdomen, breasts and genitals (Figure 5.7). The increased internal pressure causes the eyes and tongue to protrude

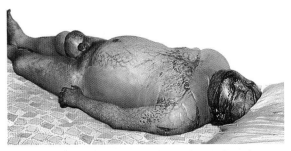

Figure 5.7 Putrefaction/decomposition of approximately 1 week in temperate summer conditions. Note the 'bloating' of soft tissues, distortion of facial features and 'purge fluid' emanating from the mouth and nose.

and forces blood-stained fluid up from the lungs which often 'leaks out' of the mouth and nose as 'purge fluid'. Such fluid is frequently misinterpreted by those inexperienced with decomposition-related changes as representing injury-associated haemorrhage.

The role of flies and maggots and other animals is discussed below and in Chapter 24, p. 236; domestic animals and other predators are not excluded from this process. As decomposition continues, soft tissues liquefy; however, the prostate and the uterus are relatively resistant to putrefaction and they may survive for months, as may the tendons and ligaments. Eventually, skeletalization will be complete and unless the bones are destroyed by larger animals, they may remain for years.

No reliable 'timetable' for decomposition can be constructed because environmental factors may favour enhanced or delayed decomposition, and such factors will generally be unknown to those investigating the death.

Immersion and burial

Immersion in water or burial will slow the process of decomposition. Casper's Law (or Ratio) states that: if all other factors are equal, then, when there is free access of air, a body decomposes twice as fast than if immersed in water and eight times faster than if buried in earth.

Water temperatures are usually lower than those on land. A body in water may adopt a number of positions, but the most common in the early stage is with the air-containing chest floating uppermost and the head and limbs hanging downwards. Hypostasis follows the usual pattern and affects the head and limbs, and these areas may also be

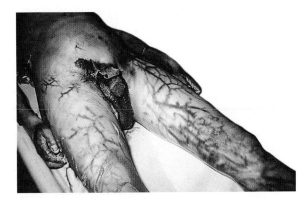

Figure 5.6 Early decomposition with skin slippage and discoloration. Note the 'marbling' representing discoloration owing to decomposition within superficial blood vessels.

damaged by contact with the bottom if the water is shallow (Figure 5.8).

The first change that affects the body in water is the loss of epidermis. Gaseous decomposition progresses and the bloated body is often, but not always, lifted to the surface by these gases, most commonly at about 1 week but this time is extremely variable. Marine predators will replace the animals found on land and they can cause extensive damage (Figure 5.9). Exposure to water can, in some cases, predispose to the formation of adipocere (see below), but this is unusual unless a body lies underwater for many weeks.

The effects and the time-scale of the changes following burial are so variable that little can be said other than buried bodies generally decay more slowly, especially if they are buried deep within the ground. The level of moisture in the surrounding soil and acidity of the soil will both significantly alter the speed of decomposition.

Adipocere

Adipocere is a chemical change in the body fat, which is hydrolysed to a waxy compound not unlike soap. The need for water means that this process is most commonly seen in bodies found in wet conditions (i.e. submerged in water or buried in wet ground) but this is not always the case and some bodies from dry vaults have been found to have adipocere formation, presumably the original body water being sufficient to allow for the hydrolysis of the fat (Figure 5.10).

In the early stages of formation, adipocere is a pale, rancid, greasy semi-fluid material with a most unpleasant smell. As the hydrolysis progresses, the material becomes more brittle and whiter and, when fully formed, adipocere is a grey, firm, waxy compound that maintains the shape of the body. The speed with which adipocere can develop is variable; it would usually be expected to take weeks or months, but it is reported to have occurred in as little as 3 weeks. All three stages of adipocere formation can coexist and they can also be found with areas of mummification and putrefaction if the conditions are correct.

Mummification

A body lying in dry conditions, either climatic or in a microenvironment, may desiccate instead of putrefy – a process known as mummification

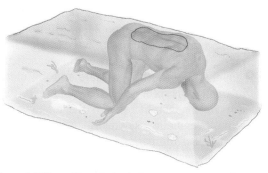

Figure 5.8 Disposition of a body floating in water. Typically the head and limbs hang down, resulting in superficial injuries to the head/ face, back of the arms and hands, knees and top of the feet.

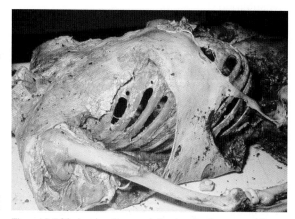

Figure 5.9 Marine creature predation in a body recovered from the North Sea after 3 months. Much of the skin has been removed by crustaceans, and the arm muscles by larger fish who have cleaned out most of the body cavity.

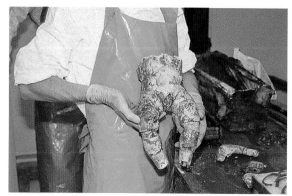

Figure 5.10 Adipocere formation. Following burial for 3 years, waxy adipocere forms a shell around the skeleton of this infant.

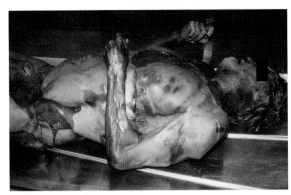

Figure 5.11 Mummification. The skin is dry and leathery following recovery from a locked room for 10 weeks.

(Figure 5.11). Mummified tissue is dry and leathery and often brown in colour. It is most commonly seen in warm or hot environments such as desert and led to the spontaneous mummification of bodies buried in the sand in Egypt. However, it is not only bodies from hot dry climates that can be mummified, as the microenvironment necessary for mummification may exist anywhere.

Mummification of newborn infants whose bodies are placed in cool dry environments (e.g. below floor boards) is common, but adults may also be mummified if they lie in dry places, preferably with a draught. Mummification is, however, much more likely in the thin individual whose body will cool and desiccate quickly.

Mummification need not affect the whole body, and some parts may show the normal soft tissue decomposition changes, skeletalization or formation of adipocere, depending on the conditions. Mummified tissues are not immune to degradation and invasion by rodents, beetles and moths, especially the brown house moth, in temperate climates.

Skeletalization

The speed of skeletalization will depend on many factors, including the climate and the microenvironment around the body. It will occur much more quickly in a body on the surface of the ground than in one that is buried. Generally speaking, in a formally buried body, the soft tissues will be absent by 2 years. Tendons, ligaments, hair and nails will be identifiable for some time after that.

At about 5 years, the bones will be bare and disarticulated, although fragments of articular cartilage may be identified for many years and for several years the bones will feel slightly greasy and, if they are cut with a saw, a wisp of smoke and a smell of burning organic material may be present. Examination of the bone marrow space may reveal residual organic material that can sometimes be suitable for specialist DNA analysis. Examination of the cut surface of a long bone under UV light may assist in dating, as there are changes in the pattern of fluorescence over time.

Dating bones, as with all post-mortem dating, is fraught with difficulty. The microenvironment in which the bone has lain is of crucial importance and the examination and dating of bones is now a specialist subject. If in doubt, the forensic pathologist should enlist the assistance of a forensic anthropologist or archaeologist who have the specialist skills and techniques to manage this type of material.

In the UK, the medico-legal interest in bones fades rapidly if a bone has been dead for more than 70–80 years, because even if it was from a criminal death, it is most unlikely that the killer would still be alive. Carbon-14 dating is of no use in this short time-scale, but examination of the bones for levels of strontium-90, which was released into the atmosphere in high levels only after the detonation of the nuclear bombs in the 1940s, may allow for the differentiation of bones from before and after that time.

Post-mortem injuries

Dead bodies are not immune to injuries and can be exposed to a wide range of trauma, and it is important to bear this possibility in mind when examining any body so that these injuries are not confused with injuries sustained during life.

Predation by land animals and insects can cause serious damage to the body: if there is any doubt about bite marks, an odontologist should be consulted (Figure 5.12). In water, fish, crustaceans and larger animals can also cause severe damage, but there is the added damage caused by the water-logging of the skin and the movement of the body across the bottom or against the banks. Contact with boats and propellers will generally lead to patterns of injuries that should be easily recognizable.

It is not true to say that post-mortem injuries do not bleed because many do leak blood, especially those on the scalp and in bodies recovered from water. The confirmation that a wound is post mortem in origin may be extremely difficult because injuries

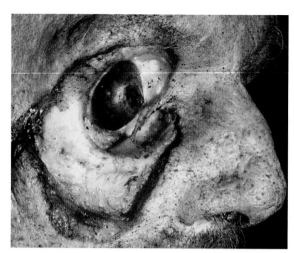

Figure 5.12 Post-mortem animal predation. The wound margins of these rat bites are free from haemorrhage or reddening. Such injuries are commonly present around the eyes, ears and nose.

inflicted in the last few minutes of life and those that were caused after death may appear exactly the same. In general, post-mortem injuries do not have a rim of an early inflammatory response in the wound edges, but the lack of this response does not exclude an injury inflicted in the last moments of life.

■ Estimation of the post-mortem interval

The pathologist is often asked for an opinion on PMI (the 'time since death') based on the pathological findings. While none of the changes after death is capable of providing a precise 'marker' of PMI, the most reliable would appear to be related to the cooling of the body after death.

Body temperature

Traditionally, the temperature of the body was taken rectally using a long, low-reading thermometer (0–50°C was considered to be adequate). However, there are problems with using this site because any interference with the anus or rectum before a full forensic examination of the area in a good light may confuse or contaminate later investigations into the presence of biological materials such as semen, blood or hair.

The development of small electronic temperature probes with rapid response times and digital

readouts has revolutionized the taking of body temperatures. These probes have allowed the use of other orifices, including the nose and ear, although it must be remembered that these areas are unlikely to register the same temperature as the deep rectum or the liver.

Currently, the most useful method of estimating the time of death is Henssge's Nomogram (which is explained in some detail in Box 5.2). Crucially, the 95 per cent accuracy claimed for this method is, at best, only 2.8 hours on either side of the most likely time (a total spread of over 5.5 hours). Henssge's Nomogram relies on three measurements – body temperature, ambient temperature and body weight – and lack of accuracy in any one of these will degrade the final result. In addition, there is the application of empirical corrective factors to allow for clothing, air movement and/or water (Table 5.1) and it should be noted that application of these empirical factors can significantly lengthen the time spans that lie within the 95 per cent confidence limits.

The need to record the ambient temperature poses some problems because pathologists are seldom in a position to do this at the time of discovery and, as their arrival at the scene is often delayed by some tens of minutes or hours, it is most unlikely that the temperature at that time will still be of relevance. Therefore, the first police officers or scientists at the scene should be encouraged to take the ambient temperature adjacent to the body and to record the time that they made their measurement. This, however, may give rise to concerns about interpretation of physical findings (dependent on how and by what route the temperature is taken). An alteration of 5°C in the ambient temperature may lead to, at least, a 1-hour alteration in the most likely time of death.

Many pathologists have in the past used various 'rules of thumb' to calculate the time of death from the body temperature but these are generally so unreliable that they should not now be used.

Sometimes the perceived warmth of the body to touch is mentioned in court as an indicator of the time of death; this assessment is so unreliable as to be useless and is even more so if the pathologist is asked to comment upon the reported perceptions of another person.

Various other methods have been researched in as yet unsuccessful attempts to find the hands of the post-mortem clock. Biochemical methods,

BOX 5.2 The rectal temperature–time of death relating nomogram

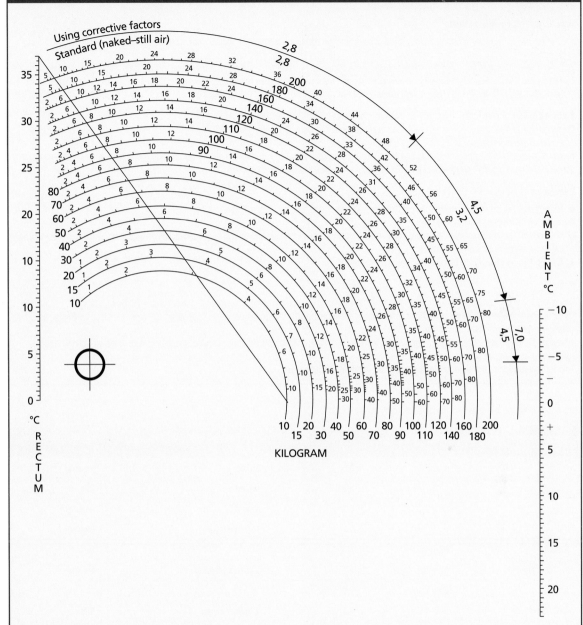

This nomogram is for ambient temperatures up to 25°C. Permissible variation of 95% (+/−h). The Henssge nomogram expresses the death-time (t) by:

$$\frac{T_{rectum} - T_{ambient}}{37.2 - T_{ambient}} = 1.25 \exp(Bt) - .25 \exp(5Bt); B = -1.2815 (kg^{-.625}) + .0284$$

The nomogram is related to the chosen standard; that is, a naked body extended lying in still air. Cooling conditions differing from the chosen standard may be proportionally adjusted by corrective factors of the real body weight, giving the corrected body weight by which the death-time is to be read off. Factors above 1.0 may correct thermal isolation conditions and factors below 1.0 may correct conditions accelerating the heat loss of a body.

(Continued)

BOX 5.2 continued

How to read off the time of death

1. Connect the points of the scales by a straight line according to the rectal and the ambient temperature. It crosses the diagonal of the nomogram at a special point.
2. Draw a second straight line going through the centre of the circle, below left of the nomogram, and the intersection of the first line and the diagonal. The second line crosses the semicircle of the body weight and the time of death can be read off. The second line touches a segment of the outermost semicircle. Here can be seen the permissible variation of 95%.

Example: temperature of the rectum 26.4°C; ambient temperature 12°C; body weight 90 kg.

Result: time of death 16 ± 1.8 hours. Statement: the death occurred within 13.2 hours and 18.8 hours (13 hours and 19 hours) before the time of measurement (with a reliability of 95%).

Note: If the values of the ambient temperature and/or the body weight are called into question, repeat the procedure with other values which might be possible (see Table 5.1 for 'corrective factors'). The range of death-time can be seen in this way.

Requirements for use

- No strong radiation (e.g. sun, heater, cooling system).
- No strong fever or general hypothermia.
- No uncertain[a] severe changes of the cooling conditions during the period between the time of death and examination (e.g. the place of death must be the same as where the body was found).
- No high thermal conductivity of the surface beneath the body[b].

Notes

[a] Known changes can be taken into account: a change of the ambient temperature can often be evaluated (e.g. contact the weather station); use the mean ambient temperature of the period in question. Changes by the operations of the investigators (e.g. taking any cover off) since finding the body are negligible: take the conditions before into account.

[b] Measure the temperature of the surface beneath the body too. If there is a significant difference between the temperature of the air and the surface temperature, use the mean.

This representation of the nomogram should not be used for actual cases

Table 5.1 Empirical corrective factors of body weight

Dry clothing/covering	In air	Corrective factor	Wet-through clothing/covering wet body surface	In air/water
		3.5	Naked	Flowing
		0.5	Naked	Still
		0.7	Naked	Moving
		0.7	1–2 thin layers	Moving
Naked	Moving	0.75		
1–2 thin layers	Moving	0.9	2 or more thicker	Moving
Naked	Still	1.0		
1–2 thin layers	Still	1.1	2 thicker layers	Still
2–3 thin layers		1.2	More than 2 thicker layers	Still
1–2 thicker layers	Moving or still	1.2		
3–4 thin layers		1.3		
More thin/thicker layers	Without influence	1.45		
Thick bedspread + clothing		1.8		
Combined		2.4		

For the selection of the corrective factor of any case, only the clothing or covering of the lower trunk is relevant! Personal experience is needed, nevertheless this is quickly achieved by the consistent use of the method.

including vitreous humour potassium levels and changes in enzyme and electrolyte levels elsewhere in the body, have been researched; some remain as interesting research tools but none has been successful in routine work.

Other techniques used in estimating or corroborating PMI

Of considerable value is the work of the forensic entomologist, who can determine a probable time of death – in the region of days to months – from examination of the populations and stages of development of the various insects that invade a body. Initially, the sarcophagus flies – the bluebottle (*Calliphora*), the greenbottle (*Lucilla*) and houseflies (*Musca*) – lay their eggs on moist areas, particularly the eyes, nose, mouth and, if exposed, the anus and genitalia. The eggs hatch into larvae, which grow and shed their skins a number of times, each moult being called an instar (Figure 5.13). Finally, they pupate and a new winged insect emerges. The time from egg laying through the instars to pupation depends on the species and on the ambient temperature, but in general it is about 21–24 days.

Other animals, both large and small, will arrive to feed on the body, with the species and the rapidity of their arrival depending on the time of year and the environment. The examination of buried bodies or skeletal remains will usually require the combined specialist skills of the forensic pathologist, an anthropologist and an entomologist.

Analysis of gastric contents – other than for toxicological purposes – may occasionally assist in an investigation, where such analysis identifies food components capable of corroborating (or refuting) other evidence that suggests that a particular meal had been eaten at a particular time, but cannot reliably be used to determine time of death. It is important, where time of death may be an issue that all stomach contents are retained for subsequent analysis.

Forensic mycology, the assessment of fungi, is the other area where some assistance may be gained in determining the time of death in some cases. The use of a range of techniques can all assist the investigator in narrowing down the possible time of death.

■ Further information sources

Amendt J, Richards CS, Campobasso CP, Zehner R, Hall MJ. Forensic entomology: applications and limitations. *Forensic Sci Med Path* 2011; (Jun) (epub).

Brown A, Marshall TK. Body temperature as a means of estimating time of death. *Forensic Sci* 1974; **4:** 125–33.

Haglund WD, Sorg MH (eds). *Forensic Taphonomy: the Postmortem Fate of Human Remains*. Boca Raton, FL: CRC Press, 1997.

Hawksworth DL, Wiltshire PE. Forensic Mycology: the use of fungi in criminal investigations. *Forensic Sci Int* 2010; (July) (epub).

Henssge C. [Precision of estimating the time of death by mathematical expression of rectal body cooling]. *Z Rechtsmed* 1979; **83:** 49–67 (in German).

Henssge C. [Estimation of death-time by computing the rectal body cooling under various cooling conditions]. *Z Rechtsmed* 1981; **87:** 147–8 (in German).

Henssge C, Brinkmann B, Püschel K. [Determination of time of death by measuring the rectal temperature in corpses suspended in water]. *Z Rechtsmed* 1984; **92:** 255–76 (in German).

Henssge C, Knight B, Krompecher T *et al*. The Estimation of the Time Since Death in the Early Post-Mortem Period, 2nd ed. London : Arnold, 2002.

Marshall TK. The use of body temperature in estimating the time of death and its limitations. *Med Sci Law* 1969; **3:** 178–82.

Marshall TK, Hoare FE. Estimating the time of death. *J Forensic Sci* 1962; **7:** 56–81, 189–210, 211–21.

Saukko P, Knight B. *Knight's Forensic Pathology*, 3rd edn. London UK: Arnold, 2004.

Shkrum MJ, Ramsay DA. *Forensic Pathology of Trauma*. Totowa, NJ: Humana Press, Inc., 2007.

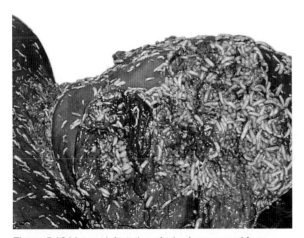

Figure 5.13 Maggot infestation of a body recovered from heated premises approximately 2 weeks after death. Forensic entomology may assist in estimating post-mortem interval (PMI) in such cases.

Chapter 6

Unexpected and sudden death from natural causes

- ■ Introduction
- ■ Cardiovascular system
- ■ Respiratory system
- ■ Gastrointestinal system
- ■ Gynaecological conditions
- ■ Deaths from asthma and epilepsy
- ■ Further information sources

■ Introduction

In countries where deaths have to be officially certified, the responsibility for certification falls either to the doctor who attended the patient during life or one who can reasonably be assumed to have sufficient knowledge of the clinical history to give a reasonable assessment of the cause of death. This is an 'honest opinion, fairly given', but many studies have shown that there is a large error rate in death certificates and that in 25–60 per cent of deaths there are significant differences between the clinician's presumption of the cause of death and the lesions or diseases actually displayed at the autopsy.

Unfortunately, it seems that there has been little or no improvement in the problems of certification of death over the years and as a result the raw epidemiological data gathered by national statistical bureaux must be treated with some caution. All doctors should take the task of certifying the cause of death very seriously but, regrettably, it is a job usually delegated to the most junior and least experienced, member of the team.

Changes to the legislation applicable to death certification are expected in the UK following several reviews, and it is expected that all death certificates will be scrutinized by a medical practitioner (a Medical Examiner) who will be in a position to advise doctors on the wording of the cause of death given on the certificate, advise the Coroner of medical matters pertaining to death certification and identify trends in deaths in their area.

There is a different approach to sudden and unexpected deaths, as these deaths are usually reportable to the authorities for medico-legal investigation. In England and Wales, doctors should only issue a death certificate if they are satisfied that they know the cause of death and that it is from natural causes. Before completing the death certificate, the body must be examined after death, unless the patient had been examined by that doctor in life within the previous 14 days; changes proposed to the death certification process are likely to remove this 'time-limit', instead relying on the doctor's ability to certify the cause of death 'with confidence'.

The World Health Organization (WHO) definition of a sudden death is death within 24 hours of the onset of symptoms, but in forensic practice most sudden deaths occur within minutes or even seconds of the onset of symptoms. Indeed, it is very likely that a death that is delayed by hours will not be referred to the Coroner or other medico-legal authority, as a diagnosis may well have been made, and a death certificate can be completed by the attending doctors.

It is crucial to remember that a sudden death is not necessarily unexpected and an unexpected death is not necessarily sudden, but these two facets are often combined.

■ Cardiovascular system

Disease of the heart

When a natural death is very rapid, the most common cause of irreversible cardiac arrest is a cardiovascular abnormality. While some degree of geographical variation is to be expected, the following lesions are the most significant as causes of sudden unexpected death.

Coronary artery disease

Narrowing of the lumen of a coronary artery (stenosis) by atheroma may lead to chronic ischaemia of the muscle supplied by that artery. If the myocardium becomes ischaemic, it may also become electrically unstable, predisposing to the development of an abnormal heart rhythm (i.e. an arrhythmia). The oxygen requirement of the myocardium is dependent upon the heart rate; an increase in heart rate – for example during exercise, following a large meal or as a consequence of a sudden adrenaline response to stress, anger, fear or other such emotion – will lead to an increase in myocardial oxygen demand. If the increased oxygen demand cannot be met, owing to restriction of blood flow through the stenotic vessel, the myocardium distal to the stenosis will become ischaemic. Ischaemia does not invariably lead to myocardial infarction, it just has to be sufficiently severe to initiate a fatal arrhythmia and, if the region rendered ischaemic includes one of the pace-making nodes or a major branch of the conducting system, the risk that rhythm abnormalities will develop is greatly increased.

Complications of atheromatous plaques may worsen the coronary stenosis and subsequent myocardial ischaemia. Bleeding may occur into a plaque and this can be seen as sub-intimal haemorrhage at autopsy. Sudden expansion of the plaque may lead to

rupture, which may also occur if the plaque ulcerates. When a plaque ruptures, the extruded cholesterol, fat and fibrous debris will be 'washed downstream' in the coronary artery and impact distally, often causing multiple mini-infarcts. The endothelial cap of a ruptured plaque may act as a flap valve within the vessel and cause a complete obstruction.

An atheromatous plaque is a site for the development of thrombus, which will further reduce the vessel lumen without necessarily fully blocking the vessel.

Coronary thrombosis underlies most of the complications of coronary artery atherosclerosis, including unstable angina, acute myocardial infarction and sudden cardiac death but such thrombi are found with variable frequency at autopsy – between 13% and 98% (Figure 6.1).

Myocardial infarction occurs when there is severe stenosis or complete occlusion of a coronary artery so that the blood supply is insufficient to maintain

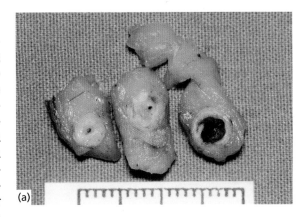

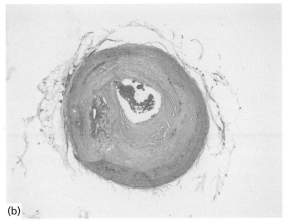

Figure 6.1 Significant coronary artery atherosclerosis and acute thrombosis. Macroscopic **(a)** and microscopic **(b)** appearance.

oxygenation of the myocardium. However, if there is adequate collateral circulation, blood can still reach the myocardium by other routes. The fatal effects of an infarct may appear at any time after the muscle has become ischaemic (Figure 6.2).

The area of muscle damaged by a myocardial infarction is further weakened by the process of cellular death and the inflammatory response to these necrotic cells. The area of the myocardial infarct is weakest between 3 days and 1 week after the clinical onset of the infarct and it is at this time that the weakened area of myocardium may rupture, leading to sudden death from a haemopericardium and cardiac tamponade. The rupture occasionally occurs through the interventricular septum, resulting in a left–right shunt. If a papillary muscle is infarcted, it may rupture, which will allow part of the mitral valve to prolapse, which may be associated with sudden death or may present as a sudden onset of valve insufficiency (Figure 6.3).

An infarct heals by 'scarring' (fibrosis), and fibrotic plaques in the wall of the ventricle or septum may interfere with physical or electrical cardiac function. Cardiac aneurysms may form at sites of infarction; they may calcify and they may rupture.

Physical lesions in the cardiac conducting system have been studied intensively in recent years, especially in relation to sudden death. Many different abnormalities have been found; it may be difficult to determine if conduction system lesions are the cause of a fatal arrhythmia or merely an incidental finding but, in the absence of any other abnormality, it may be reasonable to conclude that they were a significant factor in causing the death.

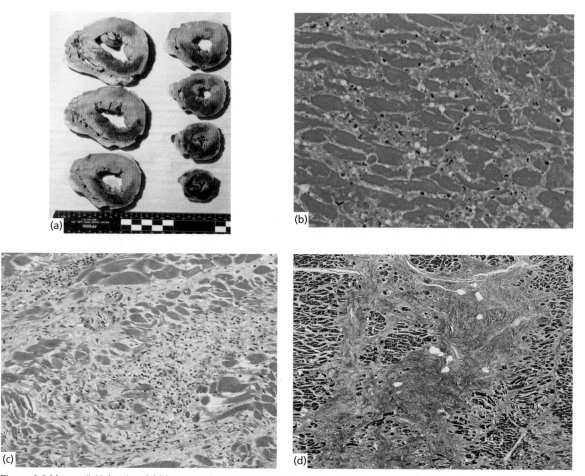

Figure 6.2 Myocardial infarction. **(a)** Macroscopic appearance of acute left-ventricular myocardial infarction. **(b–d)** Microscopic appearance of myocardial infarction with early necrosis **(b)**, organization including residual haemosiderin-laden macrophages and fibroblasts **(c)**, and extensive replacement fibrosis **(d)**.

6 *Unexpected and sudden death from natural causes*

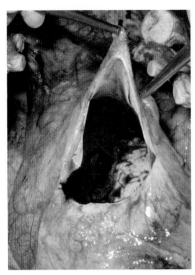

Figure 6.3 Haemopericardium causing cardiac tamponade. The distended pericardial sac has been opened to reveal fluid and clotted blood.

Hypertensive heart disease

Long-standing hypertension can result in cardiac remodelling, manifested by left-ventricular hypertrophy (and cardiomegaly). Although the 'normal heart weight' (approximately 400 g for the 'average man') is dependent on body size/weight, an enlarged heart predisposes an individual to chronic myocardial hypoxia and electrical instability which, when combined with a 'trigger', can result in a fatal arrhythmia. Some authors consider a heart weight of greater than 500 g to represent an inherently unstable heart. Hypertensive heart disease frequently coexists with coronary artery atherosclerosis, increasing the potential for the development of fatal arrhythmias at times of cardiovascular 'stress'.

Aortic stenosis

Aortic stenosis is a disease that classically affects older individuals with calcified tricuspid aortic valves, but may also be seen in younger people who have a congenital bicuspid aortic valve. The accompanying myocardial hypertrophy is similar to that caused by hypertension – leading to left ventricular hypertrophy – which may, in some cases, produce heart weights of over 700 g.

In aortic stenosis, myocardial perfusion is worsened by the narrow valve, which results in a lower pressure at the coronary ostia and hence in the coronary arteries. Sudden death is common in these patients.

Senile myocardial degeneration

Senescence is a well-accepted concept in all animals, and few humans survive beyond 90–100 years. The cause of a sudden death in these elderly individuals can be very difficult to determine. The senile heart is small, the surface vessels are tortuous and the myocardium is soft and brown owing to accumulated lipofuscin in the cells.

Primary myocardial disease

Primary diseases of the myocardium are much less common than the degenerative conditions described above and they commonly affect a significantly younger age group. They include conditions where there is a structural abnormality of the heart that is visible to the 'naked eye' and/or under the microscope (myocarditis and the 'cardiomyopathies') and those conditions having no recognizable morphological/structural abnormality (the 'channelopathies').

Myocarditis occurs in many infective diseases, such as diphtheria and viral infection, including influenza. Complications, including sudden death, associated with the infection may occur some days or even weeks after the main clinical symptoms. Myocarditis may sometimes be suspected macroscopically because of the presence of pale or haemorrhagic foci in the myocardium (having a 'mottled' appearance), although histological confirmation of multifocal inflammatory cell infiltrates and associated myocyte necrosis requires extensive sampling at post-mortem examination.

The cardiomyopathies comprise a group of disorders including:

- hypertrophic cardiomyopathy (HCM), which is an inherited disease of cardiac muscle sarcomeric proteins, characterized by symmetrical or asymmetrical hypertrophy, a sub-aortic mitral 'impact lesion' and myocyte disarray;
- dilated cardiomyopathy (DCM), which may be a primary disorder, or a secondary phenomenon (for example to chronic alcohol misuse); and
- arrhythmogenic right ventricular cardiomyopathy (ARVCM) – an inherited condition increasingly being recognized — which is characterized by

predominantly right-ventricular thinning with fibro-fatty myocyte replacement.

The cardiomyopathies are an important group of conditions linked to sudden death in the young, and are of particular importance in deaths occurring during exercise, or on the athletic field.

The channelopathies are a group of disorders receiving increasing interest because of the advent of sophisticated molecular pathology techniques. They represent a relatively small proportion of sudden deaths, presumed to be of cardiac origin, where investigations – including toxicology – have failed to identify an alternative explanation for death. These sudden deaths are often 'triggered' by a stimulus, including exercise, sudden loud noises or even during sleep. Such deaths are often characterized as falling into the broad category of sudden adult death syndrome (SADS).

New entities are continually being discovered in this group of conditions, but the main syndromes currently recognized include Wolff–Parkinson–White, Long QT, Short QT, Brugada and Catecholaminergic Polymorphous Ventricular Tachycardia and Idiopathic Ventricular Fibrillation.

Pathologically, there are no 'naked eye' or microscopic abnormalities in the heart as the defects are at a molecular level. Defects in genes encoding myocyte 'contractile units' have been characterized, and these affect the function of sodium, potassium and calcium channels (hence 'channelopathies') and the ryanodine receptor, for example. Molecular investigations are likely to form an increasing role in the post-mortem investigation of such presumed sudden cardiac deaths with a structurally normal heart.

Diseases of the arteries

The most common lesion of (extracardiac) arteries associated with sudden death is the aneurysm. Several varieties must be considered as they are very commonly found in sudden unexpected death autopsies.

Atheromatous aneurysm of the aorta

These aneurysms are most commonly found in elderly individuals in the abdominal region of the aorta (Figure 6.4).

They are formed when the elastic component of the aortic wall underlying an atheromatous plaque is

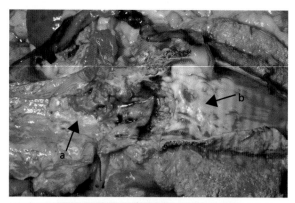

Figure 6.4 Atherosclerotic abdominal aortic aneurysm. As the aneurysm dilates, there is an increased risk of leakage and frank rupture, leading to fatal intra-abdominal or retroperitoneal haemorrhage. **a** Ulcerated atherosclerotic plaque; **b** Site of previous aneurysm repair.

damaged and blood under pressure is able to 'balloon' the weakened wall. The aneurysms may be saccular (expanding to one side) or fusiform (cylindrical). The wall of the aneurysm is commonly calcified and the lumen is commonly lined by old laminated thrombus.

Many aneurysms remain intact and are found as an incidental finding at autopsy, but others eventually rupture. The rupture may be repaired surgically if diagnosed in time, but many individuals die too quickly for any help to be given. Because the aorta lies in the retroperitoneal space, that is where the bleeding is found; it may lie to one side and envelop a kidney. Rarely, the aneurysm itself, or the retroperitoneal haematoma, ruptures through the retroperitoneal tissues to cause a haemoperitoneum.

Dissecting aneurysm of the aorta

The damage caused by an atheromatous plaque can also result in an intimal defect and weakening of the media, allowing blood from the lumen to 'dissect' into this weakened arterial wall. Once the dissection has started, the passage of blood under pressure extends the dissection along the aortic wall. The commonest site of origin of a dissecting aneurysm is in the thoracic aorta and the dissection usually tracks distally towards the abdominal region, sometimes reaching the iliac and even the femoral arteries. In fatal cases, the track may rupture at any point, resulting in haemorrhage into the thorax or abdomen. Alternatively, it can dissect proximally around the arch and into the pericardial sac, where it can produce a haemo-pericardium, cardiac tamponade and sudden death.

Dissecting aneurysms (Figure 6.5) are principally found in individuals with hypertension, but may also be seen in younger individuals with connective tissue defects, such as Marfan syndrome.

Syphilitic aneurysms

These are now relatively rare in developed countries because of the effective treatment of primary and secondary syphilis, but they are still encountered in routine autopsies on old people and in individuals from areas without an established healthcare system. The aneurysms are thin walled;

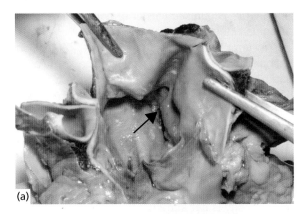

(a)

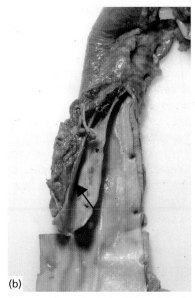

(b)

Figure 6.5 Thoracic aortic dissection. The origin of the dissection is in the aortic root, just above the tricuspid aortic valve **(a)** with a plane of dissection in the aortic media **(b)**.

they are most common in the thoracic aorta and especially in the arch. They may rupture, causing torrential haemorrhage.

Intracranial vascular lesions

Several types of intracranial vascular lesion are important in sudden or unexpected death.

Ruptured berry aneurysm

A relatively common cause of sudden collapse and often rapid death of young to middle-aged men and women is subarachnoid haemorrhage as a consequence of rupture of a 'congenital' (berry) aneurysm of the basal cerebral arteries, either in the circle of Willis itself or in the arteries that supply it. Whether berry aneurysms can be described as 'congenital' depends on the interpretation of the word: strictly speaking, they are not present at birth, but the weakness in the media of the vessel wall (usually at a bifurcation) from which they develop is present at birth. The aneurysms may be a few millimetres in diameter or may extend to several centimetres; they may be single or multiple and they may be found on one or more arteries (Figure 6.6).

The aneurysms may be clinically silent or they may leak, producing a severe headache, neck stiffness, unconsciousness and sometimes paralysis or other neurological symptoms. The rupture of a berry aneurysm on the arterial circle of Willis allows blood to flood over the base of the brain or, if the aneurysm is embedded in the brain, into the brain tissue itself. The precise mechanism of sudden death following subarachnoid haemorrhage is not understood: bathing the brain-stem in blood may

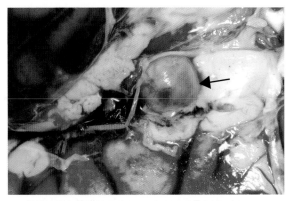

Figure 6.6 Berry aneurysm of the proximal middle cerebral artery and associated subarachnoid haemorrhage.

invoke vascular spasm resulting in critical ischaemia of cardiorespiratory control centres or the presence of subarachnoid blood under pressure may directly affect such brain-stem cardiorespiratory control.

An area of controversy in forensic pathology is the role of assault in the development of subarachnoid haemorrhage from a ruptured 'congenital' aneurysm. Particular difficulties arise when rupture of an intracerebral aneurysm follows an altercation not attended by any physical evidence of blunt force head injury; a causative role for a transient elevation of blood pressure, owing to the 'stress' of the altercation, is controversial and may be further complicated by alcohol intoxication.

An additional entity frequently encountered in forensic pathology practice is that of 'traumatic basal subarachnoid haemorrhage'. The 'classical scenario' in such cases is of an individual, often intoxicated by alcohol, receiving a blow to the head or neck, which results in a rapid extension and rotation of the head on the neck. The individual collapses rapidly following such a blow – and suffers a cardiac arrest – and is subsequently found to have a basal subarachnoid haemorrhage associated with a 'tear' in an intracranial blood vessel, frequently a vertebral artery. Microscopy of the culprit artery reveals no evidence of an intrinsic vascular abnormality and toxicological analysis reveals no evidence of stimulant drugs, such as cocaine or amphetamine. Issues that may become relevant in court relate to whether the death was caused by, for example, a punch or by the impact of the head on the ground after the punch. Criteria for ascribing such basal subarachnoid haemorrhage to trauma have been proposed, but such cases are often complicated by a lack of independent witness evidence to the incident, although the wider usage of CCTV has enabled clear links between mechanisms and pathological outcome to be confirmed in some cases. The post-mortem demonstration of such intracranial vascular injury requires careful *in situ* dissection techniques, preferably under operating microscopy, in order to exclude artefactual vascular disruption.

Cerebral haemorrhage, thrombosis and infarction

Sudden bleeding into brain tissue is common, usually in old age and in those with significant hypertension and, together with cerebral thrombosis and

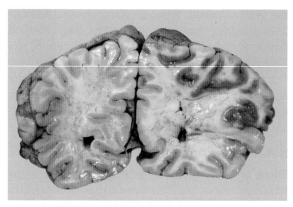

Figure 6.7 Acute cerebral infarction (predominantly middle cerebral artery territory).

resulting brain infarction, is the commonest cause of the well-recognized cluster of neurological signs colloquially termed a 'stroke'.

The term cerebrovascular accident (CVA) is in common usage in such circumstances, both as a clinical diagnosis and as a cause of death. Occasionally, it is misinterpreted by the public, and sometimes also by legal officials, as indicating an unnatural cause of death because of the use of the word 'accident'. To avoid this small risk, it is much more satisfactory, if the exact cause is known, to use the specific term that describes the aetiology (cerebral haemorrhage or cerebral infarction) or, if the aetiology is not known, to use the generic term cerebrovascular lesion (Figure 6.7).

Spontaneous intracerebral haemorrhage is most often found in the external capsule/basal ganglia of one cranial hemisphere and arises from rupture of a micro-aneurysm of the lenticulo-striate artery, sometimes called a Charcot–Bouchard aneurysm. The sudden expansion of a haematoma compresses the internal capsule and may destroy some of it, leading to a hemiplegia (Figure 6.8).

Death in such circumstances is not usually sudden, although there is a complex interaction between the brain and the heart, and thus a 'stroke' affecting a region of the brain important in such control can precipitate a cardiac arrest.

■ Respiratory system

The major cause of sudden death within the respiratory organs is again vascular. Pulmonary embolism is very common and is the most

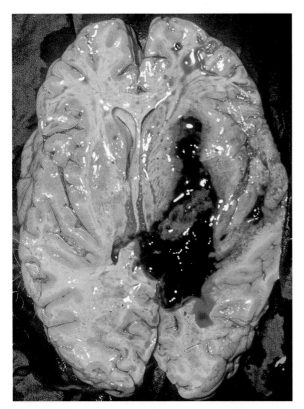

Figure 6.8 Recent intracerebral haemorrhage in a hypertensive individual.

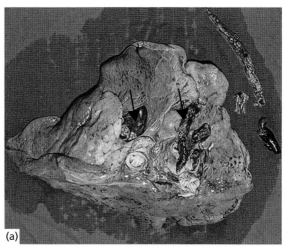

(a)

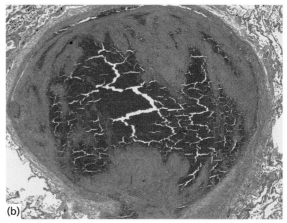

(b)

Figure 6.9 Fatal pulmonary thromboembolism. Macroscopic **(a)** and microscopic **(b)** appearance.

clinically under-diagnosed cause of death. In almost every case, the source of the emboli is in the deep leg or pelvic veins (Figure 6.9). Tissue trauma, especially where it is associated with immobility or bed rest, is a very common predisposing factor in the development of deep vein thrombosis. Most thromboses remain silent and cause no problems, but a proportion embolize and block pulmonary arteries of varying size. Large thromboemboli can occlude the origin of the pulmonary arteries (saddle emboli), resulting in massive acute right-heart strain and failure as a result of mechanical blockage, whereas smaller thromboemboli become lodged in smaller-calibre pulmonary blood vessels where they interfere with pulmonary function and lead to myocardial ischaemia and cardiac arrest.

A predisposing cause for pulmonary thromboembolism can be identified in a significant proportion of such deaths, including immobility following surgery or trauma, use of the oral contraceptive, smoking or where there is a history of metastatic cancer or a blood clotting abnormality. However,

the remainder occur unexpectedly in normal, ambulant people who have reported no clinical symptoms. This sometimes makes establishing the causal relationship between death and an injurious event difficult. For the purposes of civil law (where the standard of proof for causation is 'on the balance of probabilities') the embolism can often be linked to the trauma, but in a criminal trial in which a higher standard of proof ('beyond reasonable doubt') is required, it may be much harder to demonstrate a causal link between the two events.

Other rare causes of sudden death in the respiratory system (excluding bronchial asthma which is covered separately below) include massive haemoptysis from cavitating pulmonary tuberculosis or from an invasive tumour (Figure 6.10). Rapid (but

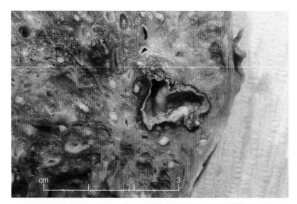

Figure 6.10 Disseminated pulmonary tuberculosis (TB). Note also the cavitating (secondary TB) lesion.

not sudden) deaths can also occur from fulminating chest infections, especially virulent forms of influenza.

Gastrointestinal system

The main causes of sudden death in the gastrointestinal system are predominantly vascular in nature; severe bleeding from a gastric or duodenal peptic ulcer can be fatal in a short time, although less torrential bleeding may be amenable to emergency medical/surgical intervention (Figure 6.11).

Mesenteric thrombosis and embolism, usually related to aortic or more generalized atherosclerosis, may result in infarction of the gut; a rapid but not sudden death is expected if the infarction remains undiagnosed. Intestinal infarction owing to a strangulated

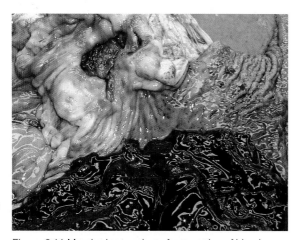

Figure 6.11 Massive haemorrhage from erosion of blood vessels in the base of this peptic gastric ulcer.

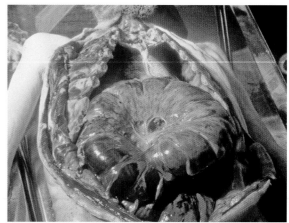

Figure 6.12 Intestinal infarction following volvulus of the sigmoid colon.

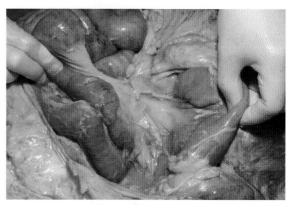

Figure 6.13 Peritonitis. Note the fibrinous deposits on the surface of loops of intestines.

hernia, or obstruction owing to torsion of the bowel as a consequence of adhesions can also prove rapidly fatal (Figure 6.12).

Peritonitis, following perforation of a peptic ulcer, diverticulitis or perforation at the site of a colonic tumour for example, can be rapidly fatal if not treated (Figure 6.13).

Many of these conditions present as sudden death in elderly people because they cannot, or will not, seek medical assistance at the onset of the symptoms, and are then unable to do so as their condition worsens.

Gynaecological conditions

When a female of childbearing age is found deceased, a complication of pregnancy must be considered to be the most likely cause of death until

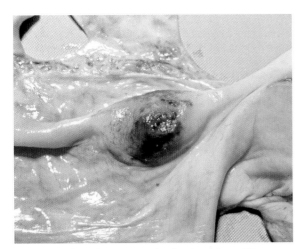

Figure 6.14 Ectopic pregnancy leading to rupture of the Fallopian tube and massive intra-abdominal haemorrhage.

other causes have been excluded. Abortion remains one possibility anywhere in the world, but especially in countries where illegal abortion is still very common.

A ruptured ectopic pregnancy, usually in a Fallopian tube, is another grave obstetric emergency that can end in death from intraperitoneal bleeding unless rapidly treated by surgical intervention (Figure 6.14).

Maternal deaths (occurring during pregnancy or within 12 months of parturition in the UK) can be classified into 'direct' deaths (caused by diseases specifically related to pregnancy, such as pulmonary thromboembolism, pre-eclampsia, obstetric haemorrhage, amniotic fluid embolism, acute fatty liver of pregnancy or ectopic gestation), 'indirect' deaths (from pre-existing disease exacerbated by pregnancy such as congenital heart disease or a cardiomyopathy) or 'coincidental' deaths. Maternal deaths are the subject of anonymous review in the UK as part of an ongoing 'Confidential Enquiry'.

■ Deaths from asthma and epilepsy

Deaths from acute bronchial asthma are infrequent with increasingly effective pharmacological control of this chronic condition. Asthma 'attacks' may be triggered by a number of common and household allergens, as well as commonly abused drugs such as heroin and crack cocaine (particularly when it is smoked). The 'naked eye' autopsy findings include hyper-inflated lungs and mucus plugging of the airways by tenacious, viscous mucus. Microscopy of the lungs commonly reveals chronic airway remodelling, with basement membrane thickening, goblet cell and smooth muscle hyperplasia, and super-imposed airway inflammation with eosinophils (Figure 6.15). An anaphylactic component may be responsible for a fatal outcome, and post-mortem blood sampling for mast cell tryptase is often rewarding.

Epilepsy – recurrent unprovoked seizures – is associated with an increased risk of mortality and, while there may be specific reasons why a person with epilepsy may die (e.g. drowning as a result of a seizure while swimming), there are approximately 500 sudden and unexpected deaths in epileptics each year in the UK where the precise cause of death is not identified. Such deaths have been classified as Sudden Unexpected Deaths in

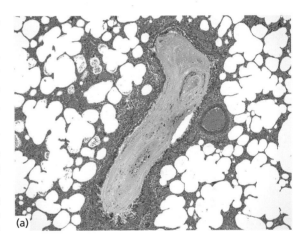

(a)

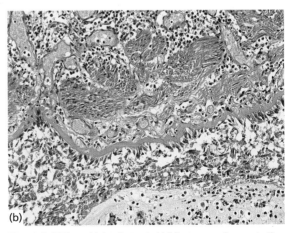

(b)

Figure 6.15 Bronchial asthma. (a,b) Microscopy demonstrating airway 'remodelling', mucus distension and inflammatory cell infiltration, including neutrophils and eosinophils.

Epilepsy (SUDEP), defined as a 'sudden unexpected, witnessed or unwitnessed, non-traumatic and non-drowning death in epilepsy, with or without evidence of a seizure, and excluding documented status epilepticus, where post-mortem examination does not reveal a toxicological or anatomic cause of death'.

The mechanism of death in such cases is uncertain, but may be related to a seizure-induced arrhythmia, seizure-mediated inhibition of respiratory centres or a complication of anti-epileptic treatment. Post-mortem findings in SUDEP are non-specific (for example pulmonary oedema and congestion) and the utility of the presence of a tongue injury in diagnosing a seizure is controversial.

Neuropathological examination of the brain is important in order to exclude the presence of a lesion capable of providing an explanation for seizure activity, such as, for example, an old brain injury or arteriovenous malformation, although the presence of more subtle changes in the brain, thought to represent evidence of seizure activity, cannot be taken as evidence of seizure activity at the time of death.

■ Further information sources

Arbustini E, Dal Bello B, Morbini P *et al*. Plaque erosion is a major substrate for coronary thrombosis in acute myocardial infarction. *Heart* 1999; **82**: 269–72.

Fornes P, Lecompte D, Nicholas G. Sudden out-of-hospital coronary death in patients with no cardiac history. An analysis of 221 patients studied at autopsy. *J Forensic Sciences* 1993; **38**: 1084–91.

Friedman M, Manwaring JH, Rosenman RH *et al*. Instantaneous and sudden deaths. Clinical and pathological differentiation in coronary artery disease. *Journal of the American Medical Association* 1973; **225**: 1319–28.

Hill SF, Sheppard MN. Non-atherosclerotic coronary artery disease associated with sudden cardiac death. *Heart* 2010; **96**: 1084–5.

Hinkle LE Jr, Thaler HT. Clinical classification of cardiac deaths. *Circulation* 1982; **65**: 457–64.

Leadbeatter S. Extracranial vertebral artery injury – evolution of a pathological illusion? *Forensic Science International* 1994; **67**: 33–40.

Libby P. Current concepts of the pathogenesis of the acute coronary syndromes. *Circulation* 2001; **104**: 365–72.

Millward-Sadler GH. Pathology of maternal deaths. In: Kirkham N, Shepherd N (eds). *Progress in Pathology 2003*, Vol 6. London: Greenwich Medical Media, 2003; 163–85.

Nashef L. Sudden unexpected death in epilepsy: terminology and definitions. *Epilepsia* 1997; **38**(Suppl 11)**:** S6–8.

Sidebotham HJ, Roche WR. Asthma deaths; persistent and preventable mortality. *Histopathology* 2003; **43**: 105–17.

Soilleux EJ, Burke MM. Pathology and investigation of potentially hereditary sudden cardiac death syndromes in structurally normal hearts. *Diagnostic Histopathology* 2008; **15**: 1–26.

Tomson T, Nashef L, Ryvlin P. Sudden unexpected death in epilepsy: Current knowledge and future directions. *Lancet Neurol* 2008 **11**: 1021–31.

Chapter 7

Deaths and injury in infancy

- ■ Introduction
- ■ Stillbirths
- ■ Infanticide
- ■ The estimation of maturity of a newborn baby or fetus
- ■ Sudden infant death syndrome
- ■ Child abuse
- ■ Further information sources

■ Introduction

The outcomes of disease and trauma are, in general terms, the same in individuals of all ages, but there are some special features of injuries to infants and children that require specific consideration. Some relate to the law, and some to medical and pathological factors. Newborns, infants, toddlers, younger children and adolescents have their own unique problems, such as stillbirth and sudden infant death syndrome, which are different from those of fully developed adults. They are also dependent, vulnerable and may encounter abuse, whether emotional, physical or sexual. This chapter emphasizes the pathologically relevant issues while Chapter 13 focuses more on the issues of the living.

■ Stillbirths

A significant number of pregnancies that continue into the third trimester fail to deliver a live child and result in a stillbirth. The definitions of a stillbirth vary from country to country, but the definition in England and Wales, which is perhaps typical, is that the child must be of more than 24 weeks' gestational age and, after being completely expelled from the mother, did not breathe or show any signs of life (Births and Deaths Registration Act 1953, as amended by the Still-Birth [Definition] Act 1992). These 'signs of life', in addition to respiration and heartbeat, are taken to mean movement, crying or pulsation of the umbilical cord.

If death occurs more than a couple of days before birth, the fetus is commonly macerated because of the effects of early decomposition combined with exposure to fluid (Figure 7.1). The infant is discoloured, usually a pinkish-brown or red, with extensive desquamation of the skin; the tissues have a soft, slimy translucence and there may be partial collapse of the head with overriding of the skull plates. The appearance of the child is quite different from that seen in an infant that has died following a live birth and then begun to putrefy. Because many, if not most, of these deaths occur after the onset of labour and during the process of birth itself, no evidence of maceration will be present.

In England and Wales a child does not have a legally-recognized 'separate existence' (and thus

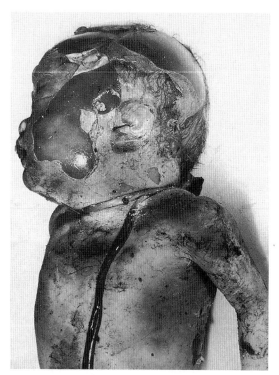

Figure 7.1 Maceration following intrauterine death. Note the widespread skin slippage and the umbilical cord around the neck.

intrauterine infections (viral, bacterial or fungal), congenital defects (especially in the cardiovascular or nervous system) and birth trauma.

■ Infanticide

The term infanticide has a very specific meaning in the many countries that have introduced legislation designed to circumvent the criminal charge of murder when a mother kills her child during its first year of life. In England and Wales, Section 1 of the Infanticide Act 1938 states that:

> Where a woman by any wilful act or omission causes the death of her child ... under the age of twelve months, but at the time ... the balance of her mind was disturbed by reason of her not having fully recovered from the effect of giving birth to the child or by reason of the effect of lactation consequent upon the birth of the child, then ... she shall be guilty of ... infanticide, and may ... be dealt with and punished as if she had been guilty of the offence of manslaughter of the child.

Because manslaughter is a less serious charge than murder and does not result in the mandatory penalty of life imprisonment that is attached to murder, a verdict of infanticide allows the court to make an appropriate sentence for the mother, which is more likely to be probation and psychiatric supervision than custody. The Infanticide Act indicates that the law recognizes the special nature of infanticide.

In England and Wales, there is a legal presumption that all deceased babies are stillborn and so the onus is on the prosecution, and hence the pathologist, to prove that the child was born alive and had a separate existence. In order to do this, it must be shown that the infant breathed or showed other signs of life, such as movement or pulsation of the umbilical cord, after having been completely expelled from the mother.

In the absence of eyewitness accounts, pathologists can make no comment about the viability or otherwise of a baby at the moment of complete expulsion from the mother; one way that they may be able to comment on the possibility of separate existence is if they can establish that the child had breathed. However, establishing that breathing had taken place is still not absolute evidence of a

does not become a legal person, capable of acquiring legal rights such as inheritance and title) until he or she is completely free from the mother's body, although the cord and placenta may still be within the mother.

The Infant Life (Preservation) Act 1929 made it an offence to destroy a baby during birth; however, an exception was made in the Act for doctors acting 'in good faith' who, to save the life of the mother, have to destroy a baby that becomes impacted in the pelvis during birth.

As babies that are stillborn have never 'lived' in the legal sense, they cannot 'die' and so a death certificate cannot be issued. In England and Wales, a special 'stillbirth certificate' may be completed either by a doctor or a midwife if either was present at the birth or by either one of them if they have examined the body of the child after birth.

The causes of stillbirth are varied and may be undeterminable, even after a full autopsy. Indeed, it may be impossible to determine on the pathological features alone if the death occurred before, during or after birth. Recognized conditions leading to intrauterine or peri-mortem death include prematurity, fetal hypoxia, placental insufficiency, 'separate existence', as a baby in a vertex delivery can breathe after the head and thorax have been delivered but before delivery of the lower body.

The 'flotation test', which used to be the definitive test for breathing, and hence separate existence, and which was depended upon for many centuries, is now considered to be unreliable, although it still appears in some textbooks. All that can be said with regard to flotation of the lungs is that if a lung or piece of lung sinks in water, the baby had not breathed sufficiently to expand that lung and so the child may have been stillborn. The converse is definitely not true, as the lungs of babies who are proven to have been stillborn sometimes float. This test is useless in differentiating between live-born and stillborn infants and should no longer be used (Figure 7.2).

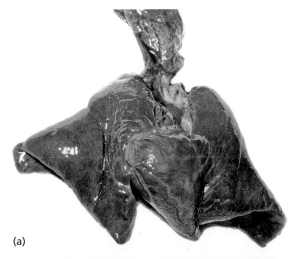

(a)

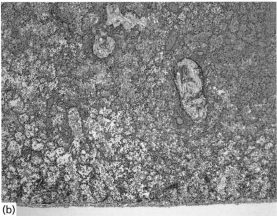

(b)

Figure 7.2 **(a)** Thoracic organs from a stillbirth. The lungs are firm and heavy with no crepitation when squeezed. **(b)** Microscopy of lungs from stillbirths showing partial expansion of terminal air spaces as a consequence of hypoxia-induced inspiratory efforts. Note also meconium aspiration.

To complicate matters further, many dead newborn babies are hidden shortly after birth and may not be discovered until decomposition has begun, which precludes any reliable assessment of the state of expansion of the lungs. Even with fresh bodies, the problems are immense and any attempt at mouth-to-mouth resuscitation or even chest compression will prevent any reliable opinion being given on the possibility of spontaneous breathing.

Conversely, if there is milk in the stomach or if the umbilical cord remnant is shrivelled or shows an inflammatory ring of impending separation, the child must have lived for some time after birth.

Establishing the identity of the infant and the identity of the mother is often a matter of great difficulty, as these babies are often found hidden or abandoned (Figure 7.3). When the baby is found in the home, there is seldom any dispute about who the mother is. DNA may be used to confirm identity and parentage.

In those cases where the mother is traced, further legal action depends on whether the pathologist can definitely decide if the baby was born alive or was stillborn. If live-born, no charge of infanticide can be brought in English law unless a wilful act of omission or commission can be proved to have caused the death. Omission means the deliberate failure to provide the normal care at birth, such as tying and cutting the cord, clearing the air passages of mucus and keeping the baby warm and fed. The wilful or deliberate withholding of these acts, as opposed to simple ignorance and inexperience, is hard to prove. Acts of commission are more straightforward for the doctor to demonstrate as

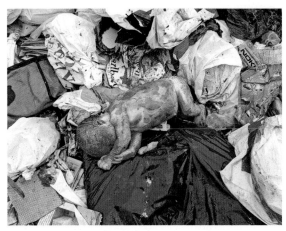

Figure 7.3 Newborn infant disposal with decompositional/putrefactive skin changes.

they may include a range of trauma, including head injuries, stabbing, drowning and strangulation.

The maturity of the infant is rarely an issue as most infants found dead after birth are at or near full term of 38–40 weeks. The legal age of maturity in Britain is now 24 weeks, although medical advances have allowed fetuses of only 20 weeks or less gestation to survive in specialist neonatal units. In infanticide, the maturity is not legally material as it is the deliberate killing of any baby that has attained a separate existence, and this does not depend directly upon the gestational age.

The estimation of maturity of a newborn baby or fetus

Legal requirements may need an estimation of gestational age of the body of a baby or fetus in relation to an abortion, stillbirth or alleged infanticide. The following are considered 'rule of thumb' formulae for estimating maturity (and should be considered to provide very rough estimates):

1 Up to the twentieth week, the length of the fetus in centimetres is the square of the age in months (Haase's rule);
2 After the twentieth week, the length of the fetus in centimetres equals five times the age in months.

There is considerable variation in any of the measured parameters owing to sex, race, nutrition and individual variation, but it is considered possible to form a reasonable estimate of the maturity of a fetus by using the brief notes in Box 7.1.

Box 7.1 Estimation of fetal maturity

- 4 weeks – 1.25 cm, showing limb buds, enveloped in villous chorion
- 12 weeks – 9 cm long, nails formed on digits, placenta well formed lanugo all over body
- 20 weeks – 18–25 cm, weight 350–450 g, hair on head
- 24 weeks – 30 cm crown–heel, vernix on skin
- 28 weeks – 35 cm crown–heel, 25 cm crown–rump, weight 900–1400 g
- 32 weeks – 40 cm crown–heel, weight 1500–2000 g
- 36 weeks – 45 cm crown–heel, weight 2200 g
- 40 weeks (full term) – 48–52 cm crown–heel, 28–32 cm crown – rump, 33–38 cm head circumference, lanugo now absent or present only over shoulders, head hair up to 2–3 cm long, testes palpable in scrotum/vulval labia close the vaginal opening, dark meconium in large intestine

---

Development can also be assessed using the femur length, ossification centres and the histological appearances of the major organs. It may be necessary to seek expert advice, from radiologists and forensic anthropologists, when determining gestational age.

Sudden infant death syndrome

The incidence of sudden infant death syndrome (SIDS) – also known as 'cot death' or 'crib death' – has declined in many developed countries from approximately 2 to 0.5 per 1000 live births, and was 0.28 per 1000 live births in England and Wales in 2007. This decline has coincided with social and housing improvements as well as a worldwide 'Back to Sleep' campaign in the early 1990s, which encouraged mothers to place babies on their back to sleep rather than face down or on their side. Publicity campaigns have also advised mothers to refrain from smoking during pregnancy or near to their babies after birth and to avoid overheating babies by wrapping them up too closely. However, despite this significant decline, SIDS still forms the most common cause of death in the post-perinatal period in countries with a relatively low infant mortality rate.

SIDS has been defined as 'the sudden unexpected death of an *infant* <1 year of age, with onset of the fatal episode apparently occurring during sleep, that remains unexplained after a thorough investigation, including the performance of a complete autopsy and a review of the circumstances of death and the clinical history'. The following are the main features of the syndrome.

- Most deaths take place between 1 month and 6 months, with a peak at 2 months.
- There is little sex difference, although there is a slight preponderance of males similar to that seen in many types of death.
- The incidence is markedly greater in multiple births, whether identical or not. This can be partly explained by the greater incidence of premature and low birth-weight infants in multiple births.
- There is a marked seasonal variation in temperate zones: SIDS is far more common in the colder and wetter months, in both the northern and southern hemispheres.

There are apparent social, racial and ethnic differences, but these are explained by fundamental underlying socio-economic factors, which show that there is a higher incidence in any disadvantaged families such as those with poor housing, lower occupational status, one–parent families, etc. However, no class, race or creed is exempt from these devastating deaths.

The essence of SIDS is that the deaths are unexpected and autopsy reveals no adequate cause of death. The history is usually typical: a perfectly well child – or one with trivial symptoms – is put in the sleeping place at night only to be found dead in the morning. At autopsy, nothing specific is found in the true SIDS death, although in about 70 per cent of cases the autopsy reveals intrathoracic petechiae on the pleura, epicardium and thymus, which formerly gave rise to the misapprehension that SIDS was caused by to mechanical suffocation. These are now believed to be agonal phenomena and not a cause of death (Figure 7.4).

The true aetiology of SIDS is unknown, but it is likely that there are many different causes, often multifactorial, which act via a final common pathway of cardiorespiratory failure. Theories about possible 'causes' of SIDS abound and include allergy to cow's milk or house-mites, botulism, prolonged sleep apnoea, spinal haemorrhages, deficiencies of liver enzymes, selenium or vitamin E, various metabolic defects, vaccinations, hyperthermia, hypothermia, carbon monoxide or dioxide poisoning, viral bronchiolitis, muscle hypotonia, abnormal development of key cardiorespiratory control areas in the brainstem and many others. As yet, none of these has been substantiated.

One persistent claim is for a possible role of deliberate mechanical suffocation by the wilful action of a parent. Speculation that up to 10 per cent of SIDS is caused in this way is difficult to refute but has never been substantiated by confessions, statistics or research.

As with sudden unexplained death in the adult, it is likely that causes not detectable by macroscopic or microscopic means, but by molecular biological techniques, may be found to be relevant in at least some cases.

Any healthcare professional must certainly be vigilant in any infant death, but the dangers of reinforcing the inevitable guilt in the great majority of innocent parents must be weighed against the chance of detecting a deliberate suffocation. The main concern in the management of SIDS is to support the family by explanations and to make sure that the counselling services established in many developed countries are made available to the parents.

Child abuse

Child abuse is a major social problem, which involves many medical specialties including paediatricians, general practitioners, psychiatrists and forensic practitioners. Child abuse is a generic term that includes all forms of physical and emotional ill-treatment, sexual abuse, neglect and exploitation that results in actual or potential harm to the child's health, development or dignity. See also Chapter 13.

Child physical abuse/non-accidental injury

The syndrome of physical abuse was recognized in the middle of the twentieth century in which limb fractures and subdural haemorrhages were described in infants. Subsequently, this combination of injuries was shown to result from ill-treatment by the carers. In fact, Caffey and his co-workers had only rediscovered a syndrome, as similar features

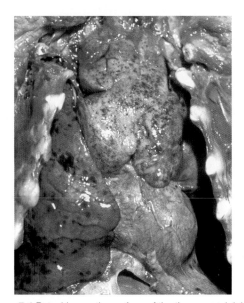

Figure 7.4 Petechiae on the surface of the thymus and right lung in a sudden infant death.

had been described by Tardieu in Paris during the middle of the nineteenth century.

In England and Wales, a more recent development in the law relating to child abuse is the introduction of the concept of 'familial homicide', in which an offence of 'causing or allowing the death of a child' is committed under section 5 of the Domestic Violence, Crime and Victims Act 2004 by a 'responsible adult household member' when failing to take reasonable steps to protect a child at significant risk of serious physical harm from members of the household.

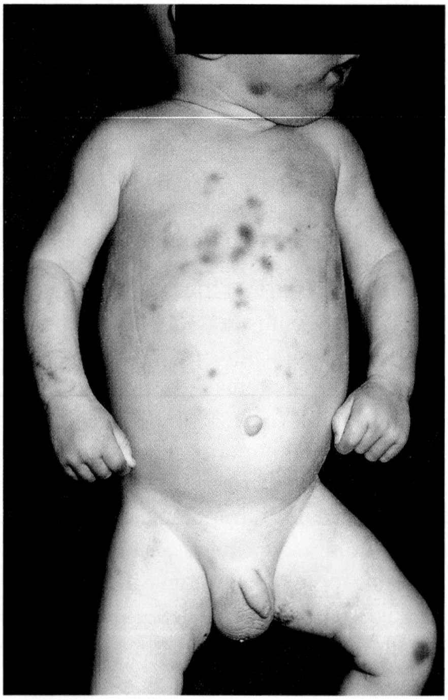

Epidemiology

The physically abused child can be of either sex and of any age. Fatalities are more common in children under the age of 2 years and the most common mode of death is head injury. Sexually abused children tend to be slightly older, although this may reflect the problems in perceiving and reporting sexual abuse in very young children. The upper age limit is very difficult to define: physical abuse is more likely to stop at a younger age, whereas sexual abuse commonly continues into the teens and even older.

Injuries in the deceased
Bruising

The features of bruises that are important can be summed up as site, age and multiplicity. Bruising of the arms and legs, especially around the upper arms, forearms, wrists, ankles and knees, may be evidence of gripping by an adult. Bruises on the face, ears, lips, neck, lateral thorax, anterior abdomen, buttocks and thighs require an explanation, as these sites are less likely to be injured in childhood falls (Figures 7.5 and 7.6). The following are suggestive of abuse: bruises over soft tissue areas in non-mobile infants, bruises that carry an imprint of an implement and multiple bruises of uniform shape.

The explanation given by the carers of how all of the injuries present on the child were caused must be noted with great care for two reasons: first, so that the doctor understands exactly what happened, allowing for a good interpretation of the injuries; and second, so that any changes in the explanation given by the carers over time or to different individuals can be compared.

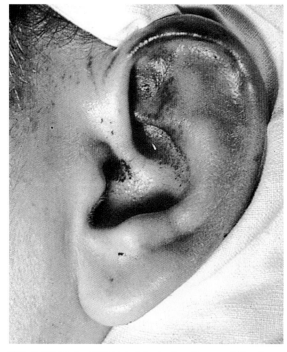

Figure 7.5 Multiple 'fingertip' bruises on the front of the trunk in an abused infant.

Figure 7.6 Ear bruising in an infant raises the possibility of non-accidental injury. Radiology revealed multiple rib fractures.

Skeletal injury

Fractures have been associated with physical child abuse for a considerable time, but it has only been relatively recently that an attempt has been made to study the pattern of skeletal injury in abuse in a more critical manner.

The investigation of all cases of suspected child abuse under the age of 2 years requires a detailed whole-body radiological survey, performed to a standard protocol (for example that set out by the British Society of Paediatric Radiology) and reported by a paediatric radiologist.

Healing fractures (representing previous traumatic episodes) can be visualized by radiological means although histological assessment post mortem is more precise.

Rib fractures are rarely accidental in children. They may occasionally be associated with birth trauma, but in general they are a feature of the application of substantial force. One particular pattern that may be seen on X-ray or at autopsy comprises areas of callus on the posterior ribs, often lying in a line adjacent to the vertebrae, and giving a 'string-of-beads' appearance. This pattern is interpreted as indicating an episode or episodes of forceful squeezing of the chest by adult hands. The possibility that such posterior rib fractures can be caused by cardiopulmonary resuscitation is thought unlikely on biomechanical grounds, as such fractures occur as a result of anterior–posterior compression during 'squeezing' of the chest. Anterolateral rib fractures as a consequence of cardiopulmonary resuscitation are rare (Figure 7.7).

A skull fracture is a marker of significant trauma to the head, and skull fractures are common in fatal cases of physical child abuse, but they are not necessarily accompanied by brain damage. Abusive skull fractures are more likely to be multiple, bilateral or cross sutures. Less often, fractures of the occipital or frontal bones are present and basal fractures are uncommon (Figures 7.8 and 7.9).

Research demonstrated that skull fractures in dead children 'dropped' from a height can be caused by passive falls from only 80 cm onto carpeted floors. For comparison, the seat of a 'standard' settee or chair is about 40 cm from the floor, the mattress of a 'standard' bed about 60 cm from the floor, and a 'standard' tabletop is about 70 cm from the floor. These figures would suggest that, unless the furniture was unusually high, or some

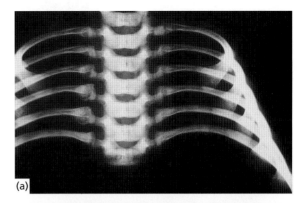

(a)

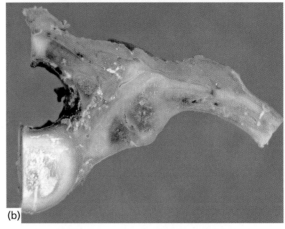

(b)

Figure 7.7 Rib fractures in infancy. **(a)** X-ray of ribs and part of the thoracic spine removed at autopsy. Note the right-sided posterior rib fractures showing evidence of healing (callus formation). Non-accidental injury should be suspected in such cases, and thoroughly investigated by a multi-disciplinary team. **(b)** A posterior rib fracture, with callus, following post-mortem removal and fixation. Microscopy of fractures assists in their 'ageing'.

other factors have to be considered, falls from furniture onto the floor are unlikely to be the cause of a skull fracture in a child. The ability for 'short-fall' events to result in subsequently fatal head injury remains controversial.

Head injuries

Head injuries are the most frequent cause of death in child abuse and, even when they are non-fatal, they may result in severe and permanent neurological disability.

There is continued controversy in the clinical, pathological and legal communities regarding the ability of 'shaking', in the absence of blunt force impact to the head, to cause fatal head/neck injury in an infant, and to cause the 'triad' of the so-called

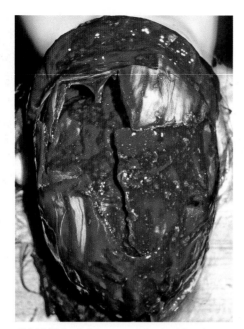

Figure 7.8 Multiple skull fractures following blunt force impacts against the floor.

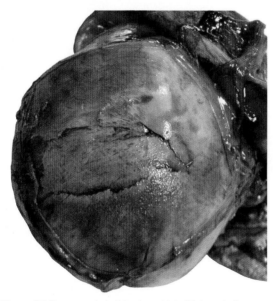

Figure 7.9 Depressed skull fracture. Not all infant skull fractures are non-accidental in origin; instrumentation and manual dis-impaction from the birth canal led to this fracture.

'shaken baby syndrome' (i.e. encephalopathy, subdural haemorrhage and retinal haemorrhage). This is an area of intense research and dispute and, while the concept of the 'shaken baby syndrome triad' was upheld by the Court of Appeal in R v Harris and others, the existence of that triad

does not automatically and necessarily lead to a diagnosis of non-accidental head injury – all of the circumstances of an individual case must be evaluated before excluding potential explanations other than abuse.

Whether from direct blows or from 'shaking', it is clear that if sufficient force is applied to the head of a child, the ultimate effects are brain injury and that injury carries with it a substantial risk of disability or death.

Ocular injuries

The significance of ocular lesions – such as retinal haemorrhages, retinoschisis and orbital content haemorrhage – is a further area of controversy in the medical and scientific community. All children suspected of being physically abused should have their eyes examined by an ophthalmologist, and the eyes should be examined as an integral component of the post-mortem examination following the death of a child suspected of being abused. The interpretation of the significance of such lesions remains controversial, but it is essential that a multi-professional team review all aspects of findings in the context of the known facts of the case and of the current state of the medical evidence base. (Figure 7.10).

Oral injuries

The lips may be bruised or abraded by blows to the face and, if the child is old enough to have teeth, the inner side of the lips may be bruised or lacerated by contact with the tooth edges. A lesion frequently seen in physical child abuse is a torn frenulum inside the lip; this can be damaged either by a tangential blow across the mouth or by an object, sometimes a feeding bottle, being rammed forcibly into the mouth between lip and gum (Figure 7.11). Current review of available data does not support the diagnosis of abuse simply based on a torn labial frenulum in isolation. The intraoral hard and soft tissue should be examined in all suspected abuse cases, and a dental opinion sought where abnormalities are found.

Visceral injuries

Visceral injuries are the second most frequent cause of death and it is the organs of the abdomen – the intestine, mesentery and liver – that are most

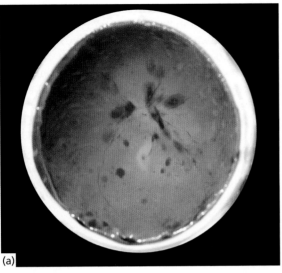

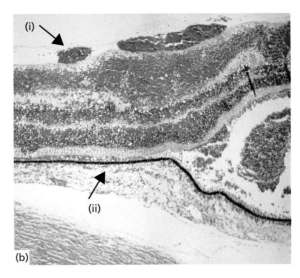

Figure 7.10 Retinal haemorrhages (a) macroscopic post-mortem appearance and (b) microscopy showing widespread haemorrhage within multiple layers of the retina. (i) Vitreous body; (ii) retinal pigment epithelium.

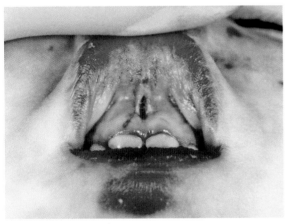

Figure 7.11 Bruising and laceration of the upper oral frenulum.

commonly injured. The anterior abdominal wall of a child offers little or no protection against direct trauma from fist or foot, and blows from the front can trap the duodenum, the jejunum or the mesentery between the compressed abdominal wall and the anvil of the lumbar spine. This compression crushes the tissues and may even result in transection of the bowel, with the obvious consequences of peritonitis and shock (Figure 7.12). Crushing or rupturing of the mesentery may lead to bruising or to frank intraperitoneal bleeding.

The liver is relatively large in a child and protrudes below the rib cage, and it can be ruptured by direct blows to the abdomen. However, the spleen is rarely damaged in physical child abuse because of its relatively sheltered position.

Other injuries

Other injuries in physical child abuse include burns and bites. Burns can be caused in many ways: from the application of heated metal objects or cigarettes to the hands, legs, buttocks or torso or to scalding due to immersion in hot water or from splashing from hot water that is thrown (see Chapter 17, p. 169). Cigarette burns have a typical appearance: they are commonly circular and, when fresh, are pink or red in colour and have an excavated appearance; ash may be see at the base of the burn crater. When healing, they tend to be silvery in the centre with a narrow red rim. A single scar left by a cigarette burn is non-specific, but multiple round scars on the body in association with a history of these burns can be diagnostic.

Bites also occur in child abuse and they are commonly multiple. They must be differentiated from bites from siblings, other children or even domestic pets. Swabs from a fresh bite should be taken as soon as possible, as they may recover saliva, which can be subjected to DNA analysis. The advice of a forensic odontologist, should also be sought as soon as possible, as the shape of the bite can be matched (by measurement, photography or latex casts) to the dentition of a suspected assailant.

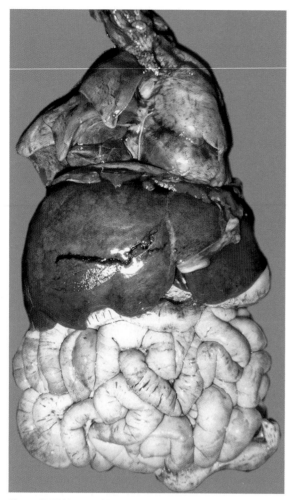

Figure 7.12 Non-accidental, blunt force, intra-abdominal visceral injury (same infant as in Figure 7.5). Note the liver laceration leading to intra-abdominal haemorrhage.

Genuine accidents to children are far more frequent than acts of child physical abuse. However, it can be extremely difficult to distinguish between them. Any doctor who examines children must always bear in mind the possibility of physical child abuse, and although it is vital that innocent parents are not unjustly accused of ill-treating their children, it is equally important that abuse is recognized, as the next time the child or a sibling, presents for treatment may be when they are fatally injured or dead.

Child sexual abuse

The problem of the sexual abuse and exploitation of children is global and thousands of children are sexually abused every day around the world. Sexual abuse has come to prominence more recently than physical abuse, although sexual contact between adults and children has been recorded in many situations and many countries for centuries. The modern definition of child sexual abuse may be expressed as 'the involvement of dependent, developmentally immature children and adolescents in sexual activities they do not truly comprehend, to which they are unable to give informed consent or which violate social taboos or family roles'.

The diagnosis and management of child sexual abuse are multidisciplinary, involving not only doctors but also social agencies and sometimes law enforcement agencies.

■ Further information sources

A Local Authority v S [2009] EWHC 2115 (Fam) (08 May 2009). http://www.familylawweek.co.uk/site.aspx?i=ed53850 (accessed 22 November 2010).

Anon. Unexplained deaths in infancy, England and Wales, 2007. Office for National Statistics Statistical Bulletin, August 2009; http://www.statistics.gov.uk/pdfdir/uinfmort0809.pdf (accessed 11 February 2011).

Barbet JP, Houette A, Barres D, Durigon M. Histological assessment of gestational age in human embryos and fetuses. *American Journal of Forensic Medicine and Pathology* 1988; **9:** 40–4.

Births and Deaths Registration Act 1953. http://www.legislation.gov.uk/ukpga/1953/20/pdfs/ukpga_19530020_en.pdf (accessed 22 November 2010).

Berry PJ. Pathological findings in SIDS. *Journal of Clinical Pathology* 1992; **45:** 11–16.

Bilo RAC, Robben SGF, van Rijn. *Forensic Aspects of Paediatric Fractures – Differentiating Accidental Trauma from Child Abuse.* Berlin: Springer-Verlag, 2010.

British Society of Paediatric Radiology. Standard for skeletal surveys in suspected non-accidental injury (NAI) in children. http://www.bspr.org.uk/nai.htm (accessed 17 April 2010).

Busuttil A, Keeling JW. *Paediatric Forensic Medicine and Pathology.* London: Hodder Arnold, 2009.

Caffey J. Multiple fractures in the long bones of infants suffering from chronic subdural hematoma. *AJR American Journal of Roentgenology* 1946; **56:** 163–73.

Case ME, Graham MA, Handy TC *et al.* Position paper on fatal abusive head injuries in infants and young children. *American Journal of Forensic Medicine and Pathology* 2001; **22:** 112–22.

Cooper N, Dattani N. Trends in cot deaths. *Health Statistics Quarterly* 2000; **5:** 10–16. (http://www.statistics.gov.uk/articles/hsq/HSQ5SIDs.pdf).

Domestic Violence, Crime and Victims Act 2004 C.28. http://www.legislation.gov.uk/ukpga/2004/28/contents (accessed 22 November 2010).

Gilliland MG, Luthert P. Why do histology on retinal haemorrhages in suspected non-accidental injury? *Histopathology* 2003; **43:** 592–602.

Goudge ST. Inquiry into paediatric forensic pathology in ontario Report 2008. www.attorneygeneral.jus.gov. on.ca/inquiries/goudge/policy_research/pdf/Limits_and_Controversies-CORDNER.pdf

Infant Life (Preservation) Act 1929 C.34. http://legislation. data.gov.uk/ukpga/Geo5/19-20/34/enacted/data.htm (accessed 22 November 2010).

Infanticide Act 1938 C.36. http://www.statutelaw.gov.uk/ content.aspx?activeTextDocId=1085464 (accessed 22 November 2010).

Kellogg ND; American Academy of Pediatrics Committee on Child Abuse and Neglect. 2007. Evaluation of suspected child physical abuse. *Pediatrics* **119:** 1232–41.

Kemp AM, Dunstan F, Harrison S *et al*. Patterns of skeletal fractures in child abuse: systematic review. *British Medical Journal* 2008; **337:** a1518.

Kemp AM, Butler A, Morris S *et al*. Which radiological investigations should be performed to identify fractures in suspected child abuse? *Clinical Radiology* 2006; **61:** 723–36.

Kleinman PK. Diagnostic imaging in infant abuse. *AJR American Journal of Roentgenology* 1990; **155:** 703–12.

Knight B. The history of child abuse. *Forensic Science International* 1986; **30:** 135–41.

Krous HF, Beckwith JB, Byard RW *et al*. Sudden infant death syndrome and unclassified sudden infant deaths: a definitional and diagnostic approach. *Pediatrics* 2004; **114:** 234–8.

Maguire S, Mann MK, Sibert J, Kemp A. Are there patterns of bruising in childhood which are diagnostic or suggestive of abuse? A systematic review. *Archives of Disease in Childhood* 2005; **90:** 182–6.

Maguire S, Mann MK, Sibert J, Kemp A. Can you age bruises accurately in children? A systematic review. *Archives of Disease in Childhood* 2005; **90:** 187–9.

Maguire S, Mann M, John N *et al*. Does cardiopulmonary resuscitation cause rib fractures in children? A systematic review. *Child Abuse & Neglect* 2006; **30:** 739–51.

Maguire S, Hunter B, Hunter L *et al*. Diagnosing abuse: a systematic review of torn frenum and other intra-oral injuries. *Archives of Disease in Childhood* 2007; **92:** 1113–17.

Maguire S, Pickerd N, Farewell D *et al*. Which clinical features distinguish inflicted from non-inflicted brain injury? A systematic review. *Archives of Disease in Childhood* 2009; **94:** 860–7.

Malcolm AJ. Examination of fractures at autopsy. Chapter 2. In: Rutty GN (ed), *Essentials of autopsy practice. New advances, trends and developments*. London: Springer-Verlag, 2008; p. 23–44.

Meservey CJ, Towbin R, McLaurin RL *et al*. Radiographic characteristics of skull fractures resulting from child abuse. *AJR American Journal of Roentgenology* 1987; **149:** 173–5.

Piercecchi-Marti MD, Adalian P, Liprandi A *et al*. Fetal visceral maturation: a useful contribution to gestational age estimation in human fetuses. *Journal of Forensic Sciences* 2004; **49:** 1–6.

Prosser I, Maguire S, Harrison SK *et al*. How old is this fracture? Radiological dating of fractures in children: a systematic review. *AJR American Journal of Roentgenology* 2005; **184:** 1282–6.

R v Harris, Rock, Cherry and Foulder (2005) EWCA Crim 1980. http://www.bailii.org/ew/cases/EWCA/Crim/2005/1980.html (accessed 22 November 2010).

Saukko P, Knight B. 'Infanticide and stillbirth (Chapter 20). In: Saukko P, Knight B. *Knight's Forensic Pathology*, 3rd edn. London: Hodder Arnold, 2004; p. 439–50.

Saukko P, Knight B. 'Sudden death in infancy (Chapter 21). In: Saukko P, Knight B. *Knight's Forensic Pathology*, 3rd edn. London: Hodder Arnold, 2004, p. 451–60.

Saukko P, Knight B. Fatal child abuse (Chapter 22) In: Saukko P, Knight B. *Knight's Forensic Pathology*, 3rd edn. London: Hodder Arnold, 2004, p. 461–79.

Scheuer JL, Musgrave JH, Evans SP. The estimation of late fetal and perinatal age from limb bone length by linear and logarithmic regression. *Annals of Human Biology* 1980; **7:** 257–65.

Still-Birth (Definition) Act 1992 C.29. http://www.legislation. gov.uk/ukpga/1992/29/contents (accessed 22 November 2010).

World Health Organization. Child maltreatment. Geneva, Switzerland: WHO, 2010; http://www.who.int/topics/ child_abuse/en (accessed 9 April 2010).

Weber MA, Risdon RA, Offiah AC *et al*. Rib fractures identified at post-mortem examination in sudden unexpected deaths in infancy (SUDI). *Forensic Science International* 2009; **189:** 75–81.

Weber W. [Experimental studies of skull fractures in infants]. *Zeitschrift für Rechtsmedizin* 1984; **92:** 87–94 (in German).

Worn MJ, Jones MD. Rib fractures in infancy: establishing the mechanisms of cause from the injuries – a literature review. *Medicine, Science, and the Law* 2007; **47:** 200–12.

Chapter

8

Assessment, classification and documentation of injury

■ Introduction

One of the most important aspects of forensic medicine – both clinical and pathological – is the assessment, classification and documentation of injury. Any healthcare professional should be able to appropriately document injury in a way that can be understood and interpreted by others. Most non-forensic healthcare professionals will not be trained in the interpretation of injuries and wound causation, but accurate documentation can greatly assist the legal process at a later stage.

Offences against individuals of a physical nature that may result in criminal prosecutions have a great variety of types and origins, not all of which may cause visible evidence (e.g. poisoning, infection). The role of the forensic pathologist and forensic physician is to ensure that the medical relevance of findings, or lack of them, is understood by the investigating authority.

■ Terminology of injury

Words to describe injury or harm are used non-specifically by lay persons and non-forensic healthcare professionals. In a legal setting the use of the word may have a specific meaning that can influence the nature of the charge and the penalties related to an offence.

Perhaps the most frequent error is the use of the word 'laceration' used in the context of a cut to the skin. In the forensic setting – as discussed below – a laceration is a split or tear in the skin caused by blunt impact. If the word laceration is used wrongly to described a cut caused by a knife (an incised wound) this may have implications with regard to the credibility of the witnesses.

Every jurisdiction will have its own legal classification of injury or wounding, and again the use of such terms may have specific relevance. Forensic practitioners must be familiar with such classifications in order to assist the courts in determining the seriousness of an injury.

Most harm or injury can be embraced by one of the following broad groups, using terms used within the England and Wales jurisdiction:

- Those with a fatal outcome
  - Murder
  - Manslaughter
- Those without a fatal outcome
  - Assault, assault occasioning actual bodily harm
  - Common assault
  - Battery, or common battery
  - Wounding or wounding with intent
  - Poisoning
  - Inflicting grievous bodily harm or causing grievous bodily harm with intent
- Sexual offences (see Chapter 12)
  - Penetrative
  - Non-penetrative (both with or without extra-genital injury).

Law of injury

In the England and Wales setting a 'wound' (used by most people interchangeably with 'injury') can have a specific legal meaning. In the legal context, a wound is an injury that breaks the continuity of the skin. There must be a division of the whole skin structure and not merely a division of the cuticle or upper layer. As the skin is not broken, a bruise or internal rupturing of blood vessels is not a wound. A broken bone is not considered a wound, unless it is a comminuted fracture.

The Offences against the Person Act 1861 ('the Act'), which has been amended over the years, sets out a range of offences for which an individual, in England and Wales, can be prosecuted when that individual is alleged to have caused injury to another person. This statute excludes homicide and sexual offences (which are covered by the Sexual Offences Act 2003).

As may be expected the terminology used in a law whose origins go back almost one and half centuries can sometimes be a little unclear. The main offences relevant to injury assessment by forensic practitioners are found in the following sections of the Offences Against the Person Act.

Section 18

This section creates the offences of wounding and causing grievous bodily harm, with intent to cause grievous bodily harm, or to resist arrest. It is punishable with life imprisonment, the specific wording being

> Whosoever shall unlawfully and maliciously by any means whatsoever wound or cause any grievous bodily harm to any person ... with intent ... to do some ... grievous bodily harm to any person, or with intent to resist or prevent the lawful apprehension or detainer of any person, shall be guilty of felony, and being convicted thereof shall be liable ... to be kept in penal servitude for life ... .

The key element of this offence is intent. Types of injury would include stabbings or shootings.

Section 20

This section creates the offences of wounding and inflicting grievous bodily harm. They are less serious than the offences created by Section 18 and carry a maximum prison sentence of 5 years. The key element of this offence is the causing of grievous bodily harm, but without the intent to do so.

Section 47

This section creates the offence of assault occasioning actual bodily harm. It encompasses those assaults that result in substantial injuries, typically requiring a degree of medical treatment for the victim and provides the penalty to which a person is liable on conviction of that offence on indictment. A periorbital haematoma with a superficial laceration after a punch, or a broken tooth, are the types of injury that may be considered a Section 47 assault.

Types of injury

Injury caused by the application of physical force can be divided into two main groups: blunt force and sharp force. There are a number of other types of injury caused by non-physical forces, which can be thermal, chemical, electrical or electromagnetic which are referred to in other Chapters.

Blunt-force injury

Blunt-force trauma is that trauma not caused by instruments, objects or implements with cutting edges. The nature of the force applied may include blows (impacts), traction, torsion and oblique or shearing forces. Blunt-force trauma may have a number of outcomes:

- no injury
- tenderness
- pain

- reddening (erythema; Figure 8.1)
- swelling (oedema; Figure 8.2)
- bruising (contusion; Figure 8.3)
- abrasions (grazes; Figure 8.4)
- lacerations (Figure 8.5)
- fractures (Figure 8.6).

Blunt impact injuries can be described (in terms of force applied) as being weak (for example a 'gentle'

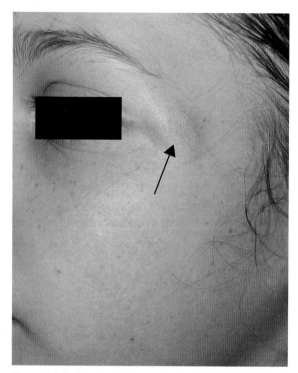

Figure 8.1 Reddening (erythema) related to blunt impact at outer aspect of left eye.

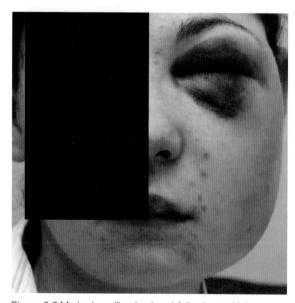

Figure 8.2 Marked swelling (oedema) following multiple punches to left side of face.

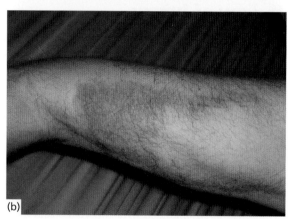

(a)

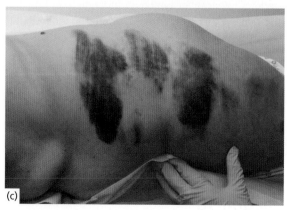

(b)

(c)

Figure 8.3 Bruising (contusion) to thigh **(a)** following direct blunt force impact (fall between iron girders). **(b)** Shows resolution of bruising 5 days after injury as seen in 8.3(a). **(c)** Bruising to leg from multiple blunt impacts with a piece of wood.

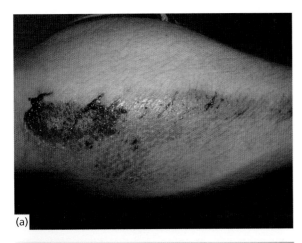

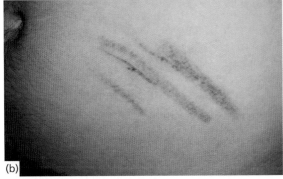

Figure 8.4 **(a)** Variable depth abrasions (grazes) caused by impact against concrete surface. **(b)** Linear abrasions caused by fingernail scratching on torso.

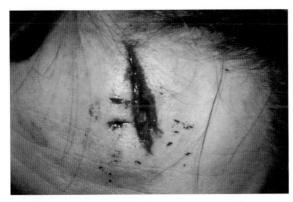

Figure 8.5 Laceration, with irregular edges, maceration and skin bridging caused by direct impact to forehead with wooden pole.

slap on the face), weak/moderate, moderate, moderate/severe or severe (for example a full punch as hard as possible). The more forceful the impact the more likely that visible marks will be evident.

Tenderness is pain or discomfort experienced on palpation by another of an area of injury. Both pain

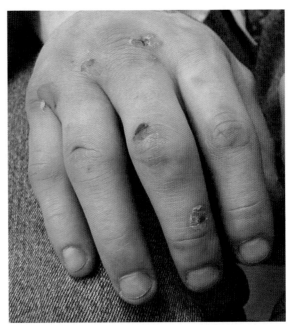

Figure 8.6 Hand with abrasions, swelling, reddening and underlying fracture of 5th metacarpal caused by repeated punching of cell door.

and tenderness are subjective findings and are thus dependent on (1) the pain threshold of the individual and (2) their truthfulness. The other features of blunt-force injury are visible effects of contact. Reddening describes increased blood flow to areas that have been subject to trauma, but not to the extent that the underlying blood vessels are disrupted. Reddening must be distinguished from red bruises by its ability to blanch from finger pressure.

Bruises

Bruises are discoloration of skin surface caused by leakage of blood into underlying tissues from damaged blood vessels.

Two events must occur before a bruise can form: damage to a blood vessel (usually small-calibre blood vessels such as veins and arterioles) from which blood leaks, and the leakage of that blood into surrounding tissues. Bruising is most commonly seen in the skin, but it can also occur in the deeper tissues, including muscle and internal organs. The extent of damage to the blood vessels is generally proportionate to the force applied: the greater the force, the more blood vessels are damaged, the greater the leakage of blood and the bigger the bruise.

Once outside the confines of the blood vessel, blood is broken down, resulting in the various colour changes seen. Eventually, all of the blood is removed and the overlying skin returns to its normal colour.

Bruises are one of the areas where a number of terms have been used in the past, which complicate the understanding of their nature. The term 'ecchymosis' has been used for specific types of bruise but should not now be used as it does not assist in understanding the type or mechanism of injury. Bruising is best used to describe visible external marks caused by leakage of blood into skin and subcutaneous tissues, while contusion can be used for leakage of blood into tissues in body cavities. The term 'haematoma' can be used to refer to a palpable collection of blood under the skin (and one which, if a needle aspiration were to be undertaken, would show liquid blood in a cavity). 'Petechiae' are small bruises, often described as 'pin-point haemorrhages', that have been said to be < 2 mm in size. However, that is an arbitrary figure and, like all bruises, petechiae can develop and evolve and coalesce, and the use of a rigid size measurement is inappropriate (Figure 8.7).

Direct blunt force, in addition to unambiguous impacts such as strikes with fists, kicks or weapons, also includes mechanisms such as poking, squeezing and gripping. Indirect blunt force may be represented by suction (as in 'love bites'; Figure 8.8) or following compression. Compression may produce petechiae at the level of or above the compressing force (e.g. in ligature strangulation). Bruises evolve and can 'migrate'. Gravity and tissue planes are two of the factors that may determine how the appearance of a bruise might change (Figure 8.9). Thus the presence of a bruise at a particular site does not necessarily imply that the blunt impact was applied at that site. Some very superficial bruises (often called intradermal bruises), caused by leakage of blood confined to the epidermis and the upper strata of the dermis, can remain in the position in which the impact occurred, and 'patterned' bruises, which reproduce the nature of the object that caused them, often have such an 'intradermal' element. Intradermal bruises are often

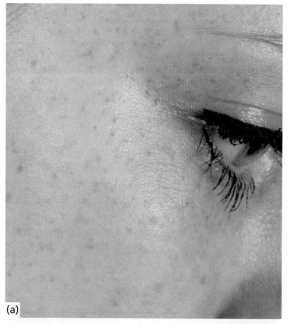
(a)

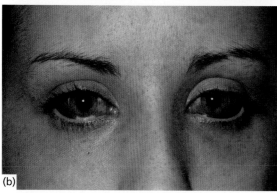
(b)

Figure 8.7 **(a)** Close-up of face after manual strangulation 2 hours after compression with multiple petechial bruising over facial skin. **(b)** Scleral blood, caused by coalescence of multiple petechiae, 36 hours after manual strangulation.

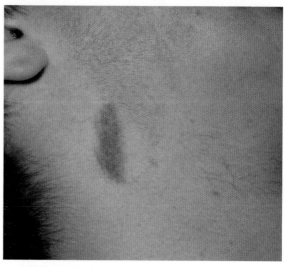

Figure 8.8 Classical love or 'hickey' bite – bruising to neck caused by suction.

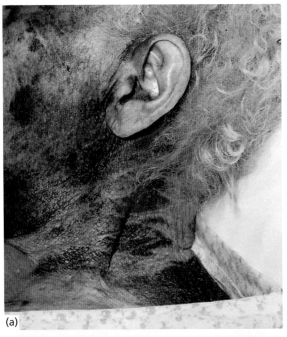

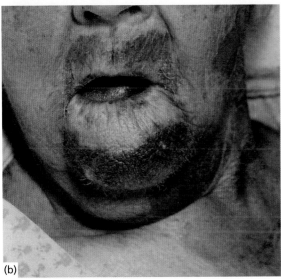

Figure 8.9 Extensive bruising following tissue planes and contours, one week after multiple blunt force impacts to (a) head and (b) face (neck was spared impacts).

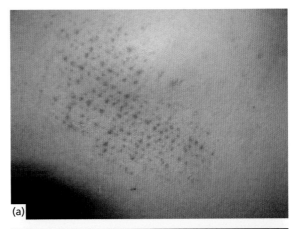

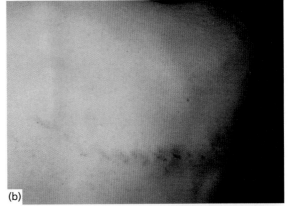

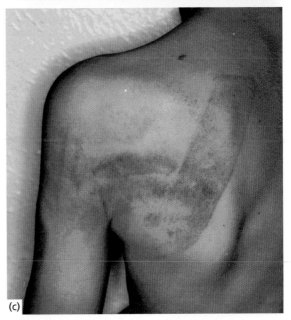

Figure 8.10 (a) Patterned bruise – intradermal bruising caused by stamping on back with textured clothing intervening. (b) Patterned bruise caused by impact of dog chain. (c) Patterned bruise (bruise obliquely towards midline) caused by impact of 2 × 2 length of wood.

associated with diffuse compression forces such as pressure from a car tyre or from a shoe during a stamp or a kick (Figure 8.10).

Certain types of blunt injury commonly cause evidentially useful patterns. Single patterned bruises may indicate the nature of the impacting object. 'Tramline' bruises (Figure 8.11) are those caused by impacts from longitudinal, generally cylindrical

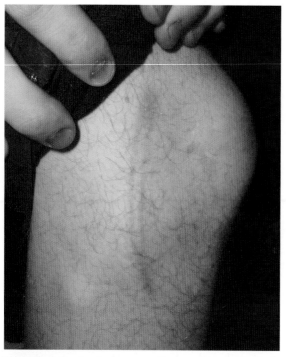

Figure 8.11 Tramline bruise caused by impact from cylindrical firm object (in this case, a police baton).

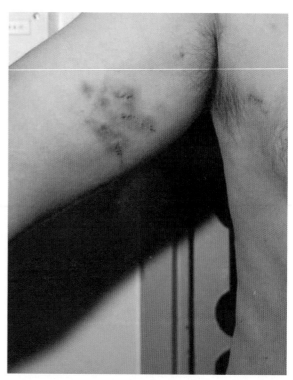

Figure 8.13 Grip marks from fingers on assailant bruises from grip and abrasions from fingernails seen on upper inner arm.

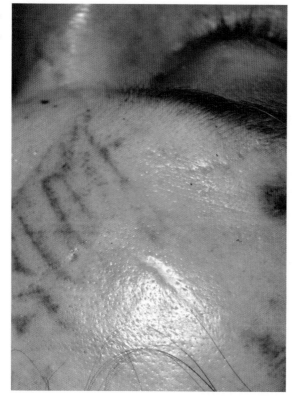

Figure 8.12 Shoeprint bruise following stamping injury to face.

or rod-like, objects (where blood is forced laterally from the point of impact, rupturing blood vessels either side of the impacting object) and footprint imprint bruises may be seen from stamp injuries (Figure 8.12).

Patterns of a number of bruises may also help corroborate the nature of the causative force. For example a row of four 1–2 cm oval or round bruises may be caused by the impact of knuckles in a punch; groups of small oval or round bruises are also indicative of fingertip pressure, as in gripping, and there is sometimes a single, larger, thumb bruise on the opposite side of the limb (Figure 8.13). Fingertip bruises on the neck or along the jaw line are commonly seen in manual strangulation.

Examination of injuries must be undertaken in good light and, in the case of bruises, such is required in order to ensure that small or subtle skin colour changes are not missed. Even with darker skin tones, a proper examination will be able to identify areas of bruising.

Age estimation based on the colour of bruising is not now considered appropriate, with one exception – a yellow-coloured bruise may be more than 18 hours old. The colouring must not be taken from photographic images where colour reproduction may be inaccurate and it must also be understood that the perception of yellow colour may be influenced by the visual capability of the viewer, interobserver variation and underlying skin tone. Studies in children suggest that estimation of ageing of bruising cannot be achieved by colour interpretation, and this principle generally applies to adults also.

Bruising can occur after death: blood vessels are just as easily damaged by the application of force and, provided that there is blood with some pressure within those vessels, bruising can occur. Such pressure may exist at the lowermost vessels because of the static weight of the column of blood. Post-mortem bruises are generally small and lie on the dependent parts of the body. Bruising may also be found in areas of post-mortem dissection and care must be taken in interpreting 'new' bruises when an autopsy has been performed.

Abrasions

An abrasion or graze is a superficial injury involving (generally) outer layers of skin without penetration of the full thickness of the epidermis. They are caused when there is contact between a rough surface and the skin, often involving a tangential 'shearing' force (Figure 8.14). They can also be caused by crushing of the skin when the force is applied vertically down onto the skin. Bite marks and the grooved, and often parchmented, abrasion found in hanging, can cause typical 'crush' abrasions (Figure 8.15).

The appearance of abrasions will allow a determination of the exact point of contact and may assist in determining the direction of the impact. Specific types of abrasions include scratches (linear abrasions, e.g. caused by fingernails; Figure 8.16), scuff (brush) abrasions (very superficial abrasions, Figure 8.17) and point or gouge abrasions (deeper linear abrasions caused by objects such as metal nails; Figure 8.18).

As the epidermis does not contain blood vessels, superficial abrasions might not bleed, but the folded nature of the junction between the dermis and the epidermis, and the presence of loops of blood vessels in the dermal folds, will mean that deep abrasions have a typical punctate or spotty appearance. Deeper abrasions may therefore bleed, resulting in subsequent scabbing and possible scarring.

The size, shape and type of abrasion depends upon the nature of the surface of the object which contacts the skin, its shape and the angle at which contact is made. Contact with the squared corner of an object (e.g. a brick) may well result in a linear abrasion, whereas contact with a side of the same object will cause a larger area of 'brush' abrasion.

Contact with a rough surface, such as a road, especially when associated with the higher levels of force found in traffic accidents, will result in areas of 'gravel rash', sometimes called 'brush' abrasions (Figure 8.19).

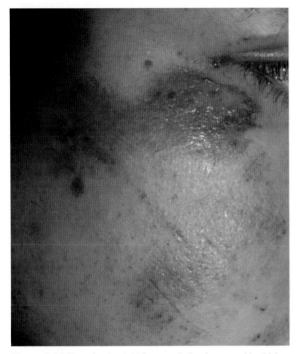

Figure 8.14 Abrasion to right face and cheek caused by kick from shod foot. Linearity of abrasion assists in determining direction of movement.

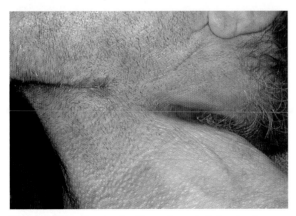

Figure 8.15 Ligature mark with parchmented abrasion in posterior part of neck.

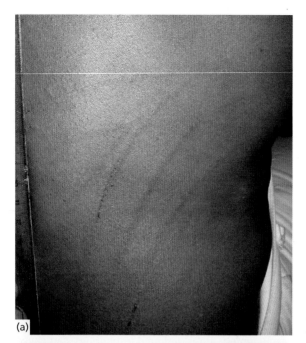

(a)

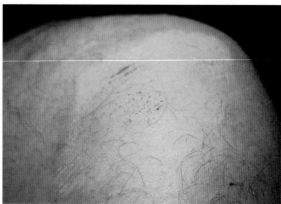

Figure 8.17 Figure 8.17 Close-up showing tags of elevated skin in scuff abrasions.

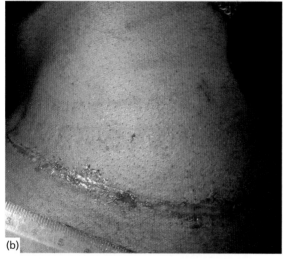

(b)

Figure 8.16a **(a)** Multiple fingernail scratches with wheal reaction and superficial abrasions. **(b)** Deeper abrasions caused by fingernails.

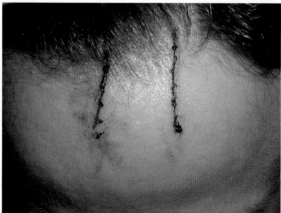

Figure 8.18 Deep linear point or gouge abrasions to forehead.

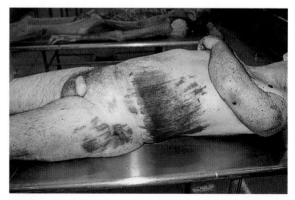

Figure 8.19 Deep and extensive abrasion ('gravel rash') caused by contact with road surface after motorcycle accident.

Tangential contact with a relatively smooth surface may well result in such fine, closely associated, linear abrasions that the skin may simply appear reddened and roughened. This may be termed a 'friction burn'; close inspection will reveal the true nature of the wound.

The direction of the causative force can be identified by close inspection of the injury (magnification of a high-resolution digital image can be useful when changes are subtle) and identifying the torn fragments of the epidermis which are pushed towards the furthest (distal) end of the abrasion (Figure 8.20).

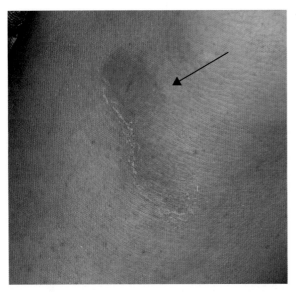

Figure 8.20 Directional scuff – note raised skin layers on left side of abrasion: arrow indicates direction of abrasive movement.

Crush abrasions – often associated with 'intradermal' bruising – are important because they may retain the pattern of the causative object. Diagrams and sketches can be extremely useful and scaled photographs should be taken in order to allow subsequent comparison to be made between the injury and a 'suspect injury-causing implement of surface'. Many different objects have been identified in this way, such as car radiator grills, the tread of escalator steps, plaited whips and the lines from floor tiles.

Lacerations

Lacerations appear as 'cuts, splits or tears' in the skin and are the result of a blunt force compressing or stretching the skin; they may extend through the full thickness of the skin and can bleed profusely. Because the skin is composed of many different tissue types, some of the more resilient tissues will not be damaged by the forces that split the weaker tissues. Those most resilient tissues are often nerves, fibrous bands of fascial planes and, sometimes, at the base of the laceration, an occasional medium-sized elastic blood vessel. These structures are seen to extend across the defect in the skin and are often referred to as 'bridging fibres'. The same blunt force causing such a laceration may also cause irregular splits, bruising and abrasion at the margins of the wound (Figure 8.21).

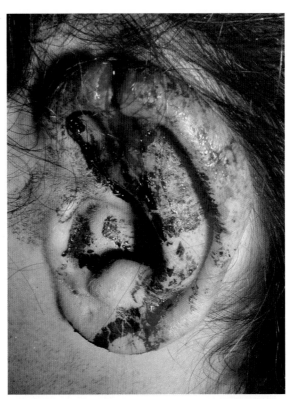

Figure 8.21 Laceration to ear following impact with baseball bat – note irregularity of laceration and associated swelling bruising masked by dry blood.

Lacerations are most common where the skin can be compressed between the applied force and underlying bone (i.e. over the scalp, face, elbows, knees, shins, etc.). They are rare (unless severe force has been applied) over the soft, fleshy areas of the body such as the buttocks, breasts and abdomen.

When significant tangential blunt force is applied to the skin, for example owing to the rolling or grinding action of a vehicle wheel, the laceration may be horizontal and result in a large area of separation of skin from the underlying tissues (often called 'flaying' or 'degloving'). The margins of a laceration are usually ragged; however, if a thin, regular, object inflicts an injury over a bony area of the body, the wound caused may look very sharply defined and can be mistaken for an incised injury. Careful inspection of the margins will reveal some crushing and bruising, and examination of the inner surfaces of the wound will reveal the presence of bridging fibres.

The shape of the laceration (e.g. linear, curvilinear or stellate) rarely reflects the nature of the impacting object (unless accompanied by other patterned blunt-force injury).

Sharp-force injury

Injuries caused by sharp force need to be distinguished from blunt-force injuries such as lacerations or gouge and point abrasions. In general, sharp-force injuries have cleanly divided, distinct wound edges, which may span irregular surfaces, and penetrate different types of tissue with the same contact (Figure 8.22).

Incised and slash wounds

Incised wounds are caused by objects with a sharp or cutting edge, most commonly a knife but examples include an axe, shards of glass,

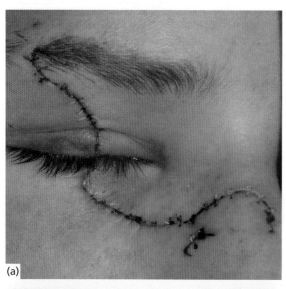

(a)

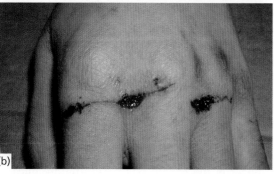

(b)

Figure 8.22 (a) Sutured incised wound caused by razor blade – note how wound follows contours. **(b)** Incised wound caused by knife drawn across surface of fingers in this case contours are spared.

broken glasses and bottles, an edge of broken pottery, a piece of metal, can also cause these wounds (Figure 8.23). An incised injury is distinguished from a stab wound by being longer on the skin surface than it is deep. A surgical operation wound is an example of an incised wound. Incised wounds caused by sharp implements moving across skin surface during an assault may sometimes be called 'slash' wounds (Figure 8.24).

The edges of the wound will give some indication as to the sharpness of the weapon causing it. A sharp edge will leave no bruising or abrasion of the wound margins. Careful inspection of the depths of the wound will reveal that no bridging fibres are present because the cutting edge divides everything in its passage through the skin.

Incised wounds, by their nature, are only life-threatening if they penetrate deeply enough to damage a blood vessel of significant size. Thus, incised wounds over the wrist or neck, where major arteries lie in more superficial tissues, can prove fatal.

Stab wounds

A stab wound is caused by a sharp implement and is deeper than it is long on the skin surface. A stab wound can, however, be created but it's progress into the body be impeded by bone, in which case the depth may not exceed wound width. This classification of such a wound is relatively straightforward in the deceased, but in the living (1) depth may not be assessed at all and (2) if it is, the measurement may be inaccurate. Forensic pathologists may also have the advantage of being able to determine direction of such wounds. The direction or depth of a wound may not be clear when interpreting medical or operative note in survivors of stab injury. Depth of the injury and the direction are of great importance when considering different accounts of causation of stab wounds and so the more information recorded at the time of treatment, the more helpful it can be to the justice system.

Any weapon with a point or tip can cause a stab wound; the edge of the blade does not need to be sharp. Stab-like wounds may also be caused by (relatively) blunt objects such as screwdrivers or car keys. For penetration of the body to occur, a variety

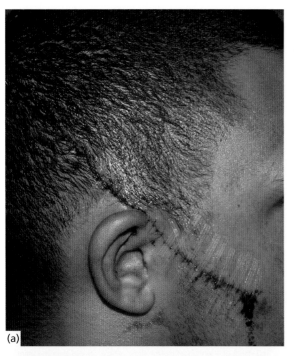

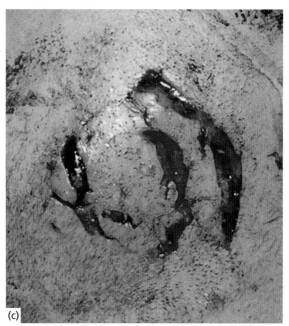

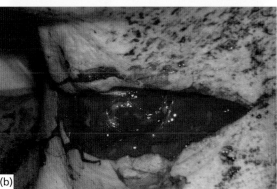

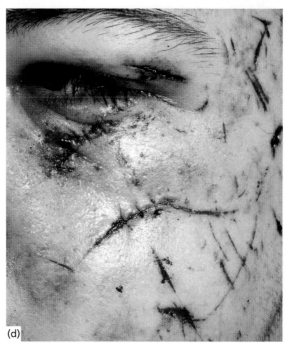

Figure 8.23 **(a)** Sutured incised wound across right side of head and face. **(b)** Incised wound to neck caused by use of knife. **(c)** Irregular incised wounds caused by glass impacted and breaking on face. **(d)** Post-treatment appearance after glassing – note multiple small superficial shard cuts in association with larger incised wounds.

of factors determine how much force is required, including:

- the sharpness of the tip of the weapon: this is often the most important factor and the sharper the tip, the easier it is to penetrate the skin
- the sharpness of the 'cutting edge' of the implement
- the nature of the force applied: stabbing incidents are usually dynamic, involving complex relative movements between victim and assailant

- whether clothing has been penetrated: some items of clothing, such as thick leather jackets, may offer significant resistance to penetration.
- whether bone has been injured: skin offers very little resistance to penetration by a sharp knife, but injury to bone tends to suggest that a greater force has been used to inflict the wound. Significant penetration of bone may also damage the knife.

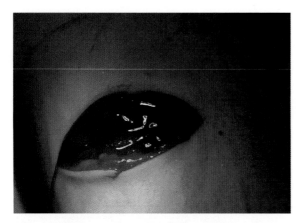

Figure 8.24 Slash-type wound to forearm: wound is wider than it is deep.

Once a knife or other sharp implement has penetrated the skin, subcutaneous tissues (except bone) offer little additional resistance to deeper penetration and, to an assailant, it may appear that the rest of the weapon 'follows through' with almost no additional effort or force being applied. The insertion of a sharp knife into the body, especially through the skin stretched across ribs, requires very little force, and pressure from a single finger may be sufficient to push a very sharp implement through the chest wall at this site. The commonest sharp weapon used in an assault is a knife of some sort, but a huge variety of weapons such as swords, shards of glass and broken bottles can be used.

The appearances of a stab wound on the skin surface can assist in determining the size and the cross-sectional shape of the weapon used (Figure 8.25). If a blade of some sort is used, the general comments in Box 8.1 apply.

Chop injury

Chop injuries may be caused by a variety of implements that are generally heavy, and relatively blunt, bladed instruments. These include some machetes, Samurai swords and axes. Because of the variability of the 'blade', injuries sustained may be a mixture of sharp- and blunt-force wounds, typically involving bruised, crushed and abraded wound margins (Figure 8.26). Fractures and amputations may also result from the use of such implements and substantial scarring may ensue.

Box 8.1 Features to consider in a possible stab wound

- A slit-like wound will distort, after removal of the weapon, because of the action of elastic fibres present in the skin. If the fibres are orientated at right angles to the skin surface wound, it will be pulled outwards and get shorter and wider; if they run parallel to the skin surface wound, it will be pulled lengthways and the edges will tend to close and the wound elongate slightly.
- Even if the edges of the wound are gently pushed together, the resulting defect is rarely the exact size as the knife.
- The size of the wound also depends on the shape/configuration of the blade and how deeply it was inserted.
- Movement of the knife in the wound, as a consequence of relative movement between the assailant and victim, may cause the wound to be enlarged. If the knife is twisted or rotated within the body, an irregularly-shaped, or even triangular, skin surface wound may be result.
- Many knives have only one cutting edge, the other being blunt. This design may be reproduced in the wound where one wound apex is sharp or 'V'-shaped, while the other is blunt, or rounded. The blunt wound apex may 'split' at each side, an appearance commonly referred to as a 'fishtail'.
- Provided that clothing has not intervened, skin adjacent to the stab wound may be bruised and/or abraded as a consequence of forcible contact between the skin and, for example, the hilt/blade guard of a knife, or the 'knife-wielding' hand of the assailant.
- The depth of a wound within the body can be greater than the length of the blade if a forceful stab is inflicted. This is because the abdomen and, to a lesser extent, the chest, can be compressed by the force of the knife hilt or knife-wielding hand against the skin.
- A blunt object such as a screwdriver or 'spike' will tend to indent, split and bruise the skin on penetration. Different types of screwdriver can cause different patterns of injury, for example 'cross-head' or 'Phillips' screwdrivers can cause very distinctive cruciate skin surface wounds.
- Unusually shaped stab wounds may be caused by implements less commonly encountered in stabbing assaults; scissors, for example, may cause a 'Z-shaped' skin surface injury, while chisels may cause rectangular-shaped stab wounds. When such injuries are encountered, it is important to consider unusual causative implements.

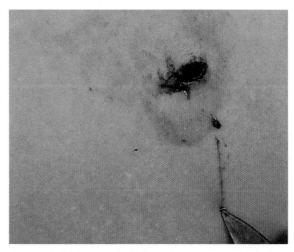

Figure 8.25 Knife wound with knife tip in bottom right of figure.

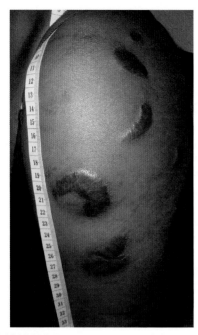

Figure 8.26 Multiple hypertrophic scars to left arm and shoulder caused by machete.

■ Other types of injury pattern

Examination of the site, orientation and pattern(s) of the wounds will often reveal useful indications about the causation of the wound. Particular actions such as punches, kicks, bites, scratching holding or gripping injuries and defence injuries can be identified by their patterns (Figure 8.27).

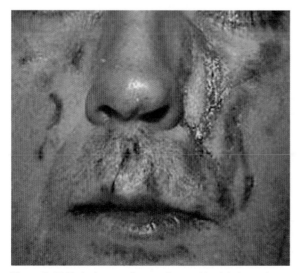

Figure 8.27 Typical severe fingernail scratching injuries to face.

Punching

A punch is a blow delivered by the clenched fist. The blow can be directed anywhere, and the effects are in part dependent on force of delivery. Visible injury is more likely to be seen over those areas of the body where the skin is closely applied to bone, as in the face and skull. The entire range of blunt force injuries can be caused, including bruises, abrasions, lacerations and fractures. These may also occur on the hand delivering the punch. On the face, the lips can also be forced back onto the teeth, resulting in bruising, abrasion and lacerations inside the lips. Any examination following a blow to the face or mouth requires intraoral examination. A single blow to the nose or forehead can cause bilateral periorbital bruising (black eyes).

Ribs may be fractured by blows of sufficient force.

Intra-abdominal injury, including mesenteric laceration, intestinal rupture and injury to the major abdominal organs, can occur if punches of adequate force are delivered to a vulnerable (i.e. unresisting) abdomen.

Kicking and stamping

Kicking and stamping injuries are caused by feet, which may be shod or unshod. Again, as with punches, the entire gamut of blunt force injury may be seen, but kicks and stamps can be more powerful than punches, and more so if delivered to an individual already vulnerable (e.g. lying on the floor or unconscious). Kicking and stamping may leave areas of intradermal bruising that reflect the pattern of the sole of the shoe and this can lead to identification of the assailant.

The victim is often on the ground when these injuries are inflicted, and blows from the foot are commonly directed towards the head and face, the chest and the abdomen. The high levels of force that can be applied by a foot mean that there are often underlying skeletal injuries. These are most common in the facial skeleton and in the ribs. Stamping injuries to the front of the abdomen may result in rupture of any of the internal organs.

Bite injuries

Bite marks are commonly associated with bruising and may be associated with lacerations if severe force is applied. Bite marks can be seen in sexual

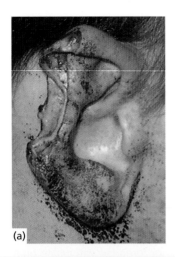

(a)

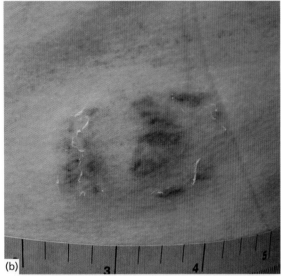

(b)

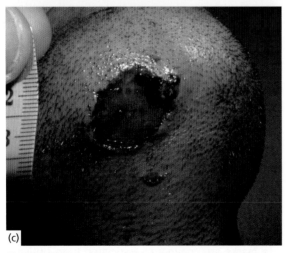

(c)

Figure 8.28 Bites. **(a)** Human bite with tissue loss to right ear. **(b)** Bite mark with bruising, skin lifts and teeth marks to chest. **(c)** Bite causing tissue loss to chin no clear teeth marks evident.

assaults, child abuse and occasionally on the sports field. A forensic odontologist should review any possible bite marks when confirmation of identity of the biter is required.

Bite marks may be found on almost any surface of the body; specific sites are associated with specific forms of assault (Figure 8.28). The neck, breasts and shoulders are often bitten in a sexually motivated attack, while in child abuse bites to the arms and the buttocks are common. Bites can also be inflicted by many common inhabitants of a house, including family pets. Odontological examination will reveal different sizes, different arch shapes and different dentition in these cases.

If a suspected bite is found at examination, a swab of the area should be taken for DNA and the bite should be photographed with a scale. Photography should be undertaken by trained forensic photographers. Photography using ultraviolet light may be of assistance in older cases but is often of limited value.

Defence injuries

In situations of assault and attack it is a normal reflex to protect oneself. In many instances the reflex involves sustaining injury but reducing the damaging results.

When a knife or a stabbing implement is directed at an individual, blows to the head and face may be defended by raising the hands and arms to cover the head and face. The hand may attempt to grab or deflect a weapon. The arms and hands sustain injuries but the head is protected. In addition, in incidents involving knives where a knife may be thrust towards an individual the individual may try and defend themselves by grabbing the knife blade and deflecting it away from, for example, the chest and abdomen. Grabbing of the cutting blade will result (if the knife is sharp enough) in cuts to the part of the hand that grabs the knife (generally the palm or gripping side of the hand and fingers; Figure 8.29). Both assailant and victim can sustain incised wounds if there has been a struggle. In general, the dominant hand may generally automatically be used to defend, but if the dominant hand (most commonly the right) is otherwise engaged, the non-dominant hand may be used. Multiple defence wounds may be sustained during an assault, and such wounds to the hands may be of variable depth, or discontinuous, as the hand is not a flat surface.

Defence-type injury after blunt weapon assault will be seen in the same regions, namely the extensor surfaces of arm and upper arm (Figure 8.30) which may be raised to protect against blows, and on the back, or the back of the legs, if an individual is taken to the ground and, for example, kicked. The victim will tend to curl up in a ball with hands and arms over the head and legs tucked up towards the chest.

Defence injuries may be absent following an assault. This may be for a number of reasons including unconsciousness from assault, or incapacity

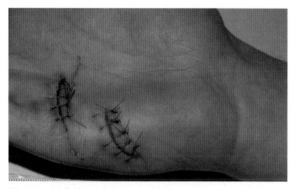

Figure 8.29 Defence injuries to right hand caused by knife.

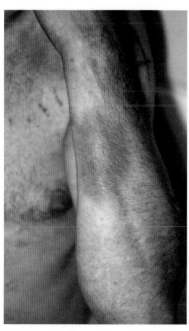

Figure 8.30 Bruising to extensor aspect of left arm – raised to ward off impact from baseball bat.

through drugs or alcohol or restraint by another person or persons.

■ Survival after injury

The length of survival following infliction of an injury is difficult to determine: every human being is different and this variability in survival and post-injury activity is to be expected. Any expression of either survival time or of the ability to move and react must be given on the basis of the 'most likely' scenario, accepting that many different versions are possible. The court should be advised of the difficulties of this assessment and should be encouraged also to consider eyewitness accounts.

It must be remembered that survival for a time after injury and long-term survival are not one and the same thing. The initial response of the body to haemorrhage is 'compensatible shock', shutting down peripheral circulation; if blood loss continues, the homeostatic mechanisms may be overwhelmed and the individual enters the phase of 'uncompensated shock', which leads inexorably to death.

Many examples exist of individuals with apparently potentially immediately fatal wounds who have performed purposeful movements/actions for some time after the 'fatal' injury. Forensic practitioners should always be very wary about allotting fixed times after which somebody could not have survived, only to be confronted with CCTV evidence showing that they clearly did.

■ Self-inflicted injury

All types of injury can be self-inflicted, accidentally inflicted or deliberately inflicted by another. Most deliberate self-inflicted injuries are caused by those with psychiatric or mental health issues, or in association with stressful situations and anxiety. Patterns of injury are well-documented in such individuals. In the forensic setting there is a small, but significant, group of individuals who self-harm for other motivations, such as staging assault for attention-seeking and similar motives, or to deliberately implicate others in criminal acts or for financial gain (e.g. insurance fraud). Such injuries will not follow the pattern of 'typical' self-arm injury.

Fatal self-inflicted blunt-force injuries may be inflicted following, for example, jumping from a height or under a train. There may be no specific features to the injuries that identify them as self-inflicted. Self-inflicted bite marks may occasionally be seen on the arms of an individual who claims to have been assaulted or blunt force injuries to the head or other parts of the body. Abrasions might be created by using objects such as abrasive pads to fabricate injury.

Self-inflicted incised or stabbing injuries, however, frequently show specific patterns that vary depending on the aim of the individual. In suicidal individuals, self-inflicted sharp-force injuries are most commonly found at specific sites on the body called 'elective sites'; for incised wounds these are most commonly on the front of the wrists and neck, whereas stabbing injuries are most commonly found over the precordium and the abdomen. In individuals who only desire to 'self-harm' or mutilate themselves, the site can be anywhere on the body that can be reached by the individual (Figure 8.31). Generally, the eyes, lips, nipples and genitalia tend to be spared.

The other features of self-inflicted injuries lie in the multiple, predominantly parallel, nature of the wounds and, in suicidal acts, the more superficial injuries are referred to as 'hesitation' or 'tentative' injuries (Figure 8.32).

The forensic practitioner has an important role in the evaluation of the nature and pattern of injuries that might be self-inflicted. In the absence of an admission of self-harm from an individual, it may be possible to come to a view as to whether injuries are likely to have been self-inflicted if the characteristics listed in Table 8.1 are considered. Some or all of these characteristics - commonly inflicted by some form of implement, such as a knife or a nail, may be present, but it is important to note that only some, and rarely all, may be present in an individual case. The absence of a particular feature listed does not preclude self-infliction; neither does its presence necessarily imply self-infliction.

In some difficult cases, it may not be possible to exclude assault, and evidence of self-harm, rather than assault, must come from alternative sources, such as other witnesses.

The staging of assault or injury may also involve other individuals complicit in the process. In such a setting, injuries that are unusual as 'self-harm' injuries (e.g. black eyes or deep abrasions) may have been inflicted by an accomplice. In such cases the detail of the accounts given (or

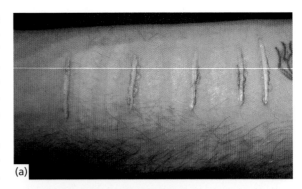

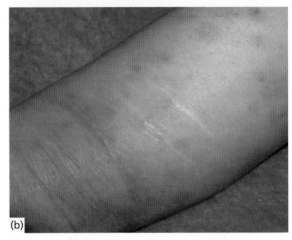

Figure 8.31 **(a)** Multiple linear burn marks (caused by heated knife blade applied to the skin) – note healed lesions between acute lesions. **(b)** Multiple incised wounds to forearm – note different ages of scars.

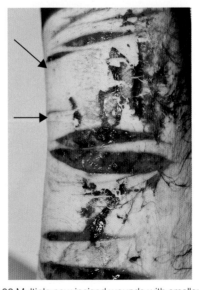

Figure 8.32 Multiple new incised wounds with smaller and more superficial tentative injuries (arrowed).

Table 8.1 Some characteristics that may be associated with self-inflicted injury

Characteristic	Additional Comments
1. On an area of the body that the individual can access themselves	Injuries in sites less accessible (e.g. the middle of the back) are less likely to have been self-inflicted
2. Superficial or minor injury	Severe self-inflicted injuries may also be caused, particularly in those with psychiatric disorder
3. If there is more than one incised wound, they are of similar appearance, style and orientation to one another (e.g. parallel with each other)	Typically, self-inflicted sharp force injuries are more superficial, numerous and similar to each other than those sustained in an assault, where the natural reaction of the injured person is to avoid repeated injury
4. If there are other types of injury (e.g. scratches, cigarette burns) these are also of similar appearance, style and orientation to each other	As above – multiple superficial, and relatively trivial injuries that are similar in nature and extent to each other should raise the possibility of self-infliction
5. Injuries grouped in a single anatomical region	As above
6. Injuries are grouped on the contralateral side to the patient's handedness	A right-handed person will tend to harm themselves on the left side of the body
7. Tentative injuries	Smaller or lesser injuries grouped with the main injuries are termed 'tentative' or 'hesitation' marks, where initial attempts at injury have been made
8. Old healed scars in similar sites	May indicate previous attempts at self-harm
9. Scars of different ages in similar sites	May indicate repeated previous attempts at self-harm
10. Slow-healing injuries	Persistence of wounds that would otherwise have been expected to heal, in the absence of any other factors
11. Psychiatric and related issues (such as eating disorders, drug and alcohol misuse)	There may be an increased incidence of self-infliction with such conditions
12. Possibility of self-inflicted injuries created to stage a crime	These may lack many of the features referred to above.

not given) can be crucial in determining the actual course of events.

◼ Torture

Article 3 of the European Convention on Human Rights states that no-one shall be subjected to torture or to inhuman or degrading treatment or punishment. Unfortunately, such treatment and punishment is still widely found throughout the world. Forensic physicians and pathologists may be asked to assess individuals claiming torture or human rights abuse. Such assessments can be complex and it may be necessary to assess and interpret physical findings for which there may be a number of explanations. The doctor's role is to assess these finding impartially. In order to make an assessment for physical evidence of torture a structured examination must take place, which involves the history, the medical history and then the physical examination. The physical examination must involve systematic

examination of the skin, face, chest and abdomen, musculoskeletal system, genitourinary system and the central and peripheral nervous systems. Specific examination and evaluation is required following specific forms of torture which include: beatings and other blunt trauma; beatings of the feet; suspension; other positional torture; electric shock torture; dental torture; asphyxiation; and sexual torture, including rape. Specialized diagnostic tests may be required to assess damage (e.g. nerve conduction studies).

The history taking should include direct quotes from the victim, establishment of a chronology, where possible backing it up, for example with old medical records and photos. A summary of detention settings, and abuses, must be obtained with details of the conditions within those settings and methods of torture and ill-treatment. Attention must also be paid to, and may require specialist assessment of, the psychological status of the victim. Specific torture techniques that may be described include:

- beating of the soles of the feet (falanga, falaka or bastinado; Figure 8.33)
- amputation (Figure 8.34)
- positional torture – e.g. cheera (legs stretched apart) or Parrot's Perch (wrists tied over knees – a pole placed under the knees)
- suspension – e.g. Palestinian hanging (arms and wrists tied and elevated behind the back; figure 8.35), which can result in disruption of shoulder joint complexes and subsequent deformity.
- electrical burns (Figure 8.36)
- wet submarine – immersing the victim's head in a container full of water until the person almost drowns
- dry submarino – placing the victim's head inside a plastic bag until nearly suffocated.

Each of these may have short and long-term sequelae.

It is important to recognize that there may be no physical evidence of torture. Where scars or marks are present it is important, for the credibility of the examination to distinguish between alleged torture scars and injuries and non-torture scars and injuries.

Istanbul protocol

In order to address the issues of torture and human rights abuses it is important that there are effective ways of documenting and comparing findings. The Istanbul Protocol is the shortened term to describe the *Manual on Effective Investigation and Documentation of Torture and Other Cruel, Inhuman or Degrading Treatment or Punishment*, a set of international guidelines for documentation of torture and its consequences. It became a United Nations official

document in 1999 and provides a set of guidelines for the assessment of persons who allege torture and ill-treatment, for investigating cases of alleged torture,

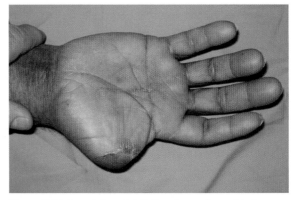
Figure 8.34 Amputation of right thumb as a form of torture.

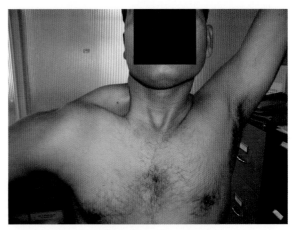
Figure 8.35 Visible abnormality subsequent to joint disruption after Palestinian hanging.

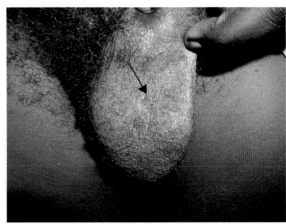
Figure 8.36 Electrical burns – scarring to scrotum as a result of application of electrodes.

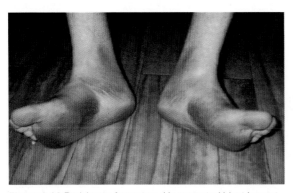
Figure 8.33 Bruising to feet caused by repeated blunt impact to feet – falanga.

and for reporting such findings to the judiciary and any other investigative body. It is the most appropriate means by which robust evidence can be presented in a standardized manner to the relevant authorities.

Interpretation of findings regarding scars or marks is undertaken using the following gradation:

- *Not consistent:* could not have been caused by the trauma described
- *Consistent with:* the lesion could have been caused by the trauma described but it is non-specific and there are many other possible causes
- *Highly consistent:* the lesion could have been caused by the trauma described, and there are few other possible causes
- *Typical of:* this is an appearance that is usually found with this type of trauma
- *Diagnostic of:* this appearance could not have been caused in any way other than that described.

Documentation of injury or marks of injury

There is a great temptation for doctors and other healthcare professionals to use medical terminology to imbue a sense of professionalism and expertise to reports and statements. This approach is generally not helpful, either to colleagues attempting to interpret their meaning or to courts unless a concurrent explanation in lay terms is provided.

Forensic pathologists have to use all available information, from police, from witnesses, from medical records, from family and many other sources to determine what may or may not have caused fatal injury. Forensic physicians dealing with the injured living person may be able to get a history directly from that person. If it is possible to take a history, then the relevance of factors such as those listed below should be considered:

- Time of injury or injuries
- Has injury been treated (e.g. at hospital or at home)?
- Pre-existing illnesses (e.g. skin disease)
- Regular physical activity (e.g. contact sports)
- Regular medication (e.g. anticoagulants, steroids)
- Handedness of victim and suspect
- Use of drugs and alcohol
- Weapon or weapons used (if still available)
- Clothing worn

This information should be easily obtainable and documented in the contemporaneous medical notes. There is often an 'evidence gap' for those seriously injured, and who require resuscitation and immediate surgery or ventilation, when compared with relatively minor interpersonal assaults, where the complainant can give a full account and injuries can be documented, and the deceased, who will have a post-mortem examination carried out by a forensic pathologist. The duty of care in the critically injured rightly outweighs the need to document injury accurately, or to retrieve crucial evidence, and lack of forensic skills mean that often hugely important evidence (e.g. nature of injury or important trace materials) is lost. There is a clear argument for (1) increasing the level of forensic skills of those involved in the care of the severely or critically injured or (2) have available forensic physicians who can (with the consent of the clinical teams) gather evidence at the earliest opportunity. The following characteristics should be recorded wherever possible for each injury:

- Location (anatomical – measure distance from landmarks)
- Pain
- Tenderness
- Reduced mobility
- Type (e.g. bruise, laceration, abrasion)
- Size (use metric values – use a ruler, do not estimate)
- Shape
- Colour
- Orientation
- Age
- Causation
- Handedness
- Time
- Transientness (of injury).

The recording of such information in the clinical setting should ideally be in three forms. First in a written form, appropriately describing the injury, second as a hand-drawn body diagram and, ideally, to supplement the first two, in digital image form. Such documentation will ensure that the opportunity for proper interpretation is maximized. Thus any clinical notes should: record the appropriate history; record accurately and clearly all findings – positive and negative; record legibly; summarize findings with clarity; use consistent terminology; and interpret within the limits of your experience.

If you cannot, or should not give opinion on your clinical findings, state this clearly.

Forensic pathologists must document and record all injuries identified at post-mortem examination in detail, sufficient to enable subsequent review of their findings, and to demonstrate the reliability of their conclusions in any legal forum.

■ Further information sources

Betz P. Pathophysiology of wound healing, Chapter 8. In: Payne-James J, Busuttil A, Smock W eds. *Forensic Medicine. Clinical and Pathological Aspects*. London: Greenwich Medical Media, 2003.

Bleetman A, Watson CH, Horsfall I, Champion SM. Wounding patterns and human performance in knife attacks: optimising the protection provided by knife resistant body armour. *Journal of Clinical Forensic Medicine* 2003; **10:** 243–8.

Bleetman A, Hughes Lt H, Gupta V. Assailant technique in knife slash attacks. *Journal of Clinical Forensic Medicine* 2003; **10:** 1–3.

Byard RW, Gehl A, Tsokos M. Skin tension and cleavage lines (Langer's lines) causing distortion of ante- and post mortem wound morphology. *International Journal of Legal Medicine* 2005; **119:** 226–30.

Chadwick EK, Nicol AC, Lane JV, Gray TG. Biomechanics of knife stab attacks. *Forensic Science International* 1999; **105:** 35–44.

Deodhar AK, Rana RE. Surgical physiology of wound healing: a review. *Journal of Postgraduate Medicine* 1997; **43:** 52–56.

Dolinak D, Matshes E. Blunt force injury, Chapter 5. In: Dolinak D, Matshes EW, Lew EO (eds). *Forensic Pathology – Principles and Practice*. London, UK: Elsevier Academic Press, 2005.

European Convention on Human Rights, Article 3. http://www.hri.org/docs/ECHR50.html#C.Art3 (accessed 22 November 2010).

Gall JAM, Boos SC, Payne-James JJ, Culliford EJ. *Forensic Medicine Colour Guide*. Edinburgh: Churchill Livingstone, 2003.

Gall J, Payne-James JJ (). Injury interpretation – possible errors and fallacies. In: Gall J, Payne-James JJ (eds) *Current Practice in Forensic Medicine*. London: Wiley, 2011.

Gall J, Payne-James JJ, Goldney RD (2011). Self-inflicted Injuries and Associated Psychological Profiles. In: Gall J, Payne-James JJ (eds) *Current Practice in Forensic Medicine*. London: Wiley, 2011.

Green MA. Stab wound dynamics – a recording technique for use in medico-legal investigations. *Journal of the Forensic Science Society* 1978; **18:** 161–3.

Henn V, Lignitz E. Kicking and trampling to death: pathological features, biomechanical mechanisms, and aspects of victims and perpetrators, Chapter 2. In: Tsokos M (ed.), *Forensic Pathology Reviews Volume 1*. Totowa, NJ, USA: Humana Press Inc., 2004.

Horsfall I, Prosser PD, Watson CH, Champion SM. An assessment of human performance in stabbing. *Forensic Science International* 1999; **102:** 79–89.

Hughes VK, Ellis PS, Langlois NE. The perception of yellow in bruises. *Journal of Clinical Forensic Medicine* 2004; **11:** 257–9.

Hunt AC, Cowling RJ. Murder by stabbing. *Forensic Science International* 1991; **52:** 107–12.

Jaffe FA. Petechial haemorrhages. A review of pathogenesis. *American Journal of Forensic Medicine and Pathology* 1994; **15:** 203–7.

Jones R. Wound and injury awareness amongst students and doctors. *Journal of Clinical Forensic Medicine* 2003; **10:** 231–4.

Karger B, Niemeyer J, Brinkmann B. Suicides by sharp force: typical and atypical features. *International Journal of Legal Medicine* 2000; **113:** 259–62.

Karger B, Rothschild MA, Pfeiffer H. Accidental sharp force fatalities – beware of architectural glass, not knives. *Forensic Science International* 2001; **123:** 135–9.

Karlsson T. Homicidal and suicidal sharp force fatalities in Stockholm, Sweden. Orientation of entrance wounds in stabs gives information in the classification. *Forensic Science International* 1998; **93:** 21–32.

Knight B. The dynamics of stab wounds. *Forensic Science* 1975; **6:** 249–55.

Langlois NE, Gresham GA The ageing of bruises: a review and a study of the colour changes with time. *Forensic Science International* 1991; **50:** 227–38.

Levy V, Rao VJ. Survival time in gunshot and stab wound victims. *American Journal of Forensic Medicine and Pathology* 1988; **9:** 215–17.

Maguire S, Mann MK, Sibert J, Kemp A. Are there patterns of bruising in childhood which are diagnostic or suggestive of abuse? A systematic review. *Archives of Diseases in Childhood* 2005; **90:**182–6.

Maguire S, Mann MK, Sibert J, Kemp A. Can you age bruises accurately in children? A systematic review. *Archives of Diseases in Childhood* 2005; **90:** 187–9.

Munang LA, Leonard PA, Mok JY. Lack of agreement on colour description between clinicians examining childhood bruising. *Journal of Clinical Forensic Medicine* 2002; **9:** 171–4.

O'Callaghan PT, Jones MD, James DS et al. Dynamics of stab wounds: force required for penetration of various cadaveric human tissues. *Forensic Science International* 1999; **104:** 173–8.

Offences against the Person Act 1861. http://www.statutelaw.gov.uk/content.aspx?activeTextDocId=1043854 (accessed 22 November 2010).

Ong BB. The pattern of homicidal slash/chop injuries: a 10 year retrospective study in University Hospital Kuala Lumpur. *Journal of Clinical Forensic Medicine* 1999; **6:** 24–9.

Ormstad K, Karlsson T, Enkler L, Law B, Rajs J. Patterns in sharp force fatalities – a comprehensive forensic medical study. *Journal of Forensic Sciences* 1986; **31:** 529–42.

Pilling ML, Vanezis P, Perrett D, Johnston A. Visual assessment of the timing of bruising by forensic experts. *Journal of Forensic and Legal Medicine* 2010; **17:** 143–9.

Polson CJ, Gee DJ. Injuries: general features. In: Polson CJ, Gee DJ, Knight B (eds). *The Essentials of Forensic Medicine*, 4th edn. Oxford: Pergamon Press, 1985.

Pretty IA. Development and validation of a human bitemark severity and significance scale. *Journal of Forensic Sciences* **52:** 687–91.

Purdue B.N. Cutting and piercing wounds. Chapter 9. In: Mason JK, Purdue BN (eds) *The Pathology of Trauma*, 3rd edn. London: Arnold, 2000.

Rutty GN. Bruising: concepts of ageing and interpretation. In: Rutty GN (ed.). *Essentials of Autopsy Practice*. London: Springer-Verlag, 2001.

Robinson S. The examination of the adult victim of assault. Chapter 10. In: Mason JK, Purdue BN (eds) *The Pathology of Trauma*, 3rd edn. London: Arnold, 2000.

Sexual Offences Act 2003. http://www.legislation.gov.uk/ukpga/2003/42/contents (accessed 22 November 2010).

Spitz W.U. Blunt force injury. Chapter 7 In: Spitz WU (ed.) *Spitz and Fisher's Medico-legal investigation of death – Guidelines to the Application of Pathology to Crime Investigation*, 3rd edn. Springfield, IL: Charles C Thomas Publishers, 1993.

Sweet D, Lorente M, Lorente JA et al. An improved method to recover saliva from human skin: the double swab technique. *Journal of Forensic Sciences* 1997; **42:** 320–2.

Thoresen SO, Rognum TO. Survival time and acting capability after fatal injury by sharp weapons. *Forensic Science International* 1986; **31:** 181–7.

Vanezis P, West IE. Tentative injuries in self stabbing. *Forensic Science International* 1983; **21:** 65–70.

Vanezis P, Payne-James JJ. Sharp force trauma, Chapter 22 In: Payne-James JJ, Busuttil A, Smock W (eds). *Forensic Medicine – Clinical and Pathological Aspects*. London: Greenwich Medical Media, 2003.

Chapter 9

Regional injuries

- Introduction
- Head injuries
- Neck injuries
- Spinal injuries
- Chest injuries
- Abdomen
- Further information sources

Introduction

Specific regions of the body may be particularly susceptible to types of trauma that may not cause serious or fatal injury elsewhere. A good example of this may the single stab wound. If this penetrates the limbs then a serious or fatal outcome is unlikely, unless a large artery is injured. If a single stab wound penetrates the heart or the abdominal aorta a fatal outcome is much more likely. Consideration of patterns of injuries according to the body region, and the potential complications of those injuries, is therefore an important component in both the clinical and pathological evaluation of trauma.

Head injuries

Any trauma to the head or face that has the potential for damaging the brain can have devastating consequences. Normally the brain is protected within the bony skull, but it is not well restrained within this compartment and injuries to the brain result from differences between the motion of the solid skull and the relatively 'fluid' brain. There are three main components of the head: the scalp, the skull and the brain.

Scalp

The scalp is vascular, hair-bearing skin; at its base is a thick fibrous membrane called the galea aponeurotica. Lying between the galea and the skull is a very thin sheet of connective tissue that is penetrated by blood vessels (emissary veins) emerging through the skull, and beneath this connective tissue is the periosteum of the outer table of the skull. Injury to the vascular scalp can lead to profuse bleeding which, although can usually be stopped by local application of pressure, in some circumstances (e.g. acute alcohol intoxication) can lead to physiological shock and death. Bleeding scalp injuries can continue to ooze after death, particularly when the head is in a dependent position.

The scalp is easily injured by blunt trauma as it can be crushed between the weapon and the underlying skull. Bruises of the scalp are associated with prominent oedema because this normal tissue response cannot spread and dissipate as easily as in other areas of the body. The easiest way to detect scalp injuries is by finger palpation, but shaving is often required for optimal evaluation, documentation and photography of injury in the deceased, and

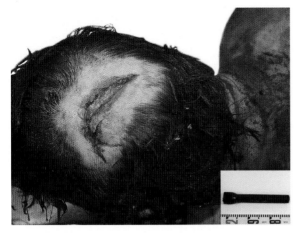

Figure 9.1 Scalp laceration caused by a heavy torch. Following shaving of hair from around the injury, the crushed and abraded wound edges can clearly be seen.

sometimes in the living. In the living a good history from the individual, and lighting, can localize any injury. It is surprisingly difficult to identify the site of profuse bleeding from the scalp in an individual with abundant head hair. In the living if there is evidence of stamping or implement assault it may also be necessary to shave the hair so that potential 'patterned injury' can be identified and recorded for overlay comparison.

Lacerations of the scalp can usually be distinguished from incised wounds; careful examination often reveals crushed, abraded or macerated wound edges and tissue bridges in the wound depths (Figure 9.1). Occasionally such a distinction is more difficult, and it may be that the nature and properties of the scalp, its relative 'thinness' and tethering to the skull, contributes to the appearance of an incised wound following blunt impact.

Tangential forces or glancing blows, either from an implement or from a rotating wheel (e.g. in a road traffic accident), may tear large flaps of tissue, exposing the underlying skull. If hair becomes entangled in rotating machinery, portions of the scalp may be avulsed. These are referred to as 'scalping' injuries.

Skull fractures

The skeleton of the human head is divided into three main parts: the mandible, the facial skeleton and the closed container that contains the brain, the calvaria. The calvaria is made up of eight plates of bone, each of varying thickness, with buttresses passing through and across the bony margins. The skull is designed in part to protect the brain and in part to provide a mobile but secure platform for the receptor organs of the special senses.

The complexity of the skull structure means that mechanisms of skull fracture can be extremely complex as a result of both direct force (e.g. direct impact to the parietal bone causing a linear fracture) and indirect force (e.g. an orbital blowout fracture caused by impact to the eyeball). These mechanisms have been studied extensively and much is known about the way the skull behaves when forces are applied to the head. The skull, although rigid, is capable of some distortion and if the forces applied exceed the ability of the skull to distort, fractures will occur. The site of fracture therefore represents that point at which the delivered energy has exceeded the capability of the skull to distort, which is not necessarily at the site of impact, unless that applied force has resulted in a localized depressed fracture. The skull's capability to distort before fracturing varies with age, and an infant skull may permit significant distortion following impact without fracturing.

Apart from depressed fractures underlying major, localized areas of trauma, skull fractures alone are not necessarily life threatening. The presence of a skull fracture indicates the application of blunt force to the head, and it is the transmission of such force to the intracranial contents – including the brain – that has the potential to cause life-threatening injury. Fatal brain injury can occur in the absence of externally visible scalp injury, or skull fracture and, conversely, scalp injury overlying skull fracture may be associated with minimal (or no recognizable) brain injury or neurological deficit. In clinical practice, however, intracranial injury should always be suspected in the presence of skull fracture.

A pathologist can only make broad comments about the possible effect upon an individual of a blow to the head. As with all injuries, a wide spectrum of effects is to be expected in a population sustaining the same injury in exactly the same way.

Scalp abrasions, bruises or lacerations represent contact injuries, and their presence will assist in the identification of the point of contact/impact. Bruises, however, may evolve, and 'move' in tissues planes, and may not precisely represent the site of contact/impact by the time the scalp is examined. Abrasions do identify sites of impact. A direct blow to the nose can cause blunt force injuries to the nose itself, but may also cause bilateral periorbital bruising, as may impacts to the central forehead, even though no impact was applied to the eyes or orbital region.

Blows to the top of the head commonly result in long, linear fractures that pass down the parietal bones and may, if the force applied was severe, pass inwards across the floor of the skull, usually just anterior to the petrous temporal bone in the middle cranial fossa. If the vault fractures extend through the skull base from both sides, they may meet in the midline, at the pituitary fossa, and produce a complete fracture across the skull base: this is known as a hinge fracture (Figure 9.2). This type of fracture indicates the application of severe force and may be seen, for example, in traffic accidents or falls from high buildings.

Falls from a height onto the top of the skull or onto the feet, where the force is transmitted to the base of the skull through the spine, may result in ring fracture of the base of the skull around the foramen magnum, whereas significant 'broad surface' blows to the skull vault, particularly the parietal bones, may result in a 'spider's web' type of fracture composed of radiating lines transected by concentric circles.

Depressed fractures will force fragments of skull inwards and, because of the bilayer construction of

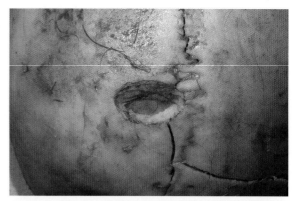

Figure 9.3 Depressed skull fracture, with rounded contours, closely replicating the dimensions of a round-headed hammer.

the skull, the degree of inner table fragmentation may be much greater than that of the outer table and fragments of bone can be driven into the underlying meninges, blood vessels and brain tissue. Blows to the head by implements, such as round-headed hammers may cause depressed vault fractures that have a curved outline with dimensions and a profile similar to that of the impacting surface of the implement (Figure 9.3).

The orbital plates, the upper surfaces of the orbits within the skull, are composed of extremely thin sheets of bone which are easily fractured, and these 'blow-out' fractures may be the only indication of the application of significant force to the skull. They are frequently seen as a consequence of a fall onto the back of the head.

Special mention must be made of skull fractures in children and infants. These fractures are extremely important forensically but their interpretation can be extremely difficult. It is self-evident that skull fractures may be the result of either deliberate or accidental acts and differentiation will depend on the consideration of as much relevant information as possible (see also Chapter 7, p. 71).

Intracranial haemorrhage

The clinical significance of any space-occupying lesion within the cranial cavity is the effect that the raised intracranial pressure caused has on brain structure and function.

Intracranial bleeding, resulting in a space-occupying lesion, is the cause of many deaths and disability following head injury, often as a result of delayed or missed diagnosis. Bleeding can compress the brain and, if it continues for sufficient time, and

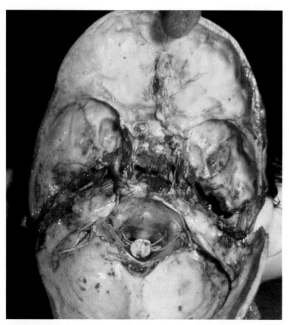

Figure 9.2 A 'hinge fracture' of the skull base caused by impact to the left side of the head after the victim was thrown to the ground, having been hit by a car.

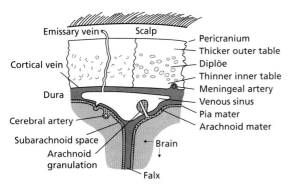

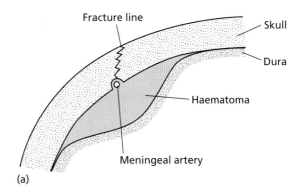

Figure 9.4 Forensic anatomy of the skull and meninges.

in sufficient quantity, can raise the pressure within the cranial cavity. As the intracranial pressure increases, blood flow to the brain decreases and, if the intracranial pressure reaches a point where it equals or exceeds arterial blood pressure, the blood flow to the brain will cease.

The anatomy of the blood vessels within the skull has a major influence on the type of bleeding that will occur following trauma (Figure 9.4). The meningeal arteries run in grooves in the inner table of the skull and lie outside the dura. They are generally protected from the shearing effect of sudden movement but are damaged by fracture lines that cross their course. The venous sinuses lie within the dura and the connecting veins pass between the sinuses and the cortical veins; these vessels are at particular risk of 'shearing' injury when there is differential movement between the brain and the skull. The true blood supply to the brain, the cerebral arteries and veins, lies beneath the arachnoid membrane and is generally protected from all but penetrating injuries.

Two main types of haemorrhage within the skull cavity, each resulting in haemorrhage in different planes, are extradural and subdural haemorrhage. Extradural haemorrhage is associated with damage to the meningeal artery, particularly the middle meningeal artery, in its course in the temporal bone (Figure 9.5). Damage to this vessel leads to arterial bleeding into the extradural space. As the blood accumulates, it separates the dura from the overlying skull and forms a haematoma. Arterial bleeding is likely to be fast, and the development of the haematoma will result in a rapid displacement of the brain and the rapid onset of symptoms. Extradural haemorrhages are ones that in the clinical setting may present with head trauma and then a 'lucid period' of half an hour or more, before rapid deterioration. Rarely, extradural haemorrhage can develop as a result of venous bleeding from

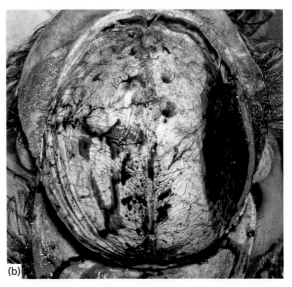

Figure 9.5 Extradural haemorrhage. Schematic representation (a) of the formation of an extradural haemorrhage and autopsy appearance (b) of a large right-sided, temporoparietal, extradural haemorrhage associated with deep scalp bruising at the site of impact. There was a linear skull fracture on the right passing through the middle meningeal artery.

damaged perforating veins or dural sinuses, in which case the development of symptoms will be slower.

The second most important cause of traumatic intracranial haemorrhage is damage to the communicating veins, as they cross the (potential) 'subdural space', causing subdural haemorrhage (Figure 9.6). This venous damage is not necessarily associated with fractures of the skull. In many instances, particularly in the very young and the very old, there may be no apparent history or evidence of any trauma to the head. These venous injuries are associated with rotational or shearing forces that cause the brain to move relative to the inner surface of the skull; this motion is thought to stretch the thin-walled veins, causing them to rupture. The venous

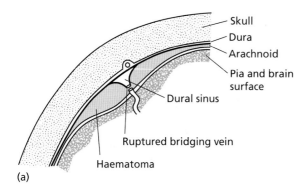

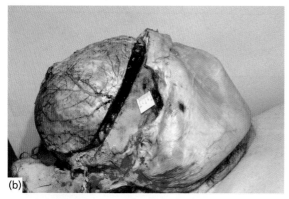

Figure 9.6 Subdural haemorrhage. Schematic representation of the formation of a subdural haematoma (a) and autopsy appearance of an acute right-sided subdural haemorrhage (b).

bleeding lies in the subdural space. Recent subdural haemorrhages are dark red in colour and shiny, but begin to turn brown after several days; microscopically, haemosiderin can be identified with Perl's stain (Figure 9.7). Older subdural collections (chronic

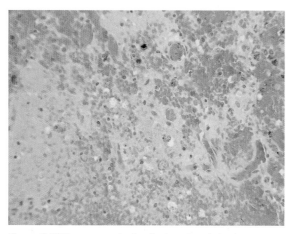

Figure 9.7 Microscopy of a 'healing' acute subdural haemorrhage, of approximately 4 days' duration, with iron-pigment-laden macrophages demonstrated by Perls' staining.

subdural haematoma) may be enclosed in gelatinous 'membranes', which can harden into a firm rubbery capsule in extreme cases. Such old collections of subdural blood are most commonly seen in the elderly, whose cerebral atrophy allows space for the formation of the haematoma without apparent significant clinical effect. Chronic subdural haematomas are also seen in those prone to frequent falls, such as those with alcohol dependencies. Occasionally, subdural haemorrhages may be present for many months or even years before diagnosis, which can be difficult because of the often non-specific neurological changes. Spontaneous subdural haemorrhages car occur.

The effects of both extradural and subdural haemorrhages are essentially the same: they can act as space-occupying lesions compressing the brain and, as discussed below, at their most severe, causing internal herniation (e.g. through the tentorium cerebelli). However, there may also be resultant brain contusion and swelling because of trauma, which accelerates the clinical deterioration and can hasten a fatal outcome.

Traumatic subarachnoid haemorrhage

Small areas of subarachnoid haemorrhage are common where there has been direct trauma to the brain, either from an intrusive injury, such as a depressed fracture, or from movement of the brain against the inner surface of the skull as a result of acceleration or deceleration injuries. These small injuries are usually associated with areas of underlying cortical contusion and sometimes laceration.

Large basal subarachnoid haemorrhages can be of traumatic origin and follow blows or kicks to the neck, particularly to the upper neck adjacent to the ear, but any blow, or even perhaps avoidance of a blow, which results in rapid rotation and flexion of the head on the neck can cause this damage. The vertebral arteries are confined within foraminae in the lateral margins of the upper six cervical vertebrae and are susceptible to trauma either with or without fracture of the foramina. It was traditionally thought that traumatic damage to the arteries occurred at the site at which they penetrate the spinal dura to enter the posterior fossa of the skull, although it is becoming increasingly evident that arterial injury leading to basal subarachnoid

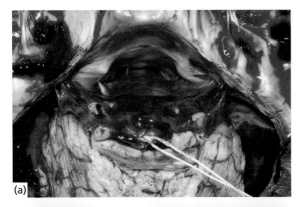

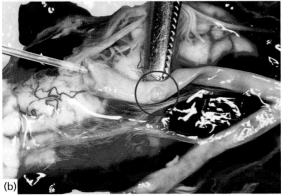

Figure 9.8 Traumatic basal subarachnoid haemorrhage.
(a) Autopsy appearance of basal subarachnoid haemorrhage,
covering the brain-stem, visualized following removal of the
cerebral hemispheres and tentorium cerebelli. The basilar
artery has been ligated. **(b)** The source of the bleeding is a tear
in a vertebral artery, confirmed following visualization of fluid
leakage from the cannulated injured vessel.

haemorrhage occurs in the intracranial portions of
the vertebral arteries (Figure 9.8).

Most basal subarachnoid haemorrhages are,
however, non-traumatic in origin and arise from the
spontaneous rupture of a berry aneurysm of one of
the arteries in the circle of Willis (see Chapter 6,
p. 59). In the deceased, particular care must be taken
to exclude this natural cause, and special autopsy
dissection techniques are required to evaluate the
integrity of the vertebral arteries.

Brain injury

Injuries that have resulted in skull fractures or
intracranial haemorrhage are clear macroscopic
markers of significant force having been applied
to the head and therefore to the brain. Sometimes,
however, these markers are absent but, as a result
of acceleration or deceleration forces, the brain has

been significantly traumatized. Whatever the precise cause of the trauma, the effects on the brain,
as a whole, are the same and, as a consequence
of the body's response to primary traumatic brain
injury, cerebral oedema develops (i.e. secondary
brain injury). The mechanism of cerebral oedema is
complex, but is in part caused by transudation of
fluid into the extracellular space.

As oedema develops, the brain swells and, as
the skull cannot expand beyond the confines of the
cranial cavity to compensate for this swelling, the
intracranial pressure rises and the brain is 'squeezed'
around meningeal folds (downwards through the
tentorium cerebelli, causing injury to the temporal
lobe unci and exerting pressure on the brain-stem,
for example), and downwards through the foramen
magnum (i.e. coning, causing injury to the cerebellar
tonsils and exerting pressure on the brain-stem) in a
process called internal herniation (Figure 9.9).

The weight of the oedematous brain is increased
and the surface of the brain is markedly flattened,
often with haemorrhage and necrosis of the unci
and the cerebellar tonsils; sectioning reveals compression of the ventricles, sometimes into thin
slits.

Direct injuries to the brain from depressed
or comminuted skull fractures result in areas of
bruising and laceration of the cortex, often associated with larger sites of haemorrhage. These
injuries can occur at any site, above or below
the tentorium. Penetrating injuries from gunshots
or from stab wounds can cause injuries deep
within the white matter, and the tissue adjacent
to the wound tracks will often be contused and
lacerated.

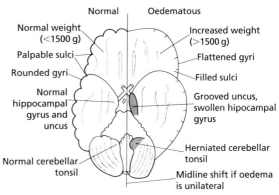

Figure 9.9 Schematic representation of the effects of brain
swelling and 'internal herniation' caused by raised intracranial
pressure.

Traumatic axonal injury

When the brain is subjected to rotational acceleration/deceleration forces, traumatic injury to axons within the brain substance can occur as a consequence of 'shearing' effects because of the differential movement of the various components of the brain which move in different ways, or at a different speeds, relative to each other. This shearing causes contusions and lacerations deep within the substance of the brain, but particularly in midline white matter structures such as the corpus callosum. Shearing is also associated with the so-called 'gliding lesions' that occur predominantly at the junction between cortical grey and white matter.

The shearing effects are also identifiable on microscopy, where damage to axons can be visualized with the aid of special staining techniques. These changes have been termed traumatic axonal injury which, when present at multiple sites throughout vulnerable areas of the cerebral hemispheres and brain-stem, may be described as diffuse traumatic axonal injury. Axonal injury takes a variable time to develop, or at least to become apparent under the microscope, and in cases of immediate or very rapid death following brain injury the microscopic changes may not be identifiable. Where there has been survival for several hours, immunohistochemical staining for β-amyloid precursor protein (ß-APP) may identify injured axons, although interpretation of such staining may be problematic, given that this stain also highlights axonal

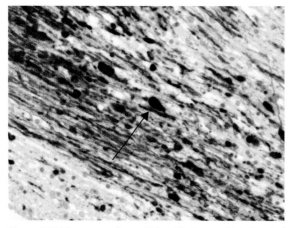

Figure 9.10 Microscopy of axonal injury. The immunohistochemical staining of β-amyloid precursor protein (β-APP) demonstrates axonal injury in white matter (corpus callosum). Discrete axonal swellings and 'axonal retraction bulbs' can be visualized following traumatic brain injury if the injured person survived for some hours after sustaining their head injury.

injury caused by non-traumatic phenomena including hypoxia-ischaemia (Figure 9.10). Progressive axonal injury, resulting in the formation of axonal retraction 'bulbs', can easily be recognized by silver staining techniques after some 12 hours following axonal injury, and subsequently on routine haematoxylin and eosin (H&E) staining.

Coup and contrecoup injuries

A coup injury to the brain occurs at the site of primary impact, when deformation of the skull contacts the underlying brain. The site of scalp injury will generally approximate the site of brain injury. Such a coup injury to the brain is usually represented by localized subarachnoid haemorrhage and cortical surface contusion with, or without, laceration.

In a 'moving head injury', such as might be experienced following a fall onto the back of the head, for example, impact causes the skull to stop moving suddenly, while movement of the brain continues momentarily before also stopping. As a consequence of such relative movement, and the effects of deceleration forces acting on the skull and the cranial contents, a distinctive pattern of head/brain injury can be recognized (Figure 9.11).

The site of impact is characterized by contact injuries to the scalp (bruising, abrasion and laceration, for example), skull (linear or depressed fractures) and sometimes cerebral contusion, although these are less commonly seen when the impact site is on the back of the head. Intracranial bleeding, particularly subdural and subarachnoid haemorrhage may be present and, of particular significance in interpreting the nature of the head injury, there are frequently cerebral contusions at sites distant from the primary impact. Such injuries, called contrecoup contusions, are most commonly seen on the under-surfaces of the frontal and temporal lobes following a fall onto the back of the head (Figure 9.12). The precise mechanism by which they are caused remains controversial, suggestions being that they represent the effects of contact against the irregular surfaces of the anterior and middle cranial fossae, or perhaps the effect of differential pressures within the brain following deceleration.

A careful evaluation of the pattern of head/brain injury is particularly important when a distinction is to be made between injuries in keeping with a fall

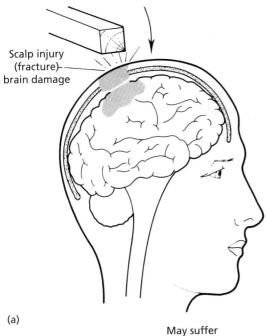

Scalp injury (fracture)— brain damage

(a)

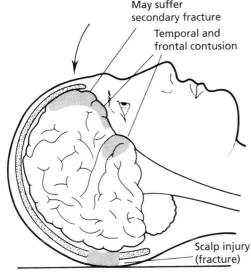

May suffer secondary fracture

Temporal and frontal contusion

Scalp injury (fracture)

(b)

Figure 9.11 Example of sclerotic representation of the formation of coup and contrecoup brain injury. **(a)** Impact to the non-moving head causing coup injuries, and **(b)** a fall onto the back of the head – a 'moving head injury' – causing contrecoup injuries.

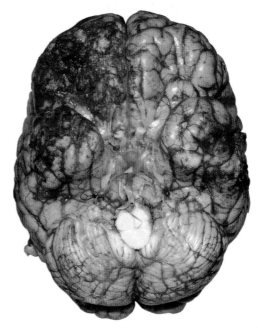

Figure 9.12 Contrecoup contusions on the under-surface of the brain.

or cerebellar hemispheres. Therefore, a definitive opinion regarding the nature of head/brain injuries in a difficult case will require close clinicopathological correlation, and an evaluation of witness evidence.

■ Neck injuries

The neck is the site of many different types of injury, some minor, some completely incapacitating. Its relevance in forensic medicine results from the presence of a large number of vital structures – the upper respiratory and gastrointestinal tracts, major blood vessels, major nerve trunks, the vertebral column and the spinal cord. It is particularly prone to injury as a consequence of assault or accidents as it can be grasped easily and the weight of the head means that rapid movement of the head on the neck (e.g. sudden deceleration in a road traffic collision) can result in substantial trauma. Protection of the integrity of the neck in the living, following traumatic insults likely to have injured it, is imperative prior to clinical and radiological assessment. Layered, dissection of the anterior (and often posterior) neck structures is an integral part of the forensic post-mortem examination.

versus assault; a head that is struck, while in contact with the ground and not moving, will not generally be accompanied by contrecoup cerebral injuries.

For reasons that are not altogether clear, but which may reflect the relative smoothness of the inner surface of the posterior cranial fossae, falls onto the front of the head are rarely accompanied by contrecoup contusions of the occipital lobes

Penetrating trauma – sharp force or ballistic – to the neck has the potential to injure a variety of complex structures and requires careful evaluation in the living as well as at post-mortem examination. Of particular forensic significance in incised wounds to the neck is the pattern of injury (self-inflicted versus assault), the presence of arterial injury capable of explaining 'arterial spray' in blood-staining at the scene of a suspicious death and venous injury raising the possibility of death having been caused by cardiac air embolism.

The application of pressure to the neck, whether it be manual or by means of a ligature, and the pattern of injury seen in such a scenario, is considered in more detail in Chapter 15, p. 152.

■ Spinal injuries

The spine is a complex structure with interlocking but mobile components. It is designed to flex to a great extent but lateral movement and extension are much more limited. The spine is very commonly injured in major trauma such as road traffic accidents or falls from a height, and severe injury with discontinuity is easily identified. However, sometimes the spinal injuries are more subtle and it is only after careful dissection that damage to the upper cervical spine and, in particular, disruption of the atlanto-occipital joint will be revealed.

For the survivors of trauma, spinal injuries may have some of the most crucial long-term effects because the spinal cord is contained within the spinal canal and there is little, if any, room for movement of the canal before the cord is damaged. The sequelae of spinal damage will depend upon the exact anatomical site and mechanism of injury.

The type of injury to the spine will depend upon the degree of force and the angle at which the spine is struck. A column is extremely strong in compression and, unless the force applied is so severe that the base of the skull is fractured, vertically applied forces will generally result in little damage if the spine is straight. Angulation of the spine will alter the transmission of force and will make the spine much more susceptible to injury, particularly at the site of the angulation.

Force applied to the spine may result in damage to the discs or to the vertebral bodies. The other major components of the vertebrae – the neural arches and the transverse processes – are more likely to be injured if the force of the trauma is not aligned with the spine.

Whiplash injuries associated with road traffic fatalities are very common and are caused by hyperextension of the neck; hyperflexion is less likely to cause damage. Hyperflexion injuries can be caused if heavy weights are dropped onto the back of a crouching individual; this scenario may be seen in roof falls in the mining industry. Hyperflexion injuries are also seen in sports – particularly rugby scrums and diving. Such injuries can cause fatalities or substantial disability such as quadriplegia.

Forceful extension of the spine can be seen, although rarely now, in the cervical injuries associated with judicial hanging where there is a long drop before the sudden arrest and forceful extension of the neck. Forceful flexion of the spine will commonly lead to the 'wedge' fracture or compression of the anterior aspect of a vertebral body (Figure 9.13). Lateral forces will lead to fracture dislocations where one vertebral body passes across its neighbour; this displacement will seriously compromise the integrity of the vertebral canal. Damage to the intervertebral discs can occur as a solitary lesion or it may be part of a more complex spinal injury.

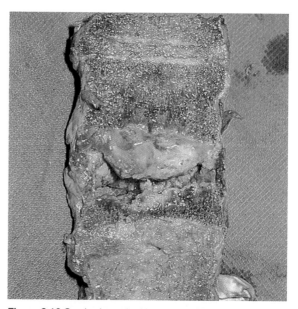

Figure 9.13 Crushed vertebral body as a result of a hyperflexion injury.

■ Chest injuries

The chest can be subject to all kinds of injury and is particularly susceptible to both blunt and penetrating injuries.

Adequate respiration requires freedom of movement of the chest, functioning musculature and integrity of the chest wall. Any injury that impairs or prevents any of these activities will result in a reduction in the ability to breathe, which may result in asphyxiation. External pressure on the chest may result in traumatic asphyxia by restricting movement; this may occur during road traffic collisions or following collapse of structures such as mine tunnels, or buildings in earthquakes. Pressure on the chest that restricts movement may also occur if the individual simply gets into, or is placed into, a position in which the free movement of the chest is restricted. This positional asphyxia occurs most commonly in individuals that are rendered immobile through alcohol or drugs and may be seen following restraint in custodial settings; it may also be seen in the healthy, for example, attempting to climb through a small window to gain access to a property.

Blunt injury may result in fractures of the ribs. The fracture of a few ribs is unlikely to have much effect, other than causing pain, in a fit adult. In an individual with respiratory disease (e.g. chronic obstructive pulmonary disease) there are greater risks for the development of respiratory compromise or infection. If there are numerous rib fractures, and particularly if they are in adjacent ribs, the functional integrity of the chest wall may be compromised, limiting respiratory capabilities even in fit individuals. Multiple rib fractures may result in the so-called 'flail' chest and, clinically, the area of chest around the fractures may be seen to move inwards on inspiration – paradoxical respiration (Figure 9.14). The clinical effects of such injuries depend on their extent and on the respiratory reserve of the individual: an elderly man with chronic lung disease may be tipped into terminal respiratory failure by injuries that would only be a painful irritant to a fit young man. Trauma that has fractured left sided 10th, 11th and 12th ribs may be substantial enough to cause injury to the underlying spleen.

Rib fractures may have other more serious consequences. If the sharp ends of the fractured bones are driven inwards, they may penetrate the underlying pleural lining of the chest wall cavity, or even

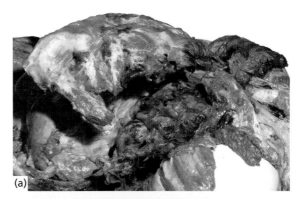

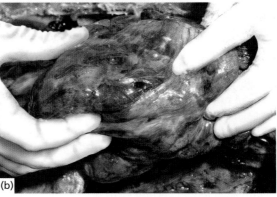

Figure 9.14 Multiple rib fractures **(a)** following a road traffic collision. There were many 'flail' segments and fractured rib ends pierced the underlying lung **(b)**.

the underlying lung itself, resulting in a pneumothorax. If subcostal, or pulmonary, blood vessels are also injured, the resulting haemorrhage associated with the leakage of air will produce a haemopneumothorax. Pneumothoraces may also develop if fractured rib margins are forced outwards through the skin.

Children are, in general, more resilient and better able to cope with rib fractures. However, rib fractures in children have a particular place in forensic medicine, as they can be a marker for non-accidental injury (see Chapter 7, p. 71 and Chapter 13, p. 137).

Rib (and sternal) fractures in adults are frequently identified at post-mortem examination following cardiopulmonary resuscitation (CPR) or cardiac massage. They are usually located anteriorly, or laterally, and involve those ribs underlying the regions that experience most compression during CPR. They are frequently symmetrical and, if there has been no survival following CPR attempts, they lack associated haemorrhage. Posterior rib fractures, or fractures of the first rib, for example would be unusual as a consequence of CPR. The nature of rib fractures, thought to be related to CPR may become the subject of argument in court and, in an individual with a history of chest trauma, who subsequently receives CPR attempts, microscopic examination of rib fractures identified at post-mortem examination – for evidence of 'healing changes' – may be of assistance.

Penetrating injuries of the chest, whether caused by sharp-force trauma (stab wounds) or gunshot wounds, may result in damage to any of the organs or vessels within the thoracic cavities. The effect of the penetration will depend mainly upon which organ(s) or vessel(s) are injured. Penetration of the chest wall can lead to the development of pneumothorax, haemothorax or a combination (haemo-pneumothorax).

Injury to the lungs will also result in the development of pneumothoraces, and damage to the blood vessels will result in haemorrhage, which may be confined to the soft tissues of the mediastinum or enter the pleural cavities. Haemorrhage from penetrating injuries to the chest may remain concealed with little external evidence of bleeding and it is not unusual to find several litres of blood within the chest cavity at post-mortem examination. Following penetrating chest injury, and when an injured person is capable of purposeful movements following infliction of such an injury, external blood loss may not be apparent at the locus of infliction of that injury, resulting in potential difficulties in the interpretation of the scene of an alleged assault. It follows that the lack of any evidence of external bleeding at such a scene does not imply that infliction of the – subsequently fatal – injury could not have occurred at that locus. The answer to the question commonly asked in court, 'Would you not have expected immediate bleeding from such a serious injury', must be 'Not necessarily'.

■ Abdomen

The anatomy of the abdominal cavity plays a major role in determining the type of injuries that are found. The vertebral column forms a strong, midline, vertical structure posteriorly, and blunt trauma, especially in the anterior/posterior direction, may result in compression of the organs lying in the midline against the vertebral column. This compressive injury may result in substantial blunt

force injury to intra-abdominal organs, including bruising (or even transection) of the duodenum or jejunum, rupture of the pancreas, rupture of the liver, and disruption of omentum and mesentery (Figures 9.15 and 9.16).

The forces required to cause these injuries in an adult must be considered to be severe and they are commonly encountered in road traffic collisions. In an otherwise healthy adult, it would be unusual for a simple punch to the abdomen to cause significant intra-abdominal injuries, but kicks and stamps are commonly the cause of major trauma. The kidneys and the spleen are attached only by their hila and are susceptible not only to direct trauma but also to rotational forces that may result in avulsion from their vascular pedicles. Blunt trauma to the spleen is sometimes associated with delayed rupture leading to haemorrhage and possibly death some hours or even days after the injury. Pancreatic trauma may

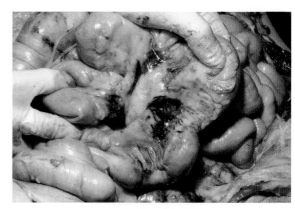

Figure 9.15 Mesenteric bruising and laceration following blunt force trauma in a road traffic collision.

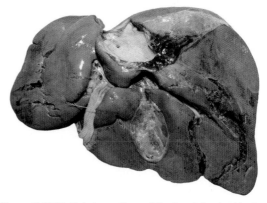

Figure 9.16 Multiple lacerations of the liver following blunt force abdominal trauma in a road traffic collision.

lead to the development of a pseudocyst, with little or no short-term or long-term sequelae. Once diagnosed the successful treatment of these conditions may be conservative or surgical.

Abdominal injuries in children may have the same causes, but the forces required to cause them will be considerably reduced, and the slower compressive forces associated with squeezing of the abdomen during abuse may also result in the injuries described above. The possibility of intra-abdominal injuries being caused by CPR is also one that is raised in court, but such instances of injury to either solid or hollow intra-abdominal organs in adults or children are very rare.

Penetrating injuries to the abdomen can be the result of either gunshots or sharp-force trauma. The effects of these injuries will depend almost entirely on the organs and vessels involved in the wound track. A penetrating injury to the aorta, or inferior vena cava, can result in severe haemorrhage and may produce rapid death. Peritonitis from a ruptured bowel or stomach may not be recognized until too late, by which time overwhelming septicaemia will have developed. The presence of peritonitis and blood clots at post-mortem are both factors which may give indications of how long before death intra-abdominal trauma had occurred.

■ Further information sources

Adams JH, Mitchell DE, Graham DI, Doyle D. Diffuse brain damage of immediate impact type. Its relationship to 'primary brain-stem damage' in head injury. *Brain* 1977; **100:** 489–502.

Adams JH, Doyle D, Ford I *et al.* Diffuse axonal injury in head injury: definition, diagnosis and grading. *Histopathology* 1989; **15:** 49–59.

Bathe Rawling L. Fractures of the skull. Lecture 1. *Lancet* 1904; **163:** 973–979.

Blumbergs P, Reilly P, Vink R. Trauma, Chapter 11. In: Love S, Louis DN, Ellison DW (eds) *Greenfield's Neuropathology*, 8th edn. London: Hodder Arnold, 2008; pp. 733–832.

Dawson SL, Hirsch CS, Lucas FV, Sebek BA. The contrecoup phenomenon. Reappraisal of a classic problem. *Human Pathology* 1980; **11:** 155–66.

Dunn LT, Fitzpatrick MO, Beard D, Henry JM. Patients with a head injury who 'talk and die' in the 1990s. *Journal of Trauma* 2003; **54:** 497–502.

Geddes JF. What's new in the diagnosis of head injury? *Journal of Clinical Pathology* 1997; **50:** 271–4.

Geddes JF, Vowles GH, Beer TW, Ellison DW. The diagnosis of diffuse axonal injury: implications for forensic practice. *Neuropathology and Applied Neurobiology* 1997; **23:** 339–47.

Geddes JF, Whitwell HL, Graham DI. Traumatic axonal injury: practical issues for diagnosis in medico-legal cases. *Neuropathology and Applied Neurobiology* 2000; **26:** 105–16.

Gennarelli TA, Thibault LE. Biomechanics of acute subdural haematoma. *Journal of Trauma* 1982; **22:** 680–5.

Gentleman SM, Roberts GW, Gennarelli TA *et al.* Axonal injury: a universal consequence of fatal closed head injury? *Acta Neuropathologica* 1995; **89:** 537–43.

Graham DI, Lawrence AE, Adams JH *et al.* Brain damage in non-missile head injury secondary to high intracranial pressure. *Neuropathology and Applied Neurobiology* 1987; **13:** 209–17.

Graham DI, Smith C, Reichard R *et al.* Trials and tribulations of using β-amyloid precursor protein immunohistochemistry to evaluate traumatic brain injury in adults. *Forensic Science International* 2004; **146:** 89–96.

Gurdjian ES. Cerebral contusions: re-evaluation of the mechanism of their development. *Journal of Trauma* 1976; **16:** 35–51.

Gurdjian ES, Webster JE, Lissner HR. The mechanism of skull fracture. *Journal of Neurosurgery* 1950; **7:** 106–14.

Hampson D. Facial injury: a review of biomechanical studies and test procedures for facial injury assessment. *Journal of Biomechanics* 1995; **28:** 1–7.

Hein PM, Schulz E. Contrecoup fractures of the anterior cranial fossae as a consequence of blunt force caused by a fall. *Acta Neurochirugica (Wien)* 1990; **105:** 24–9.

Heinzelman M, Platz A, Imhof HG. Outcome after acute extradural haematoma, influence of additional injuries and neurological complications in the ICU. *Injury* 1996; **27:** 345–9.

Le Count ER, Apfelbach CW. Pathologic anatomy of traumatic fractures of cranial bones. *Journal of the American Medical Association* 1920; **74:** 501–11.

Lee MC, Haut RC. Insensitivity of tensile failure properties of human bridging veins to strain rate: implications in biomechanics of subdural hematoma. *Journal of Biomechanics* 1989; **22:** 537–42.

Lindenberg R, Freitag E. The mechanism of cerebral contusions. A pathologic–anatomic study. *Archives of Pathology* 1960; **69:** 440–69.

Margulies SS, Thibault LE, Gennarelli TA. Physical model simulations of brain injury in the primate. *Journal of Biomechanics* 1990; **23:** 823–36.

Milroy CM, Whitwell HL. Difficult areas in forensic neuropathology: homicide, suicide or accident, Chapter 11. In: Whitwell HL (ed) *Forensic Neuropathology*. London: Arnold, 2005; p. 124–34.

Munro D, Merritt HH. Surgical pathology of subdural hematoma. *Archives of Neurology and Psychiatry* 1936; **35:** 64–78.

Ommaya AK, Grubb RL Jr, Naumann RA. Coup and contre-coup injury: observations on the mechanics of visible brain injuries in the rhesus monkey. *Journal of Neurosurgery* 1971; **35:** 503–16.

Ommaya AK, Goldsmith W, Thibault L. Biomechanics and neuropathology of adult and paediatric head injury. *British Journal of Neurosurgery* 1992; **16:** 220–42.

Preuss J, Padosch SA, Dettmeyer R *et al*. Injuries in fatal cases of falls downstairs. *Forensic Science International* 2004; **141:** 121–6.

Rizen A Jo V, Nikolić V, Banović B. The role of orbital wall morphological properties and their supporting structures in the etiology of 'blow out' fractures. *Surgical and Radiologic Anatomy* 1989; **11:** 241–8.

Reichard RR, Smith C, Graham DI. The significance of beta-APP immunoreactivity in forensic practice. *Neuropathology and Applied Neurobiology* 2005; **31:** 304–13.

Saukko P, Knight B. Gunshot and explosion deaths, Chapter 8. In: Saukko P, Knight B (eds) *Knight's Forensic Pathology*, 3rd edn. London: Hodder Arnold, 2004; p. 182.

Yoganandan N, Pintar FA, Sances A *et al*. Biomechanics of skull fracture. *Journal of Neurotrauma* 1995; **12:** 659–68.

9 Regional injuries

Chapter 10

Ballistic injuries

■ Introduction

The use of firearms as weapons of assault outside conflict or police settings continues to increase. Firearms are relatively easy to obtain, whether in jurisdictions where their possession and use is permitted or not. Legislation intended to reduce availability often seems to have an impact only on those with a lawful need or reason for possession, rather than on those intent to use firearms for criminal purposes. In whichever jurisdiction the forensic practitioner practices, he or she will encounter injury and death caused by a wide variety of firearms.

■ Types of firearms

There are two main types of firearm: those with smooth barrels, which fire groups of pellets or shot, and those with grooved or rifled barrels, which fire single projectiles or bullets. The main types are discussed further in Chapter 23, p. 232. Both of these types of weapon rely upon the detonation of a solid propellant to produce the gases that propel the projectile(s). Air guns and air rifles form a separate group of weapons that rely upon compressed gas to propel the projectiles, and these weapons, together with the more unusual forms of projectile or firearm, such as the rubber bullet, stud guns and humane killers, are considered at the end of this section.

The term 'Dum-Dum bullets' relates to the .303 centrefire rifle cartridges with a hollow-point style bullet that were made at the British arsenal in Dum-Dum, India, in the late nineteenth century. The use of Dum-Dum and other expanding bullets was forbidden in wars between signatories of the Geneva Convention in 1864. This rule was reiterated by subsequent declarations of the Hague Conferences. It should be noted that the restrictions apply to war only and that no restriction applies to the use of this type of bullet if war has not been formally declared.

Modern propellants consist of nitrocellulose or other synthetic compounds prepared as small coloured flakes, discs or balls. The process of firing a bullet or shotgun cartridge is as follows. The firing pin strikes the primer cup and the primer compound explodes; small vents between the primer cup and the base of the cartridge case allow the flame of this detonation to spread to the propellant. The propellant burns rapidly, producing large volumes of gas, which are further expanded by the very high temperatures of the ignition, and it is the pressure of this gas that propels the shot or bullet from the barrel.

The speed with which the projectile leaves the end of the barrel (the muzzle velocity) varies from a few hundred metres per second in a shotgun to a thousand or more in a high-velocity military weapon. The energy of the projectile is proportional to the speed at which it travels and is calculated from the kinetic energy ($\frac{1}{2}MV^2$) of the bullet, so higher muzzle velocities are considerably more effective at delivering energy to the target than larger bullets. The extent of injury, and wound pattern, created by a firearm is directly related to the muzzle velocity.

■ Gunshot injuries

Discharging a firearm (with the exception of an airgun) will result in the formation of smoke, flame and gases of combustion. These exit the barrel, together with portions of unburned, burning and burnt propellant and other items such as wadding and plastic containers for the pellets. These 'contaminants' will usually follow the projectile(s), but in some guns they may also precede them. The distance they will travel from the end of the muzzle is extremely variable, depending mainly on the type of weapon and the type of propellant. They can also escape from small gaps around the breech and will soil hands or clothing close to the breech at the time of discharge. The presence, location and distribution of such contaminants may have great importance in the forensic investigation of a shooting incident.

Injuries from smooth-bore guns

Discharge from a cartridge forces pellets along the barrel by the gases of detonation. The pellets will leave the muzzle in a compact mass, the components of which spread out as it travels away from the gun. The shot pattern expands as a long, shallow cone with its apex close to the muzzle of the shotgun. The further away from the gun that the victim is situated, the larger the pellet spread, and the larger the area of potential damage (Figure 10.1).

Contact wounds are created when the gun muzzle abuts the skin and usually results in a circular entrance wound that approximates the size of the muzzle (Figures 10.2 and 10.3). The wound edge will be regular and often has a clean-cut

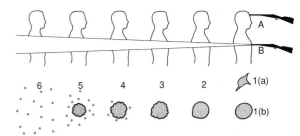

Figure 10.1 Variation in appearance of a shotgun wound at increasing range of discharge: **(a)**, split wound from contact over bone; **(b)**, usual round contact wound; 2, close but not contact range up to approximately 30 cm (variable); 3, 'rat hole' (scalloped) wound from 20 cm to approximately 1 m (variable); 4, satellite pellet holes appearing over approximately 2 m; 5, spread of shot increases, central hole diminishes; 6, uniform spread with no central hole over approximately 10 m. All these ranges vary greatly with barrel choke, weapon and ammunition.

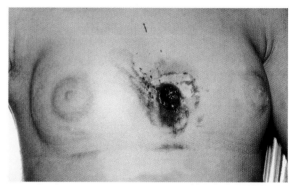

Figure 10.2 Suicidal twelve-bore shotgun entrance wound, with soot soiling. The wound shows the outline of the non-fired muzzle, indicating that the weapon was a double-barrelled shotgun pressed against the skin at discharge.

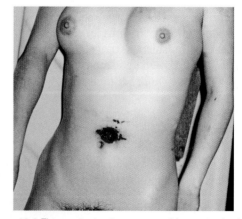

Figure 10.3 Firm contact entrance wound from a twelve-bore shotgun. Clothing prevented soot soiling, but minor peripheral abrasions were caused by impact of a belt. Gas expansion in the distensible abdomen has prevented skin splitting at the wound edges.

10 Ballistic injuries

appearance with no individual pellet marks apparent. There will commonly be smoke soiling of at least some of the margin of the wound. There may be a narrow, circular rim of abrasion around some or all of the entrance wound, caused when the gases of the discharge enter through the wound and balloon the tissues upwards so that the skin is pressed against the muzzle. If the discharge was over an area supported by bone, the gases cannot disperse as readily as they would in soft, unsupported areas such as the abdomen, and the greater ballooning of the skin results in splits of the skin, which often have a radial pattern. In contact wounds, any wadding or plastic shot containers may usually be recovered from the wound track. The tissues along the wound track may be blackened and the surrounding tissues are said to be pinker than normal as a result of the carbon monoxide contained within the discharge gases.

A close discharge, within a few centimetres of the surface, will also produce a wound with a similar appearance, but as there is now room for muzzle gases to escape, there will be no muzzle mark. More smoke soiling can occur, and burning of skin, with singeing and clubbing of melted hairs, can be seen around the wound (Figure 10.4). There is also, very commonly, powder 'tattooing' of the skin around the entry wound. This tattooing results from burnt and burning flakes of propellant causing tiny burns on the skin and cannot be washed off. As with contact discharges, wads will generally be found in the wound track.

At intermediate ranges, between 20 cm and 1 m, there will be diminishing smoke soiling and burning of the skin, but powder tattooing may persist. The spread of shot will begin, first causing an irregular rim to the wound. This is often called a 'rat-hole' because of the appearance of the wound edge; the term 'scalloping' may also be used. Separate injuries caused by the wads or plastic shot containers may be seen (Figure 10.5).

At a range of over 1 m, smoke damage and tattooing generally do not occur and injuries caused at longer ranges will depend upon the spread of the shot, which in turn is dependent upon the construction of the barrel. With a normal shotgun, satellite pellet holes begin to be seen around the main central wound at a range of about 2–3 m (Figure 10.6).

It is important to measure the spread of the shot so that if the weapon is recovered, test firings using identical ammunition can be performed to establish the range at which a particular spread of shot will occur. Estimates based on generalizations about the ratio of the diameter of this spread to the range are unreliable.

At long ranges, such as 20–50 m, there is a uniform peppering of shot, and this is rarely fatal. (Figure 10.6b)

Shotguns rarely produce an exit wound when fired into the chest or abdomen, although single-pellet exit wounds can occasionally be seen. Exit

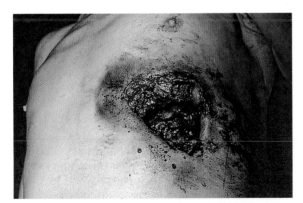

Figure 10.4 Suicidal close range discharge of a twelve-bore shotgun wound to the chest. This wound has torn a large ragged defect in the chest wall and there is soot discoloration at the medial wound edge because of the tangential orientation of the discharge.

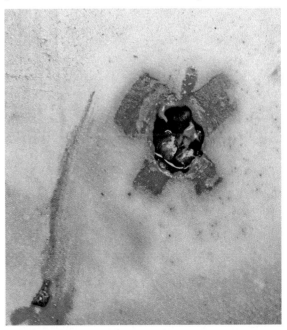

Figure 10.5 Abraded bruise surrounding an intermediate-range homicidal shotgun entrance wound, caused by impact against the skin from the opening up of the plastic pellet container. Note the scalloping of the wound edges.

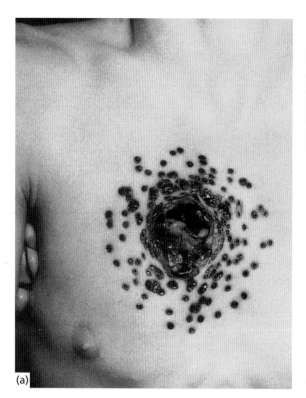

(a)

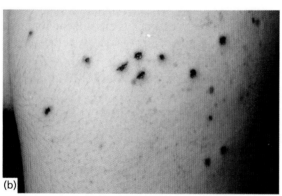

(b)

Figure 10.6 **(a)** Distant-range shotgun entrance wound, with a central hole surrounded by peripheral satellite pellet holes. This wound was caused by discharge from approximately 4 m; measurement of shot-spread can be compared with that created from test-firing the suspect weapon and ammunition to provide a more accurate assessment of range of fire. **(b)** Shotgun pellet injury to skin from discharge about 12 m away

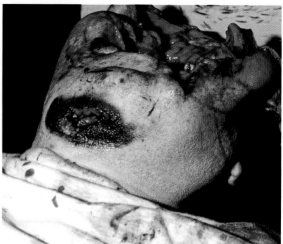

Figure 10.7 Suicidal twelve-bore shotgun entrance wound in a 'site of election' under the chin. The circular soot discoloration on the skin surface indicates a very close (or even 'loose' contact) discharge. Note the extensive destruction reflecting the explosive effect of shotgun discharges to the head.

Wounds from rifled weapons

Bullets fired from rifled weapons, generally at a higher velocity than pellets from a smooth-bore weapon, will commonly cause both an entry and an exit wound. However, many bullets are retained within the body because they did not possess enough energy to complete the passage through it, or energy was expended on contact with other structures (e.g. bone).

Entrance and exit wounds

Contact wounds from a rifled weapon are generally circular, unless over a bony area such as the head, where splitting caused by the propellant gas is common. There may be a muzzle mark on the skin surface if the gun is pressed hard against the skin, and a pattern may be imprinted from a fore-sight or self-loading mechanism. There may be slight escape of smoke, with some local burning of skin and hair, if the gun is not pressed tightly. Bruising around the entry wound is not uncommon (Figures 10.8 and 10.9).

At close range, up to about 20 cm, there will be some smoke soiling and powder burns, and skin and hair may be burnt, although this is very variable and depends upon both the gun and the ammunition used. The shape of the entry wound gives a

wounds can be seen when a shotgun is fired into the head, neck or mouth. The exit wound in these cases may be a huge ragged aperture, especially in the head, where the skull may virtually explode with the gas pressure from a contact wound, ejecting part or even all of the brain from the cranial cavity (Figure 10.7).

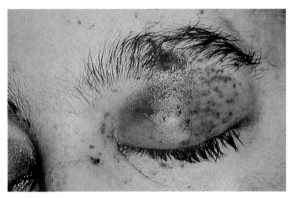

Figure 10.8 Close-range gunshot entrance wound from a pistol, with powder tattooing on the adjacent skin. The eye is blackened as a result of bleeding 'tracking' down from fracturing of the anterior cranial fossa in the skull base.

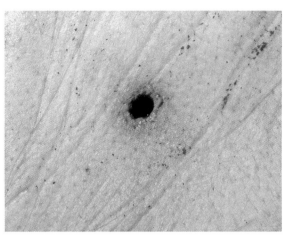

Figure 10.10 Circular distant gunshot entrance wound from a rifle bullet. There is no associated soot soiling or burning of the wound edges, with only minimal marginal abrasion and bruising.

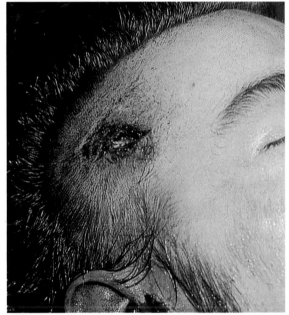

Figure 10.9 Suicidal contact gunshot entrance wound to the temple. The skin is burnt and split because of the effects of the discharge products.

guide to the angle that the gun made with that area of skin: a circular hole indicates that the discharge was at right angles to the skin, whereas an oval hole, perhaps with visible undercutting, indicates a more acute angle.

Examination of the entry wound will show that the skin is inverted; the defect is commonly slightly smaller than the diameter of the missile because of the elasticity of the skin. Very commonly, there is an 'abrasion collar' or 'abrasion rim' around the hole, which is caused by the friction, heating and dirt effect of the missile when it indents the skin during penetration. Bruising may or may not be associated with the wound.

Over 1 m or so, there can be no smoke soiling, burning or powder tattooing. At longer ranges (which may be up to several kilometres with a high-powered rifle), the entrance hole will have the same features of a round or oval defect with an abrasion collar (Figure 10.10). At extreme ranges, or following a ricochet, the gyroscopic stability of the bullet may be lost and the missile begins to wobble and even tumble, and this instability may well result in larger, more irregular wounds.

The exit wound of a bullet is usually everted with split flaps, often resulting in a stellate appearance (Figure 10.11). No burning, smoke or powder soiling will be evident. If the bullet has been distorted or fragmented, or if it has fractured bone, the exit wound may be considerably larger and more irregular, and those fragments of bullet or bone may cause multiple exit wounds, potentially leading to difficulties in interpretation.

Where skin is firmly supported, as by a belt, tight clothing or even a person leaning against a partition wall, the exit wound may be as small as the entrance and may fail to show the typical eversion. To increase the confusion, it may also show a rim of abrasion, although this is commonly broader than that of an entry wound.

The internal effects of bullets depend upon their kinetic energy. Low-velocity, low-energy missiles, such as shotgun pellets and some revolver bullets, cause simple mechanical disruption of the tissues in their path. High-velocity bullets, however, cause

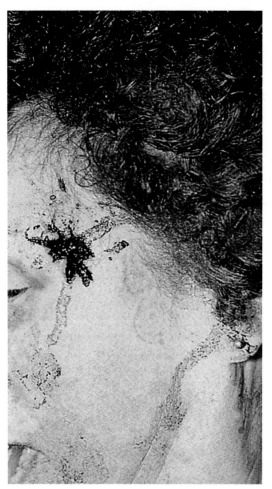

Figure 10.11 Typical exit wound with everted, split edges, with no soiling of the surrounding skin.

far more damage to the tissues as they transfer large amounts of energy, which results in the formation of a temporary cavity in the tissues. This cavitation effect is especially pronounced in dense organs, such as liver and brain, but occurs in all tissues if the energy transfer is large enough and can result in extensive tissue destruction away from the wound track itself.

■ Air weapons, unusual projectiles and other weapons

Air guns and rifles

Air weapons rely upon the force of compressed air to propel the projectile, usually a lead or steel pellet although darts and other projectiles may be used. There are three common ways in which the gas is compressed. The simplest method employs the compression of a spring which, when released, moves a piston along a cylinder; more powerful weapons use repeated movements of a lever to pressurize an internal cylinder. The third type has an internal cylinder which is 'charged' by connecting it to a pressurized external source. The barrel of an air weapon may or may not be rifled; the more powerful examples have similar rifling to ordinary handguns and rifles.

The energy of the projectile will depend mainly on the way in which the gas is compressed, the simple spring-driven weapon is low powered, while the more complex systems can propel projectiles with the same energy, and hence at approximately the same speed, as many ordinary handguns.

The injuries caused by the projectiles from air weapons will depend upon their design, but entry wounds from standard pellets are often indistinguishable from those caused by standard bullets in that they have a defect with an abrasion rim. The relatively low power of these weapons means that the pellet will seldom exit, but if it does do so, a typical exit wound with everted margins will result.

Miscellaneous firearms and weapons

A number of other implements may fulfil the criteria for firearms while others may mimic their effects. It is appropriate to have a knowledge of such implements to take their possible effects into consideration when determining injury causation.

In public disorder situations, where law enforcement or security forces are involved, plastic rounds may be fired from specially adapted guns, for crowd control purposes. The purpose of these weapons is to disable and discourage rioters but not to kill or seriously injure them (see also Chapter 11, p. 125). The plastic rounds are about 10 cm long, 3.5 cm in diameter and weigh about 130 g. They should not be fired at ranges less than about 20 m and should only be fired at the lower part of the body. Some deaths, and many serious injuries, including fractures of skull, ribs and limbs, eye damage and internal injuries have occurred, and these are usually associated with improper use. The mark left on the skin surface by a plastic round is usually distinctive.

Injuries and deaths from stud guns are well recorded. Stud guns are devices used in the building industry to fire steel pins into masonry or timber by means of a small explosive charge. They have been used for suicide and even homicide, but accidental injuries are more common. The skin injury often appears similar to many small-calibre entry wounds, although the finding of a nail will usually solve the diagnostic problem.

Humane killers are devices used in abattoirs, and by veterinary surgeons, to stun animals before slaughter. They may fire either a small-calibre bullet or a 'captive bolt', where a sliding steel pin is fired out for about 5 cm by an explosive charge. The skin injury will depend on the type of weapon used. These weapons have been used for both homicide and suicide, but accidental discharges are also recorded and may cause serious injury or death.

Bows and crossbows are used recreationally but may also be used as weapons of assault. These weapons fire arrows or bolts, which are shafts of wood or metal with a set of flights at the rear to maintain the trajectory of the projectile. The tips of these projectiles may have many shapes from the simple point to complex, often triangular, forms. The energy produced is extremely variable, depending on the construction of the weapon. The injuries caused depend on the energy of the projectile as well as on its construction. However, if the projectile has a simple pointed tip, and if it has been removed from the body, the entry wounds can appear very similar to those caused by standard bullets, with a central defect and surrounding abrasion rim.

■ Determination of accident, suicide or murder

The determination of the circumstances in which an individual has died from a firearm injury is crucial. Death investigators, including pathologists, must be aware of the potential for 'staging' of homicide in order to give the appearance of death having occurred as a result of accident or suicide. Those who have killed themselves must generally have wounds the site and range of which are within the reach of the deceased's arm, unless some device has been used to reach and depress the trigger. The weapon must be present at the scene, although it may be at a distance from the body because it may

have been thrown away from the body by recoil, or by movement of the individual if death was not immediate. It may be expected that the deceased's DNA or fingerprints will be present on the weapon (unless gloves were worn). Suicidal gunshot injuries are most commonly in the 'sites of election', which vary with the length of the weapon used.

Both long-barrelled and short-barrelled weapons can be used in the mouth, below the chin, on the front of the neck, the centre of the forehead or, more rarely, the front of the chest over the heart. Discharges into the temples are almost unique to handguns and are usually on the side of the dominant hand, but this is not an absolute rule. People almost never shoot themselves in the eye or abdomen or in inaccessible sites such as the back. It is unusual for females to commit suicide with guns and females are rarely involved in firearms accidents.

If suicide can be ruled out by the range of discharge, by absence of a weapon or by other features of the injury or the scene, a single gunshot injury could be either accident or homicide. Multiple firearm wounds strongly suggest homicide. However, there have been a number of published reports of suicidal individuals who have fired repeatedly into themselves even when each wound is potentially fatal. The distinction between homicide, suicide and accident can sometimes be extremely difficult and a final conclusion can only be reached after a full medico-legal investigation.

It is as unwise to state that a gunshot wound, as with any other sort of injury, must have been immediately fatal. It is most likely that severe damage to the brain, heart, aorta and any number of other vital internal organs will lead to rapid collapse and death; however, many forensic practitioners will have seen cases of survival (sometimes long-term) following a contact discharge of a firearm into the head.

■ Evidence recovery

In the living, all efforts must be directed to saving life but, if at all possible, the emergency medicine specialist, and surgeon, should make good notes of the original appearances of the injuries and preferably take good-quality images before any surgical cleaning or operative procedures are performed. Any foreign objects such as wads, bullets or shot, and any skin removed from the margin of a firearm wound during treatment, should be carefully preserved for the police. Ideally, the police should be contacted (with the individual's consent) should surgical intervention be required so that a 'chain of custody' for evidence can be established.

Those arrested for possible involvement in firearms offences will need detailed examination and taking of samples, including skin and hand swabs, and nasal samples, to identify any firearms residue.

The same general rules apply to the post-mortem recovery of exhibits. The skin around the wounds may be swabbed for powder residue if this is considered to be necessary, but the retention of wounds themselves is no longer considered to be essential. Swabs of the hands of the victim should be taken. The pathologist must ensure that accurate drawings and measurements of the site, size and appearance of the wound are obtained and that distant and close-up photographs are taken of each injury with an appropriate scale in view.

In many countries, all firearm wounds, whether or not they are fatal, must be reported to the police, irrespective of the consent of the injured individual.

■ Explosives

Armed conflict, and terrorist activity, leads to many deaths from explosive devices. Terrorist activity is now present in many countries and therefore there has been an increase in the experience of medical personnel in the assessment and treatment of explosive injuries.

In military bomb, shell and missile explosions, the release of energy may be so great that death and disruption from blast effects occur over a wide area. In contrast, terrorist devices, unless they contain very large amounts of explosive, rarely compare with military effectiveness and thus the pure blast effects are far more limited. However, such devices are often detonated within relatively confined spaces (e.g. subways and buses), influencing the subsequent pattern of injury caused. The energy generated by an explosion decreases rapidly as the distance from the epicentre increases.

When an explosion occurs, a chemical interaction results in the generation of huge volumes of gas, which are further expanded by the great heat that is also generated. This sudden generation of gas causes a compression wave to sweep outwards; at the origin, this is at many times the speed of sound.

The pure blast effects can cause either physical fragmentation or disruption of the victim or bomber solely from the effects of the wave of high pressure and hot gases striking the body. A minimum pressure of about 700 kPa (100 lb/inch^2) is needed for tissue damage in humans. There will also be pressure effects upon the viscera and these effects are far more damaging where there is an air–fluid interface, such as in the air passages, the lungs and the gut. Rupture and haemorrhage of these areas represent the classical blast lesion.

Although the primary effect of blast is large, in most cases many more casualties, fatal and otherwise, are caused by secondary effects of explosive devices, especially in the lower-powered terrorist bombs. These secondary effects include:

■ burns – directly from the near effects of the explosion and secondarily from fires started by the bomb;
■ missile injuries from parts of the bomb casing, contents or shrapnel or from adjacent objects;
■ peppering by small fragments of debris and dust propelled by the explosion;
■ various types of injury owing to collapse of structures as a result of the explosion;
■ injuries and death from vehicular damage or destruction, such as decompression, intrusion of occupant space, fire and ground impact of bombed aircraft and crash damage to cars, trucks, buses, etc.

The investigation of bombing is a huge, and technically complex exercise with a number of factors to be considered, including preservation of life and evacuating casualties, frequently confounding the

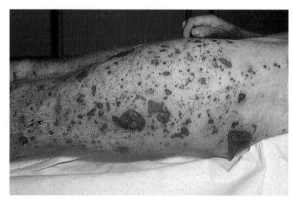

Figure 10.12 Multiple abrasions and lacerations caused by flying debris projected in a bomb blast.

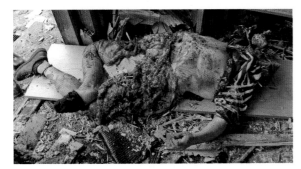

Figure 10.13 Massive disruption of the body of an individual who had constructed an explosive device.

required process of establishing a crime scene (or scenes) for the identification, sampling and preservation of evidence.

Examination of either the living or the dead following an explosion is essential, with careful documentation of the sites and sizes of all injuries. Post-mortem radiology is essential, in order to identify unexploded ordinance, and items comprising components of the explosive device. Identification of deceased individuals is important, not only ethically, but also to enable the relevant medico-legal authority to discharge their responsibilities. The identity of suicide bombers, whose bodies are frequently extensively disrupted following the explosion, may be extremely challenging (Figures 10.12 and 10.13).

■ Mass disasters and the doctor

Previously, transport incidents probably represented the most frequent setting for mass casualties and death. Increasingly, such a situation is just as likely to involve a terrorist incident. For the non-specialist doctor at the scene of a mass disaster of any kind, the first consideration is, of course, the treatment of casualties, which may involve taking difficult ethical decisions about triage. In 2006 the World Medical Association made recommendations for physicians faced with a mass disaster; these are outlined in Box 10.1.

Box 10.1 Recommended ethical principles and procedures with regard to the physician's role in disaster situations, from WMA statement 2006

1. Triage is a medical action of prioritizing treatment and management based on a rapid diagnosis and prognosis for each patient. Triage must be carried out systematically, taking into account the medical needs, medical intervention capabilities and available resources. Vital acts of reanimation may have to be carried out at the same time as triage. Triage may pose an ethical problem owing to the limited treatment resources immediately available in relation to the large number of injured persons in varying states of health.

2. Ideally, triage should be entrusted to authorized, experienced physicians or to physician teams, assisted by a competent staff.

3. The physician should separate patients into categories and then treat them in the following order, subject to national guidelines:

   a. Patients who can be saved but whose lives are in immediate danger should be given treatment straight away or as a matter of priority within the next few hours.

   b. Patients whose lives are not in immediate danger and who are in need of urgent but not immediate medical care should be treated next.

   c. Injured persons requiring only minor treatment can be treated later or by relief workers.

   d. Psychologically traumatized individuals who do not require treatment for bodily harm might need reassurance or sedation if acutely disturbed.

   e. Patients whose condition exceeds the available therapeutic resources, who suffer from extremely severe injuries such as irradiation or burns to such an extent and degree that they cannot be saved in the specific circumstances of time and place, or complex surgical cases requiring a particularly delicate operation which would take too long, thereby obliging the physician to make a choice between them and other patients may be classified as 'beyond emergency care'.

   f. As cases may evolve and thus change category, it is essential that the situation be regularly reassessed by the official in charge of the triage.

   The following statements apply to treatment beyond emergency care:

   g. It is ethical for a physician not to persist, at all costs, in treating individuals 'beyond emergency care', thereby wasting scarce resources needed elsewhere. The decision not to treat an injured person on account of priorities dictated by the disaster situation cannot be considered a failure to come to the assistance of a person in mortal danger. It is justified when it is intended to save the maximum number of individuals. However, the physician must show such patients compassion and respect for their dignity, for example by separating them from others and administering appropriate pain relief and sedatives.

   h. The physician must act according to the needs of patients and the resources available. He/she should attempt to set an order of priorities for treatment that will save the greatest number of lives and restrict morbidity to a minimum.

Reproduced from WMA Statement on Medical Ethics in the event of disasters. Revised by the WMA General Assembly, Pilanesberg, South Africa, October 2006. Copyright, World Medical Association.

The investigation of the causes of death, the causes of the incident (such as a bomb), and the identification of the dead, are specialist operations involving individuals from a wide variety of professional backgrounds, including those with expertise in the provision of emergency mortuary accommodation, pathologists, dentists, the police and the usual state agencies responsible for sudden death; in England and Wales this is the Coroner. A team of pathologists, assisted by police officers and mortuary staff, and backed up by dental and radiological facilities, inspects every body and records all clothing, jewellery and personal belongings still attached to the bodies. The body, or body part, is then carefully examined for every aspect of identity, including sex, race, height, age and personal characteristics. All these details are recorded on standard forms and charts and the information is sent back to the identification teams, who can compare this post-mortem information with ante-mortem information obtained from relatives, friends, etc. An internal post-mortem examination is usually performed to determine the cause of death, retrieve any foreign objects that, for example, may be related to an explosive device, and to seek any further identifying features, such as operation scars and prostheses.

■ Further information sources

Besant-Matthews P.E. Examination and interpretation of rifled firearm injuries, Chapter 4. In: Mason JK, Purdue BN (eds) *The Pathology of Trauma*, 3rd edn. London: Arnold, 2000; p. 47–60.

Breitenecker R. Shotgun wound patterns. *American Journal of Clinical Pathology* 1969; **52:** 258–69.

Cassidy M. Smooth-bore firearm injuries, Chapter 5. In: Mason JK, Purdue BN (eds) *The Pathology of Trauma*, 3rd edn. London: Arnold, 2000; p. 61–74.

Dana SE, DiMaio VJM. Gunshot trauma, Chapter 12. In: Payne-James JJ, Busuttil A, Smock W (eds) *Forensic Medicine – Clinical and Pathological Aspects*. London: Greenwich Medical Media, 2003; p. 149–68.

DiMaio VJM. *Gunshot Wounds: Practical Aspects of Firearms, Ballistics and Forensic Techniques*, 2nd edn, Boca Raton, FL: CRC Press, 1999.

Fackler ML. Wound ballistics. A review of common misconceptions. *Journal of the American Medical Association* 1988; **259:** 2730–6.

Karger B, Billeb E, Koops E, Brinkmann B. Autopsy features relevant for discrimination between suicidal and homicidal gunshot injuries. *International Journal of Legal Medicine* 2002; **116:** 273–8.

Marshall TK. Deaths from explosive devices. *Medicine, Science and the Law* 1976; **16:** 235–9.

Milroy CM, Clark JC, Carter N *et al*. Air weapon fatalities. *Journal of Clinical Pathology* 1998; **51:** 525–9.

Santucci RA, Chang YJ. Ballistics for physicians: myths about wound ballistics and gunshot wounds. *Journal of Urology* 2004; **171:** 1408–14.

Saukko P, Knight B. Gunshot and explosion deaths, Chapter 8. In: Saukko P, Knight B (eds) *Knight's Forensic Pathology*, 3rd edn. London: Arnold, 2004; p. 245–80.

Thali MJ, Kneubuehl BP, Zollinger U, Dirnhofer R. A study of the morphology of gunshot entrance wounds, in connection with their dynamic creation, utilising the 'skin–skull–brain' model. *Forensic Science International* 2002; **125:** 190–4.

Thali MJ, Kneubuehl BP, Dirnhofer R, Zollinger U. The dynamic development of the muzzle imprint by contact shot: high-speed documentation utilizing the 'skin–skull–brain model'. *Forensic Science International* 2002; **127:** 168–73.

Volgas DA, Stannard JP, Alonso JE. Ballistics: a primer for the surgeon. *Injury* 2005; **36:** 373–9.

Chapter 11

Use of force and restraint

Use of force

The need at certain times for restraint techniques to control groups of individuals or others who are violent or suffering from acute behavioural disturbance is one that requires a sensitive balance between duty of care and safety and security of those being restrained, and the type or means of restraint to secure that control. The term 'use of force continuum' refers to standards that provide law enforcement or security personnel (e.g. police or prison officers) with clear guidelines as to how much force may be used against a non-compliant subject in a given situation. The purpose of a defined 'use of force continuum' is to clarify for those restraining, those restrained and the public in general, the means by which control may be properly and appropriately achieved. Most police or law enforcement agencies will have a published policy which will vary in nature. Such policies will define appropriate actions in response to actual or perceived threat (e.g. verbal or physical violence) and other factors (e.g. safety of others, presence of weapons). Hand in hand with this recognition of the need for appropriate response is the development of less-lethal weapons that can incapacitate or control with less likelihood of a fatal outcome, such as baton rounds and conducted electrical weapons.

Conflict resolution

Any law enforcement officer involved in restraint control or public order setting should have an understanding of conflict resolution and the factors that will affect how individuals respond to certain threats or actions. It is important that all progression or escalation of force is seen to be reasonable in order that any adverse outcome may be justified at a later date. The offender behaviour is characterized in a number of ways from that of compliance, to verbal and gestured responses, passive resistance, active resistance, assault and aggression to the most serious category, aggravated aggression (which may involve the use of weapons). Many factors may affect the subsequent behaviour of an individual and how an officer responds (Box 11.1).

> **Box 11.1** Conflict resolution: factors affecting the behaviour of an individual and how an officer responds
>
> - Presence of an imminent danger
> - Comparative ages
> - Sex and size
> - Strength
> - Skills
> - Specialist knowledge
> - Presence of drugs or alcohol
> - Mental state
> - Relative position of disadvantage
> - Injury
> - Number of individual's involved
> - Whether weapons are present
> - Officer's overall perception of the situation

A wide variety of techniques, implements and weapons may be used for control and restraint. Some may cause injury and some, either through inappropriate use, or some other circumstance, may result in complications. Doctors, particularly forensic physicians and emergency medicine specialists may become involved in the assessment of the medical consequences of controlling or restraining people. This may be with respect to medical management and documentation of injuries. In some situations there is the potential for serious injury or even death. The principles involved in the documentation of any injury (see Chapter 8, p. 95) should apply as the techniques used may become the focus of attention in criminal or Coroner's court, civil claims or disciplinary hearings. The history from the injured person may need further clarification by direct communication with the restraining personnel concerned. Review of available CCTV or video recordings may be relevant.

■ 'Empty hands' – unarmed restraint

A variety of arm locks and holds, pressure-point control and knee and elbow strikes may be used. If excessive force is used, either directly by the officer or as a result of the restrained person moving, joints

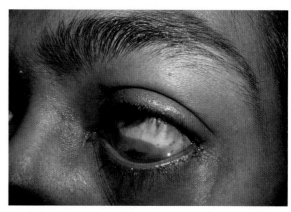

Figure 11.1 Scleral haemorrhage 2 hours after neck compression in a restraint setting.

such as the wrist, elbow or shoulder can be strained to varying degrees. Other soft tissue injuries may be found.

Neck hold and neck restraints are discouraged by law enforcement agencies in the UK, as there is believed to be a clear risk of serious injury or fatality from neck compression. This approach is not worldwide and a number of agencies train in specific types of neck hold. If an individual is restrained in such a hold the neck and head should be examined carefully for signs of injury. Examination for petechial bruising is mandatory in the skin of the head, neck, face, ears and scalp, the intraoral mucosa and the eyes (Figure 11.1; see also Chapter 15, p. 153). Clothing can be grabbed in a scuffle and the tightening, mock-ligature effect of this can cause linear or patchy type bruising around the neck.

Restraint asphyxia occurs as a result of the individual being held down and being unable to maintain adequate respiratory movement either because of the chest and/or the diaphragm being splinted. Risk factors include lying prone, inability to change position, obesity.

■ Handcuffs

Three main means of handcuffing individuals exist: traditional handcuffs with two wrist pieces connected by a short chain; rigid cuffs whereby the two wrist pieces are connected by a bar and cannot move in relation to each other; and plasticuffs – in effect larger size cable ties which are easy to store and easy to apply but less secure than the first two types. The fixed connecting bar

11 Use of force and restraint

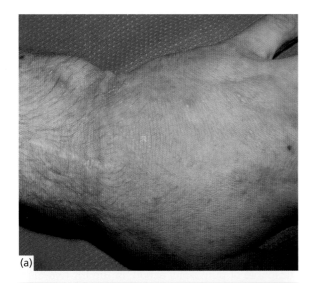

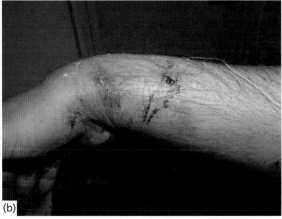

Figure 11.2 Handcuff injuries. **(a)** Imprint of handcuff following tight, prolonged application; **(b)** bruise, abrasion, laceration and underlying ulnar fracture following struggle after handcuff applied.

of the rigid handcuffs allows controlled application of force across the wrist to gain control. Once applied, simple pressure against the wrist allows the single bar of the cuffs to release over the top of the wrist and close with a ratchet mechanism. If the individual is non-compliant and continues moving the handcuffs can progressively tighten causing increasing pain and potentially increasing the risk of neurological and skin damage. A number of injuries may be caused by handcuff application. Soft tissue injuries may be produced by movement of the wrist within the handcuff, movement of the handcuff on the wrist or by the handcuff being too tight. The commonest injuries are blunt force injuries of reddening, abrasions and bruising, particularly to the radial and ulnar borders of the wrists. Superficial cuts, from the edge

of the cuff, may be present in the same locations. Numbness or hyperaesthesia in the distribution of the cutaneous nerves distal to the applied cuff are not uncommon. Specific handcuff neuropathies may be caused and single or multiple nerves may be affected, the extent being determined by a number of factors including the tightness of compression, the length of time compression has occurred and the degree of resistance by the detainee.

In most cases the damaged nerves fully recover within a few weeks. Persistence of symptoms may require nerve conduction studies.

It is rare for handcuffs to cause fractures of the wrists secondary to the use of handcuffs. However, they should be considered when there is marked tenderness, loss of movement or extensive bruising. The most vulnerable parts of the wrist are the styloid processes, particularly on the ulna (Figure 11.2).

■ Batons

Law enforcement and security agencies commonly use batons to gain control. In the UK, three baton types are in general issue: the three-part gravity friction lock baton made of steel (an expandable baton with two telescopic tubes that extend to a locked format with the flick of the user's wrists (e.g. ASP) (Figure 11.3), an acrylic patrol baton (APB), which is available in three lengths – 22, 24 and 26 inches (approximately 56, 61 and 66 cm), and rarely now, a 15-inch (38 cm) wooden patrol baton. Batons can be used for defensive and offensive activities: the long portion can be used for a direct strike, the baton can be held at both grip and long end and used to push back an individual and both ends can be used to the front and back to jab against someone else. The potential for injury will vary with the amount of energy transferred in a baton strike. The heavier, expandable baton will potentially cause more injury than the lighter standard patrol baton. Batons used in crowd control situations are heavier still and even more likely to cause significant injury.

When batons are deployed there are certain body targets that are classified into low, medium and high risk of injury areas. Areas of low injury potential (and thus primary targets) are legs (in the areas of the common peroneal, femoral and tibial nerves) and arms (in the areas of the radial and median nerves). Anticipated possible medical complications of strikes in these areas include transitory bruising

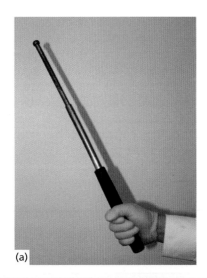

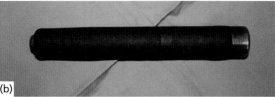

(a)

(b)

Figure 11.3 ASP baton. **(a)** Fully extended and **(b)** non-extended expandable.

of the target area and transitory motor dysfunction of the affected limb. The medium injury potential areas (and therefore not primary targets) are knees and ankles, wrist, elbow, hands, upper arms and the clavicles. Anticipated possible medical complications include bone fractures, dislocation and soft tissue damage. Higher injury potential areas (and which should not be targeted) are the head, neck/throat, spine, loins (kidneys) and abdomen (small

bowel, stomach, liver, pancreas). Anticipated complications include damage to vital organs, which could lead to serious injury or fatalities. Injuries from a baton strike will embrace the range of blunt force injury including bruising, in particular tramline bruising. Circular patterned bruising can occur as a result of someone being struck by the end of the baton (Figure 11.4). Lacerations may be caused by baton blows over bony surfaces. Fractures are rare but can occur, for example from direct impact to the ulna.

■ Incapacitant sprays

Incapacitant sprays use a variety of agents to render individuals or groups of individuals temporarily incapable of purposeful action. In the UK two main incapacitant sprays are used by police services – CS and PAVA.

The active ingredient of CS incapacitant spray, o–chlorobenzylidine malonitrile, is a solid at room temperature but is dissolved in an organic solvent – methyl iso–butyl ketone (MIBK) – to be used as a liquid aerosol. This is used to spray the face of a person from up to 3–4 m away, delivering CS to the eyes, nose and mouth causing immediate irritation to the eyes, upper respiratory tract and skin (Figure 11.5). The main symptoms are lacrimation, eye pain, blepharospasm, conjunctival reddening and photophobia; stinging or burning in the mouth; pain in the nose, sneezing, coughing, and rarely other respiratory symptoms similar to asthma attacks. The skin will experience a burning sensation and reddening. In most cases the symptoms and signs are short-lived, resolving over 15–30 minutes. About 10% of people sprayed are not

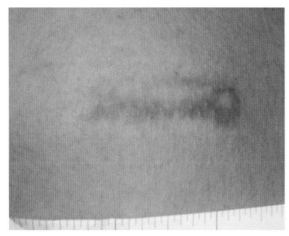

Figure 11.4 Baton imprint.

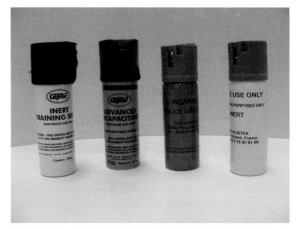

Figure 11.5 Example of CS spray containers.

incapacitated by exposure. It is not possible to predict who will respond and who will not.

PAVA (pelargonic acid vanillylamide) spray is the synthetic equivalent of capsaicin (the active ingredient of natural pepper). It is intended to be directed towards the eyes where it causes extreme discomfort and closure. Less research has been done on PAVA spray, but the effects, treatment and management are similar to those of CS spray. Effects on eyes, respiratory system, mouth or skin that last for > 6 hours should generally be referred for specialist assessment. The most important action is to stop continued exposure by removal of the effected individual from the contaminated environment to a well-ventilated area, preferably with a free flow of air and removal of contaminated clothing. Each exposed individual should be fully examined with particular reference to eyes, oral and nasal cavity, respiratory system and skin.

■ Baton rounds and plastic bullets

Baton rounds or plastic bullets (the names are used interchangeably) refer to assorted devices that are intended to incapacitate but not kill (Figure 11.6). Baton rounds have two roles: public order and as another option to the use of conventional firearms against individuals armed with bladed weapons. For use in public order role, the normal operating range is 20–40 m. For use as a less lethal alternative to firearms, it may be used at 1 m range. Because of their size and profile they are only accurate at short

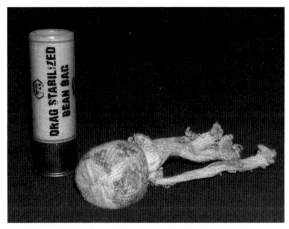

Figure 11.7 Bean bag round.

distances and the projectiles are prone to tumble after discharge, decreasing their accuracy. Deaths from baton rounds are very uncommon and principally result from head and chest trauma. Impact to the lower torso and limbs results in bruising, abrasions and occasionally skin lacerations. There is a very low reported frequency of intra-abdominal trauma. Fractures to limbs do occur occasionally. The chest is regarded as a vulnerable area and although the system has been designed to avoid impact to this region, these may occasionally occur in operational practice; rib fracture and pulmonary contusion may occur. In order to minimize serious complications guidelines on firing must be adhered to. Bean bag (flexible baton) projectiles have also been deployed (Figure 11.7). The baton round currently deployed in the UK is the Attenuating Energy Projectile. They are currently used very rarely.

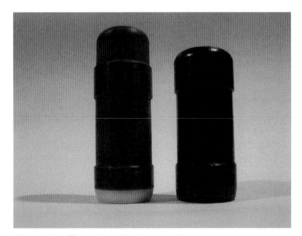

Figure 11.6 Examples of baton rounds.

■ Dogs

Trained dogs from law enforcement agencies are capable of restraining and detaining individuals who need to be controlled. In some cases dogs can bite. These all require medical assessment as there may be, dependent on the site and degree of injury, risk of infection, neurological or vascular injury. In some circumstances bites may of such a degree that soft tissue defects requiring surgical intervention may be created. On occasions, there may be dispute about the source of bite injury and a forensic odontologist may be required to provide a definitive opinion.

■ Conducted electrical weapons

Conducted electrical weapons (or conducted energy devices) have been developed and are part of the use of force continuum with a specific aim of providing a less lethal option of incapacitation. The most widely used by law enforcement agencies is the Taser (Thomas A Swift's Electrical Rifle) developed around three decades ago. The Taser® X26™ (Taser International, Inc., Scottsdale, AZ, USA) generates a 19 Hz, 5-second train of 100-µ second electrical pulses (Figure 11.8). These pulses are delivered to the body either by two propelled barbs (which embed in clothing or skin but remain connected to the handset by conductive wire) or by direct contact of the handset's electrodes (drive-stun). The effect of the discharge depends on the mode of use. Because of the small separation of the electrodes in drive-stun mode, the principal action of the Taser® is to induce pain. When the barbs are propelled, the greater barb separation allows the discharge to induce involuntary (and

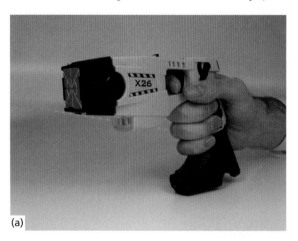
(a)

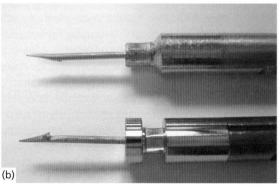
(b)

Figure 11.8 **(a)** Taser® X26™ and **(b)** barbs.

painful) contraction of skeletal muscle that results in temporary immobilization. Such effects are almost instantaneous with only a slightly slower recovery.

The neuromuscular stimulation caused by the electrical current is painful and fatiguing. The barbs can penetrate bare skin to a maximum depth of 0.6 cm and are easily removed by supporting the skin around the barb and applying gentle traction. A case has been reported which shows that a Taser® barb can penetrate the skull and injure the meninges and underlying brain. A Taser® injury around the orbits should raise the suspicion of a penetrating ocular injury. Any suspicion of such an injury requires referral to an ophthalmic surgeon as a matter of urgency. In such cases, removal of the Taser® barb may be required in an operating theatre under general anaesthesia. 'Electrical' cataract has been documented following use of Tasers. Secondary injury may result if a Tasered individual falls in a semi-controlled fashion as a result of their generalized involuntary muscular contractions. This can lead to soft tissue injuries, such as bruising or abrasions, but an uncontrolled fall from other situations or onto other objects has caused more serious injuries, including fatal head injuries. Rhabdomyolysis has been reported. Vertebral compression fractures have been documented following Taser® discharge, caused by either muscle contraction or fall. There is a potential risk of damage or disturbance to implanted electrical devices such as a pacemaker which may misinterpret electrical signals. A newer extended range device is now available – the Taser® XREP™ cartridge which is a self-contained, wireless electronic control device (ECD) that deploys from a 12-gauge pump-action shotgun. It is supposed to deliver a similar neuromuscular bioeffect as the Taser® X26™ but can be delivered to a maximum effective range of 100 feet (30.48 m), combining blunt impact force (Figure 11.9).

Such devices can assist in the safe and proper enforcement of law. However, it is important that any current and new technologies being introduced as less lethal options are appropriately and robustly tested and scrutinized in a scientifically credible manner to reassure a sometimes appropriately cynical and sceptical general public. Unfortunately, some devices are deployed without appropriate review.

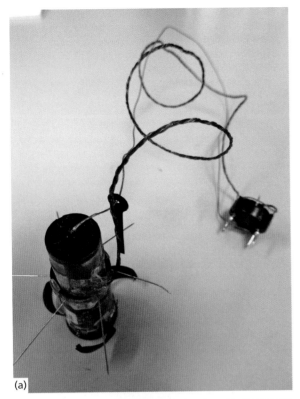

(a)

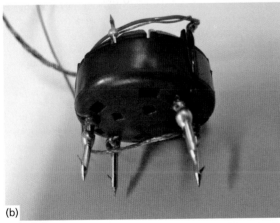

(b)

Figure 11.9 **(a)** Taser® XREP™ contact device and **(b)** projectile.

■ Further information sources

Amnesty International report no. AMR 51/146/2008. List of deaths following use of stun weapons in US law enforcement. http://www.amnestyusa.org/uploads/ListOfDeaths.pdf (accessed 28 February 2011).

Armstrong EJ. Distinctive patterned injuries caused by an expandable baton. *Am J Forensic Med Pathol* 2005; **2:** 186–8.

Blain PG. Tear gases and irritant incapacitants. 1-chloroacetophenone, 2-chlorobenzylidene malononitrile and dibenz[b,f]-1,4-oxazepine. *Toxicol Rev* 2003; **22(2):** 103–10.

Bleetman A, Steyn R, Lee C. Introduction of the Taser into British policing. Implications for UK emergency departments: an overview of electronic weaponry. *Emerg Med J* 2004; **21(2):** 136–40.

Bozeman WP, Hauda WE 2nd, Heck JJ, Graham DD Jr, Martin BP, Winslow JE. Safety and injury profile of conducted electrical weapons used by law enforcement officers against criminal suspects. *Ann Emerg Med* 2009; **53(4):** 480–9.

Bui ET, Sourkes M, Wennberg R. Generalized tonic-clonic seizure after a Taser shot to the head. *CMAJ* 2009; **180:** 625–6.

Carron P-N, Yersin B. Management of the effects of exposure to tear gas. *BMJ* 2009; **338:** 1554–8.

Chan TC, Vilke GM, Neuman T, Clausen JL. Restraint position and positional asphyxia. *Annals of Emergency Medicine* 1997; **30:** 578–586.

Chariot P, Ragot F, Authier FJ, Questel F, Diamant-Berger O. Focal neurological complications of handcuff application. *J Forensic Sci* 2001; **46(5):** 1124–5.

Chute DJ, Smialek JE. Injury patterns in a plastic (AR-1) baton fatality. *Am J Forensic Med Pathol* 1998; **19(3):** 226–9.

Cook AA. Handcuff neuropathy among U.S. prisoners of war from Operation Desert Storm. *Mil Med* 1993; **158(4):** 253–4.

de Brito D, Challoner KR, Sehgal A, Mallon W. The injury pattern of a new law enforcement weapon: the police bean bag. *Ann Emerg Med* 2001; **38(4):** 383–90.

Emson HE. Death in a restraint jacket from mechanical asphyxia. Canadian *Medical Association Journal* 1994; **151:** 985–987.

Euripidou E, MacLehose R, Fletcher A. An investigation into the short term and medium term health impacts of personal incapacitant sprays. A follow up of patients reported to the National Poisons Information Service. *Emerg Med J* 2004; **21;** 548–552.

Forrester MB, Stanley SK. The epidemiology of pepper spray exposures reported in Texas in 1998-2002. *Vet Hum Toxicol* 2003; **45(6):** 327–30.

Grant AC, Cook AA. A prospective study of handcuff neuropathies. *Muscle Nerve* 2000; **23(6):** 933–8.

Haileyesus T, Annest JL, Mercy JA. Non-fatal conductive energy device-related injuries treated in US emergency departments, 2005-2008. *Inj Prev.* 2011; **Jan 21.** [Epub ahead of print]

Han JS, Chopra A, Carr D. Ophthalmic injuries from a Taser. *CJEM* 2009; 11: 90–93.

Ho JD, Dawes DM, Bultman LL *et al.* Respiratory effect of prolonged electrical weapon application on human volunteers. *Acad Emerg Med* 2007; **14:** 197–201.

Hughes D, Maguire K, Dunn F *et al.* Plastic baton round injuries. *Emerg Med J* 2005; **22;** 111–112.

Karagama YG et al. Short-term and long-term physical effects of exposure to CS spray. *JRSM* 2003; **96:** 172–174.

Kobayashi M, Mellen PF. Rubber bullet injury: case report with autopsy observation and literature review. *Am J Forensic Med Pathol* 2009; **30(3):** 262–7.

Kroll MW. Physiology and pathology of Taser® electronic control devices. *J Forensic Leg Med* 2009; **16:** 173–177.

Maguire K, Hughes DM, Fitzpatrick MS *et al.* Injuries caused by the attenuated energy projectile: the latest less lethal option. *Emerg Med J* 2007; **24(2):** 103–5.

McGorrigan J, Payne-James JJ. Incapacitant Sprays: Clinical Effects and management: Recommendations for Healthcare Professionals. http://fflm.ac.uk/upload/documents/1265990238.pdf (accessed 28 2 2011).

Ng W, Chehade M. Taser penetrating ocular injury. *Am J Ophthalmol* 2005; **139(4):** 713–5.

O'Brien AJ, McKenna BG, Thom K, Diesfeld K, Simpson AI. Use of Tasers on people with mental illness; a New Zealand database study. *Int J Law Psychiatry* 2011; **34**(1): 39–43.

Olivas T, Jones B, Canulla M. Abdominal wall penetration by a police "bean bag". Am Surg. 2001 May; **67**(5): 407–9.

Parkes J. Sudden death during restraint: a study to measure the effect of restraint positions on the rate of recovery from exercise. *Medicine, Science and the Law* 2000; **40:** 39–44.

Payne-James J, Sheridan B, Smith G. Medical implications of the Taser. *BMJ* 2010 22; 340.

Payne-James JJ. Restraint injuries and crowd control agents. In: Rogers D, Norfolk G, Stark M (eds). *Good Practice Guidelines for Forensic Medical Examiners* 2nd Edition. London: Metropolitan Police Service, 2008.

Pollanen MS, Chiasson DA, Cairns JT, Young JG. Unexpected death related to restraint for excited delirium: a retrospective study of death in police custody and in the community. *Canadian Medical Association Journal* 1998. **158:** 1603–1607.

Pudiak CM, Bozarth MA (1994) Cocaine fatalities increased by restraint stress. Life Science 55: 379–382.

Reay DT, Eisele JW. Death from law enforcement neck holds. *Am J Forensic Med Pathol* 1982; **3**(3): 253–8.

Reay DT, Holloway GA Jr. Changes in carotid blood flow produced by neck compression. *Am J Forensic Med Pathol* 1982; **3**(3): 199–202.

Rehman TU, Yonas H, Marinaro J. Intracranial penetration of a Taser dart. *Am J Emerg Med* 2007; **25:** 733.

Rezende-Neto J, Silva FD, Porto LB *et al.* Penetrating injury to the chest by an attenuated energy projectile: a case report and literature review of thoracic injuries caused by "less-lethal" munitions. *World J Emerg Surg* 2009; **26:** 4–26.

Roberts A, Nokes L, Leadbeatter S, Pike H. Impact characteristics of two types of police baton. *Forensic Sci Int* 1994; **67**(1): 49–53.

Roggla G, Roggla M. Death in a hobble restraint. *Canadian Medical Association Journal* 1999; **161:** 21.

Ross DL. Factors associated with excited delirium deaths in police custody. *Modern Pathology* 1998; **11:** 1127–1137.

Ross EC. Death by restraint: horror stories continue, but best practices are also being identified. *Behavior and Health Tomorrow* 1999; **8:** 21–23.

Smith J, Greaves I. The use of chemical incapacitant sprays: a review. *J Trauma* 2002; 52(3): 595–600.

Southward RD. CS incapacitant spray. *J Accid Emerg Med* 2000; **17:** 76.

Strote J, Range Hutson H. Taser use in restraint-related deaths. *Prehosp Emerg Care* 2006; **10**(4): 447–50.

Strote J, Walsh M, Angelidis M, Basta A, Hutson HR. Conducted electrical weapon use by law enforcement: an evaluation of safety and injury. *J Trauma* 2010; **68(5):** 1239–46.

Vilke GM, Sloane CM, Suffecool A *et al.* Physiologic effects of the TASER after exercise. *Acad Emerg Med* 2009; **16:** 1–7.

Wahl P, Schreyer N, Yersin B. Injury pattern of the Flash-Ball, a less-lethal weapon used for law enforcement: report of two cases and review of the literature. *J Emerg Med* 2006; **31**(3): 325–30.

Walter RJ, Dennis AJ, Valentino DJ *et al.* TASER X26 discharges in swine produce potentially fatal ventricular arrhythmias. *Acad Emerg Med* 2008; **15:** 66–73.

Watson K, Rycroft R. Unintended cutaneous reactions to CS spray. *Contact Dermatitis* 2005; **53**(1): 9–13.

Weir E. The health impact of crowd control agents. *Canadian Medical Association Journal* 2001; **164(13):** 1889–1890.

Worthington E, Nee Patrick A. CS- exposure – clinical effects and management. *J Accid Emerg Med* 1999; **16:** 168–170.

Chapter 12

Sexual assault

Introduction

Adults and children, males and females may all be victims of sexual assault. Most victims are female but a large minority, perhaps 10%, are male. Sexual assault occurs within families or may be by strangers and may be associated with crimes against humanity, war crimes and genocide. Over 40 000 serious sexual crime (rape, sexual assault and sexual offences against children) were identified by the British Crime Survey 2009–10. These figures almost certainly underestimate the true incidence of such events and represent an increase on the previous survey period.

Examination requirements

It is important the complainants of sexual assault are examined by competent, sympathetic sexual offence examiners; these are generally physicians with a special interest in forensic aspects of medicine. Complainants (and suspects of sexual assault) should be offered the choice of a doctor of their own gender. Sexual Assault Referral Centres (SARCs) – specialist centres for assessment of complainants of rape and other forms of sexual assault – are being created in most countries. They provide appropriate assessment and sampling following the initial assault, and post-assault care with regard to issues such as genitourinary health, contraception and counselling. Emergency contraception may involve use of the oral contraceptive or insertion of an intrauterine device. Prevention of sexually transmitted infection, for which there is a huge range of potential risk, will require appropriate prescribed medication for which standard prophylactic/therapeutic regimens will apply. Infection by the human immunodeficiency virus (HIV) is of great concern and specialist advice may need to be sought regarding post-exposure prophylaxis. Hepatitis B is a significant risk following male rape and that risk increases with additional factors such as multiple assailants, intravenous (IV) drug use, or high prevalence area.

Many SARCs also allow complainants who do not wish to involve the authorities immediately to provide anonymized assessment and collection of samples, so that a complainant may later proceed with police investigation if they change their mind.

Definitions and the law

Each jurisdiction had its own laws or statutes relating to sexual assault. In England and Wales the Sexual Offences Act 2003 applies. Key definitions and offences from this Act are listed in Box 12.1. The Act defines numerous other offences including, for example 'rape and other offences against a child under 13' (see also Chapter 13, p. 138).

Box 12.1 Key definitions of offences under the Sexual Offences Act 2003 (England and Wales)

Section 1: definition of the act of 'rape'

A person (A) commits an offence [of rape] if:
- he intentionally penetrates the vagina, anus or mouth of another person (B) with his penis,
- B does not consent to the penetration, and
- A does not reasonably believe that B consents.

A person found guilty of rape under this section is liable, on conviction on indictment, to imprisonment for life.

Section 2: definition of the offence of 'assault by penetration'

A person (A) commits an offence if:
- he intentionally penetrates the vagina or anus of another person (B) with a part of his body or anything else,
- the penetration is sexual,
- B does not consent to the penetration, and
- A does not reasonably believe that B consents.

A person guilty of an offence under this section is liable, on conviction on indictment, to imprisonment for life.

Section 3: definition of 'sexual assault'

A person (A) commits an offence if:
- he intentionally touches another person (B),
- the touching is sexual,
- (B) does not consent to the touching, and
- (A) does not reasonably believe that (B) consents.

A person guilty of an offence under this section is liable:
- (a) on summary conviction, to imprisonment for a term not exceeding 6 months or a fine not exceeding the statutory maximum, or both;
- (b) on conviction or indictment, to imprisonment for a term not exceeding 10 years.

Medical assessment

Medical assessments of sexual assault complainants and suspects are to identify and treat injury or other risk issues (e.g. infection), and to identify and collect evidence that may assist the courts to establish the facts of the case. The medical and scientific evidence may help confirm, or corroborate, the account of either the complainant or suspect. In many cases the medical evidence is neutral and the issue of consent is the determination the court has to make.

In some cases the need for urgent medical care because of injury overrides the immediate need for a sexual assault examination. Healthcare aspects have priority. Wherever possible, examinations should be undertaken at the earliest opportunity in order to ensure best opportunities for evidential sampling.

It is essential that the examining doctor explains the nature, purpose and process of the assessment in order that consent is fully informed and that chaperones are used when appropriate. An assessment requires a detailed history and examination. The history of the alleged assault from the complainant is an extremely important part of the assessment. The doctor should ensure that they record the briefing details from the referring police team, and then record verbatim the account of the complainant themselves, as discrepancies may become very significant at a later stage of any legal proceedings. Apart from a general medical history, detail of the full history of events and any specific physical contacts must be identified (e.g. penis to mouth, mouth to genitalia, penis to anus, penis to vulva/vagina, ejaculation, object/implement penetration of mouth/vulva/vagina/anus, kissing/licking/biting/sucking/spitting).

Recent drug and alcohol intake must be recorded in as much detail as possible and this may be relevant in terms of ability to recall events appropriately or if there is a possibility of drugs or alcohol having been administered in possible cases of drug-facilitated sexual assault.

Specific questions are also asked about events after the assault as these may affect subsequent findings or recovery of evidence. Such questions include 'Since the assault have you... noted pain... noted bleeding... brushed teeth... passed urine... defaecated... douched?' A full medical history must include past medical history, past surgical history, past gynaecological history, menstrual history and past psychiatric history so that, if necessary, any influence of these on examination findings can be considered. Previous sexual history should not generally be relevant, but it is important to enquire sensitively about recent sexual activity before the alleged assault and sexual activity after the assault. The appropriateness of the need for this information is still subject to some debate. Based on this history, an appropriate examination can be undertaken to collect appropriate evidential samples.

The nature of the examination of the adult in sexual assault cases is determined in part by the history elicited, in that certain points may direct an examiner to areas of particular interest. The following should always be documented: weight, height, general appearance, skin abnormalities of changes (e.g. scars, tattoos, piercing) and appearance of the hair (e.g. dyed, shaved).

A standard general physical examination will be done and a detailed physical, external examination identifying injury or abnormality and recording absence of injury and abnormality. This examination will be documented on body diagrams and images of abnormalities should be taken. The external examination will focus on those areas that the history indicated as having been in general or particular physical contact, as these are particular areas where trace evidential materials that may provide DNA or other links may be found.

The genito-anal examination may be undertaken by naked eye, or with the assistance of specialist lighting, magnification or colposcopes. Examination of a female complainant (dependent in part on the history) will record the presence of any abnormalities or the absence of any findings in the following anatomical sites: thighs, buttocks and perineum; pubic area; pubic hair; labia majora; labia minora; clitoris; posterior fourchette; fossa navicularis; vestibule; hymen; urethral opening; vagina and cervix. For the male (suspect or complainant) the buttocks, thighs, perineum, anus, perianal area, testes, scrotum and penis (including shaft, glans and coronal sulcus) will be examined.

■ Evidential samples and documentation of findings

Appropriate samples in sexual assault will assist in determining the nature of sexual contact, the gender and possibly identity of the assailant and possible links with other offences. Samples that may be required include blood (for DNA and drugs and alcohol), urine; hair (head and pubic), nails and swab samples from body orifices, mouth, ears, nose and genitalia, including vulva, vagina, cervix, penis, anal canal and rectum. Appropriate sample kits, assembled with appropriate quality control, for particular areas of the body should be used wherever possible (Figure 12.1). Sampling must conform

to agreed protocols and a clear chain of custody (see Chapter 23, p. 218) established.

Table 12.1 summarizes the type of sample and what may be achieved from analysis of such a sample. In all cases if uncertain, confirm with forensic science laboratories (1) the type of specimen required and (2) how it should be stored to ensure optimum preservation. Samples should be taken in the light of the known history and accounts of events. If there is any doubt whether a particular sample may be relevant it is better to take a sample and retain it for later analysis. In the case of a suspect the doctor should advise the police investigators regarding samples as legal requirements will need to be observed in order to appropriately request samples. Control swabs may be required, depending on local laboratory protocols and standard operating procedures.

The persistence of evidentially relevant materials is variable and advice should be sought from a forensic scientist or forensic toxicologist when considering whether a sample is relevant to take. In general, foreign biological fluids (e.g. semen) can be detected in the mouth up to about 48 hours after contact, in the anus or rectum up to about 3 days and in the vagina or endocervix up to about 7 days.

As with all forensic assessments, documentation should be thorough, legible and meticulous, recording relevant positive and negative findings. Documentation of finding should be in written form (ideally using standardized proforma), with body diagrams accompanying all written notes. Wherever possible, photographic images should be taken of all abnormalities, under the direction of the doctor, with colour bars and rules in all images. If colposcopy has been used for genito-anal assessment, photographic

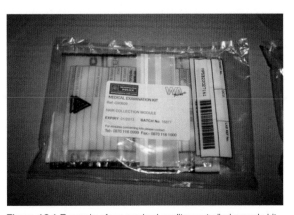

Figure 12.1 Example of pre-packed quality controlled sample kit.

Table 12.1 Type of sample taken and what may identified by analysis

Sample type	What may be identified by analysis
Blood	Presence and amount of alcohol and drugs; identify DNA
Urine	Presence and amount of alcohol and drugs
Hair (head), cut and combed	Identify biological fluids (wet and dry); foreign material (e.g. vegetation, glass, paint, fibres); comparison with other hairs found on body; past history of drug use
Hair (pubic), cut and combed	Identify biological fluids (wet and dry); foreign material (e.g. vegetation, glass, fibres); comparison with other hairs found on body; past history of drug use (prescribed; licit and illicit)
Buccal scrape	DNA profiling
Skin swabs (at sites of contact)	Identify biological fluids (e.g. semen, saliva – wet and dry); cellular material; lubricant (e.g. KY, Vaseline)
Mouth swabs	Identify semen
Mouth rinse	Identify semen
Vulval swab	Identify biological fluids (e.g. semen, saliva); foreign material (e.g. hairs, vegetation, fibres)
Low vaginal swab	Identify body fluids (e.g. semen, saliva); foreign material (e.g. hairs, vegetation, fibres); identify biological fluids (e.g. semen, saliva); foreign material (e.g. hairs, vegetation, fibres)
High vaginal swab	Body fluids (e.g. semen, saliva); foreign material (e.g. hairs, vegetation, glass, fibres); identify biological fluids (e.g. semen, saliva); foreign material (e.g. hairs, vegetation, fibres)
Endocervical swab	Identify biological fluids (e.g. semen)
Penile swabs (shaft, glans, coronal sulcus)	Identify biological fluids (e.g. semen)
Perianal swabs	Identify biological fluids (e.g. semen)
Anal swabs	Identify biological fluids (e.g. semen)
Rectal swabs	Identify biological fluids (e.g. semen)
Fingernail swabs, cuttings or scraping	Identify foreign material (e.g. skin cells), matching of broken nails

or video recordings (e.g. DVD) may be used. Most jurisdictions will have guidelines for the safe custody and viewing of such sensitive images.

■ Medical findings after sexual contact

Interpretation of findings, unlike the assessment and documentation of findings, should only be undertaken by a doctor experienced in such assessments and fully aware of current research concerning physical findings after sexual assault. It is incorrectly assumed by many that sexual assaults will result in injury to the victim whether adult or child. This is incorrect and in the majority of cases medical abnormalities (in both adults and children) will be absent. Conversely, consensual sexual activity can result in injury to the body and genitalia. The presence or absence of injuries in association with allegations of sexual assault do not by themselves indicate whether the particular activity

was consensual or non-consensual, and it is essential that these facts are understood when reporting and interpreting findings.

Many factors may affect the severity of injury in the female. Similar injuries may be seen in both consensual and non-consensual sexual contact. Some of the factors that may influence the possibility of genital injury are age of the complainant, type of sexual activity, relative positions of the participants and degree of intoxication of either or both of the participants. Consensual insertion or attempts at insertion of a finger or fingers, penis or any other object into the vagina may result in bruises, abrasions and lacerations of the labia majora, labia minora, hymen and posterior fourchette. Consensual digital vaginal penetration may result in accidental fingernail damage or injury to parts of the female genital tract that may not be noticed at the time.

Non-genital injury of even a minor nature can often be very significant evidentially and corroborate accounts of assault. Marks of blunt contact (e.g. punches, kicks), restraint (e.g. ties around wrists or

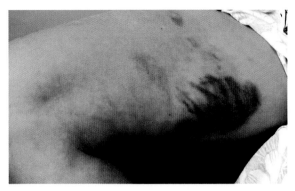

Figure 12.2 Example of non-genital injury: bruising caused by hand applied to force thighs apart.

ankles, grip marks) and bite marks are all examples of non-genital injuries seen in sexual assault complainants (Figure 12.2). Occasionally, false allegations do occur and analysis of the character and nature of the injury in the light of the accounts given is crucial in determining whether there may be any suggestion of deliberate self-harm (see Chapter 8, p. 91).

Anal intercourse is part of the normal sexual repertoire of many heterosexual and homosexual couples. Consensual anal intercourse can (in the same way as vaginal sex) be pain and discomfort free and would not normally leave any residual injury. Non-consensual anal intercourse if done without force, with or without lubrication and without physical resistance on the part of the person being penetrated may leave no residual injury and may be pain free. The effects of drugs and alcohol may make penetration easier. The likelihood of pain or injury in non-consensual anal intercourse may be increased:

- in someone who has not experienced anal intercourse
- in the absence of lubrication
- if force is used
- if there is great disparity between the size of the anus (which varies little in the adult) and the penis (which may vary a lot).

The types of injury include bruises, fissures or tears. In the absence of repeated trauma, any fissures, tears or lacerations would be expected to heal within 2 weeks or so and leave no residual marks. It is important for any examining doctor to be aware of, or to be able to distinguish, abnormalities caused by medical conditions that may mimic, or be mimicked by injury after sexual contact.

Care after sexual assault

Care of those who have been sexually assaulted is most appropriately managed by those with specialist skills such as genitourinary medicine specialists who can provide the most appropriate and up to date post-assault treatment and advice. It should be the responsibility of the examining doctor or healthcare professional to ensure that appropriate post-assault prophylaxis against pregnancy, or HIV or other genitourinary conditions are anticipated. Counselling or psychological support may also be required to support victims. Proactive support should be offered and follow-up should be provided so that vulnerable individuals do not have the problems associated with the initial assault compounded by poor or absent care later.

Further information sources

Ahmed SM, Volpellier M, Forster G. The use of the super accelerated hepatitis B vaccination regimen in a north London sexual assault referral centre. *Journal of Forensic and Legal Medicine* 2007; **14:** 72–4.

Anderson SL, Parker BJ, Bourgignon CM. Changes in genital injury patterns over time in women after consensual intercourse. *Journal of Forensic and Legal Medicine* 2008; **15:** 306–11.

Avegno J, Mills TJ, Mills LD. Sexual assault victims in the emergency department: analysis by demographic and event characteristics. *Journal of Emergency Medicine* 2009; **37:** 328–334.

Bakhru A, Mallinger JB, Fox MC. Postexposure prophylaxis for victims of sexual assault: treatments and attitudes of emergency department physicians. *Contraception* 2010; **82:** 163–73.

Bechtel LK, Holstege CP. Criminal poisoning: drug facilitated sexual assault. *Emergency Medicine Clinics of North America* 2007; **25:** 499–525.

Beh P and Payne-James JJ. Adult sexual assault. In: Gall J, Payne-James JJ (eds) *Current Practice in Forensic Medicine*. London: Wiley, 2011.

Burger C, Olson M, Dykstra D, Jones JS, Rossman L. What happens at the 72 hour mark? Physical findings in sexual assault cases when victims delay 2009 reporting. *Annals of Emergency Medicine* 2009; **54:** S93.

Eckert LO, Sugar N, Fine D. Factors impacting injury documentation after sexual assault: role of examiner experience and gender. *American Journal of Obstetrics and Gynecology* 2004; **190:** 1739–46.

Hall P, Innes J. Violent and sexual crime. In: *Crime in England and Wales 2009/10. Findings of the British Crime Survey and Police Recorded Crime*. London, Home Office, 2010;

http://rds.homeoffice.gov.uk/rds/pdfs10/hosb1210chap3.pdf (accessed 23 November 2010).

Fleming RI, Harbison S. The use of bacteria for the identification of vaginal secretions. *Forensic Science International: Genetics* 2010; **4:** 311–15.

Gallion HR, Dupree LJ, Scott TA, Arnold DH. Diagnosis of *Trichomonas vaginalis* and adolescents evaluated for possible sexual abuse: a comparison of the InPouch TV culture method and wet mount microscopy. *Journal of Pediatric and Adolescent Gynecology* 2009; **22:** 300–5.

Girardet RG, Lemme G, Biason TA, Bolton K, Lahoti S. HIV post-exposure prophylaxis in children and adolescents presenting for reported sexual assault. *Child Abuse and Neglect* 2009; **33:** 173–8.

Grossin C, Sibille I, de la Grandmaison GL, Banasr A, Brion F, Durigon M. Analysis of 418 cases of sexual assault. *Forensic Science International* 2003; **131**, 125–30.

Häkkänen-Nyholm H, Repo-Tiihonen E, Lindberg N, Salenius S, Weizmann-Henelius G. Finnish sexual homicides: offence and offender characteristics. *Forensic Science International* 2009; **188:** 125–30.

Hall JA, Moore CB. Drug facilitated sexual assault – a review. *Journal of Forensic and Legal Medicine* 2008; **15:** 291–7.

Hilden M, Schei B, Sidenius K. Genitoanal injury in adult female victims of sexual assault. *Forensic Science International* 2005; **154**, 200–5.

Hughes, H, Peters, R, Davies, G, Griffiths, K. A study of patients presenting to an emergency department having had a 'spiked drink'. *Emergency Medicine Journal* 2007; **24:** 89–91.

Ingemann-Hansen O, Sabroe S, Brink O, Knudsen M, Charles A. Characteristics of victims of assaults of sexual violence – improving inquiries and prevention. *Journal of Forensic & Legal Medicine* 2009; **16:** 182–188.

Jina R, Jewkes R, Munjanja SP *et al*. Report of the FIGO Working Group on sexual violence/HIV: guidelines for the management of female survivors of sexual assault. *International Journal of Gynecology and Obstetrics* 2010; **109:** 85–92.

Jones JG, Worthington T. Genital and anal injuries requiring surgical repair in females less than 21 years of age. *Journal of Pediatric and Adolescent Gynecology* 2008; **21:** 207–11.

Jones JS, Dunnuck C, Rossman L, Wynn BN, Nelson-Horan C. Significance of toluidine blue positive findings after speculum examination for sexual assault. *American Journal of Emergency Medicine* 2004; **222:** 201–3.

Jones JS, Rossman L, Diegel R, Van Order P, Wynn BN. Sexual assault in post menopausal women: epidemiology and patterns of genital injury. *American Journal of Emergency Medicine* 2009; **27:** 922–9.

MacLeod KJ, Marcin JP, Boyle C, Miyamoto S, Dimand RJ, Rogers KK. Using telemedicine to improve the care delivered to sexually abused children in rural, underserved hospitals. *Pediatrics* 2009; **123:** 223–8.

Maguire M, Goodall E, Moore T. Injury in adult female sexual assault complainants and related factors. *European Journal of Obstetrics & Gynecology and Reproductive Biology* 2009; **142:** 149–53.

Masho SW, Odor RK, Adera T. Sexual assault in Virginia: a population study. *Women's Health Issues* 2005; **15:** 157–66.

McCall-Hosenfeld JS, Freund KM, Liebschut JM. Factors associated with sexual assault and time to presentation. *Preventive Medicine* 2009; **48:** 593–5.

McCauley J, Ruggiero KJ, Resnick HS, Conoscenti LM, Kilpatrick DG. Forcible, drug-facilitated and incapacitated rape in relation to substance use problems: results from a national sample of college women. *Addictive Behaviours* 2009; **34:** 458–62.

Norfolk GA. Accidental anal intercourse: does it really happen? *Journal of Clinical Forensic Medicine* 2005; **12:** 1–4.

Okonkwo JEN, Ibeh CC. Female sexual assault in Nigeria. *International Journal of Gynaecology and Obstetrics* 2003; **83:** 325–6.

Palmer CM, McNulty AM, D'Este C, Donovan B. Genital injuries in women reporting sexual assault. *Sexual Health* 2004; **11:** 55–9.

Payne-James JJ, Roger DJ. Drug facilitated sexual assault, 'ladettes' and alcohol. *Journal of the Royal Society of Medicine* 2002; **95:** 326–7.

Peel M, Mahtani A, Hinshelwood G, Forrest D. The sexual abuse of men in detention in Sri Lanka. *Lancet* 2000; **355:** 2069–70.

Riggs N, Houry D, Long G, Markovchick V, Feldhaus KM. Analysis of 1076 cases of sexual assault. *Annals of Emergency Medicine* 2000; **35:** 358–62.

Rossman L, Jones JS, Dunnuck C, Wynn BN, Bermingham M. Genital trauma associated with forced digital penetration. *American Journal of Emergency Medicine* 2004; **22:** 101–4.

Saltzman LE, Basile KC, Mahendra RR, Steenkamp M, Ingram E, Ikeda R. National estimates of sexual violence treated in emergency departments. *Annals of Emergency Medicine* 2007; **492:** 10–17.

Santos JC, Neves A, Rodrigues M, Ferrão P. Victims of sexual offences: medico-legal examinations in emergency settings. *Journal of Clinical Forensic Medicine* 2006; **13:** 300–3.

Sexual Offences Act 2003. http://www.legislation.gov.uk/ukpga/2003/42/contents (accessed 23 November 2010).

Sommers MS, Zink T, Baker RB *et al*. The effects of age and ethnicity on physical injury from rape. *Journal of Obstetric, Gynecologic and Neonatal Nursing* 2006; **35:** 199–207.

Sturgiss EA, Tyson A, Parekh V. Characteristics of sexual assaults in which adult victims report penetration by a foreign object. *Journal of Forensic and Legal Medicine* 2010; **17:** 140–2.

Sugar NF, Fine DN, Eckert LO. Physical injury after sexual assault: findings of a large case series. *American Journal of Obstetrics and Gynecology* 2004; **190**, 71–6.

Templeton DJ, Williams A, Healey L, Odell M, Wells D. Male forensic physicians have an important role in sexual assault care. 'A response to "Chowdhury-Hawkins *et al*. Preferred choice of gender of staff providing care to victims of sexual assault in Sexual Assault Referral Centres (SARCs)" [J. Forensic Legal Med. 15 (2008) 363–367]'. *Journal of Forensic and Legal Medicine* 2010; **17:** 50–2.

Chapter 13

Child assault and protection

- ■ Introduction
- ■ Definitions and law
- ■ Children Act 1989
- ■ Safeguarding
- ■ Physical abuse
- ■ Sexual abuse
- ■ Neglect and emotional abuse
- ■ Factitious disorder by proxy
- ■ Management of child abuse
- ■ Further information sources

■ Introduction

Vulnerabilities of children are now recognized on a worldwide basis. Despite – or perhaps because of – the increased awareness of the extent of problems governments and other agencies seek to protect children. Roles and responsibilities of those in contact with or treating children and their duties of care are much better defined in many countries now, with a more proactive approach to intervening at early stages when concerns about a child's well-being are raised. Recognition of child abuse is not a new problem, and can occur in many forms, and be interpreted in different ways in different cultures. Child sexual abuse may be universally condemned, but use of children as cheap labour may not be seen as abuse by every society or culture.

Child abuse can cause adverse physical outcomes (death, injury), psychiatric, psychological and behavioural disorders (persisting into adulthood) may ensue, together with developmental delay, growth retardation and failure to thrive. Increased drug and alcohol misuse and self-injurious behaviour are also observed. There is also a clear increased risk of children who have been abused, becoming abusers themselves as adults. The risk factors for abuse can be classified according to the children themselves (e.g. behavioural issues, being adopted), parents (e.g. drug, alcohol or mental health issues, domestic violence) and environmental and social factors (e.g. poverty, unemployment, single parent). For many children, multiple predisposing factors for increased risks of abuse are present.

■ Definitions and law

Article 1 of the United Nations Convention on the Rights of the Child (UNCRC) defined children as persons under 18 years of age. This age limit may be applied variably in different cultures and jurisdictions may vary in how that age limit is applied. The UNCRC places a duty on the state to promote the well-being of all children in its jurisdiction. Article 3 of the Convention states that any decision or action affecting children, either as individuals or as a group should be focused on their best interests.

Child abuse can be defined in a number of ways and many governments have systems in place to ensure that health professionals recognize that they have an overriding duty to report concerns if they believe that the child may be at risk of harm. Physical abuse of a child is defined by the World Health Organization as 'that which results in actual or potential physical harm from an interaction or lack of interaction which is reasonable within the control of a parent or person in a position of responsibility, power or trust'. In 1962 Henry Kempe identified 'the battered child syndrome'. The term 'Non-Accidental Injury' (NAI) describes injury that was considered to be inflicted by another and by inference as a deliberate assault

Within the UK child abuse is classified as physical abuse, emotional abuse; sexual abuse; and neglect. All can occur concurrently.

- Examples of physical abuse include hitting, shaking, throwing, poisoning, burning or scalding, drowning, or when a parent or carer feigns the symptoms of, or deliberately causes ill-health to a child whom they are looking after (see Factitious Disorder by Proxy, p. 140).
- Emotional abuse is the persistent emotional ill-treatment or neglect of a child such as to cause severe persistent adverse effects on the child's emotional development. For example, it may involve seeing or hearing the ill-treatment of another. It may involve serious bullying, causing children frequently to feel frightened or in danger, or the exploitation or corruption of children. Emotional abuse to a greater or lesser degree is involved in all types of ill-treatment of a child, although it may occur alone.
- Sexual abuse involves forcing or enticing a child or young person to take part in sexual activities. Such activities may include physical contact, including penetrative or non-penetrative sexual acts; non-contact activities, such as involving children in looking at, or being involved in the production of, pornographic material or watching sexual activities, or encouraging children to behave in sexually inappropriate ways.

- Neglect is the persistent failure to meet a child's basic physical or psychological needs, likely to result in the serious impairment of the child's health or development. It may involve a parent or carer failing to provide adequate food, shelter and clothing, failing to protect a child from physical harm or danger, or the failure to ensure access to appropriate medical care or treatment.

Most jurisdictions now have laws, statutes or codes in place aimed at protecting children and identifying those children at risk.

■ Children Act 1989

In England and Wales, the Children Act 1989 identified a number of principles including:

- the child's welfare being the court's paramount consideration ('the paramountcy principle');
- the parents have prime responsibility for bringing up children;
- local authorities should provide supportive services to help parents in bringing up children;
- local authorities should take reasonable steps to identify children and families in need;
- every local authority should have a register of children in need;
- sensitivity to ethnic considerations in assessing a child's needs and providing services.

The Act created protection orders for children 'at-risk' including:

- Emergency Protection Orders – for which any person may apply to court and then has parental responsibility for the child;
- Police Protection Provision – by which a police officer can take a child into police protection without assuming parental responsibility;
- Child Assessment Orders – which allow proper assessment of a child up to 7 days; and
- Care and Supervision Orders – which allow the child to be placed in the care of, or under supervision of, the local authority for up to 8 weeks.

The Act used the term 'harm' to describe the effects of ill-treatment and poor care leading to injury, impairment of health or development of a child. The term 'significant harm' was used to determine the severity of the ill-treatment and is the threshold for compulsory intervention in child protection cases.

All police services within the UK should now have specialist Child Abuse Investigation Units tasked with investigating suspected cases of child abuse.

Safeguarding

In response to a number of high-profile deaths of children the Children Act 2004 imposed a duty on local authorities to establish Local Safeguarding Children Boards, which have overall responsibility for deciding how relevant organizations work together to safeguard and promote the welfare of children in their areas. Where statutory child protection proceedings have been initiated, then a local authority social care worker is tasked with taking the lead in supporting and safeguarding the child. Serious case reviews are undertaken when a child dies or is seriously injured, and abuse or neglect are known or suspected to be factors in the death. They are carried out under the auspices of Local Safeguarding Children Boards so that lessons can be learned locally.

Physical abuse

Physical abuse takes many forms. Children are prone to injury as a result of accident and play and sports, and the type and site of injury will relate to those factors as well as their age and mobility. The prevalence, number and location of bruising relates to motor development. Non-abusive bruises tend to be small, sustained over bony prominences, and found on the front of the body (Figure 13.1). In children alleged to have been subject to abuse, bruising is common. Any part of the body is vulnerable. Bruises are away from bony prominences; the commonest site is head and neck (particularly face) followed by the buttocks, trunk, and arms (Figure 13.2). Bruises are large, commonly multiple and occur in clusters. However bruising, as with other findings in suspected child abuse, must be assessed in the context of medical, social and developmental history, the explanation given and the patterns of non-abusive bruising. Examples of patterns of injury that should raise the possibility of physical abuse include multiple facial bruising, bruises to the ears, neck or abdomen, multiple old scars, cigarette burns, bite marks or torn frenulum.

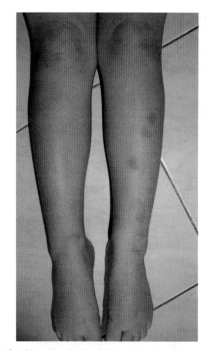
Figure 13.1 Non-abusive bruising.

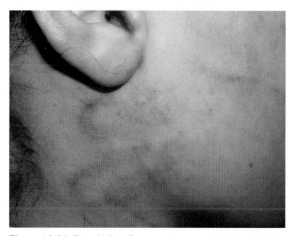
Figure 13.2 Inflicted injury-finger marks to neck from slap with hand by non-accidental injury (NAI).

Bruises in non-mobile infants, bruises over areas of soft tissues, patterned bruises and multiple similar shape bruises should raise concerns. Intentional scalds (Figure 13.3) are often immersion injuries with symmetrical, well-defined clear upper margins (tide marks). Unintentional scald injuries more commonly result from spill injuries of other hot liquids; they usually affect the upper body with irregular margins and variable depth of burn (Figure 13.4). In infants (under 18 months) physical abuse must be considered in the differential diagnosis when they present with

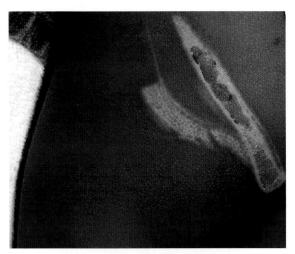

Figure 13.3 Scar caused by application of heated cutlery handle to lower limb.

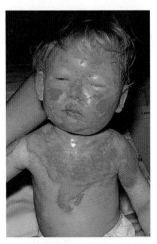

Figure 13.4 Accidental scald.

a fracture in the absence of clear history of trauma. Multiple fractures are more common after physical abuse than after accidental injury. The history is a crucial part of the assessment. Examples of features that may support abuse include discrepancies in the history, a changing account, different accounts by different carers and delays in presentation. Specific enquiry should be made regarding pre-existing conditions, which may cause excessive or easy bruising (e.g. haemophilia), or known skin disease, which may mimic or be mimicked by physical abuse. Other aspects that are essential are the emotional, behavioural and developmental history, the nutritional history, family history (e.g. genetic or inherited disorders), social history and environmental history. Physical examination requires a comprehensive head

to toe examination with appropriate consent. In addition to a full general examination all scars, healing injuries and new injuries must be noted Each injury, scar or mark must be examined and documented in appropriate detail (preferably in written form, on body diagrams, and photodocumented) so that they are capable of proper external review and interpretation (see Chapter 8, p. 96). If injury is noted, consideration should be given to repeat examination and serial photography to note the evolution of injury or scars. If physical abuse is suspected then consideration must be given to a full radiographic skeletal survey, which must subsequently be reviewed by a paediatric radiologist, and perhaps bone scintigraphy. In addition, laboratory-based investigations may also be required and include blood count, urinalysis, liver function, amylase, calcium, phosphorus, vitamin D,screen for metabolic bone disease; coagulation studies.

Interpretation of physical findings in physical abuse cases requires a full understanding of mechanisms of injury and how those mechanisms apply with respect to the accounts of causation (of which there may be several) given (Box 13.1).

Box 13.1 Types of injury in physical abuse

- Head injury – of all types; the 'shaken-baby' syndrome is an extremely complex area requiring multi-professional input and assessment to determine the relevance of clinical and radiological findings
- Skin injury – in particular it is important to recognize possible slap marks, punch marks, grip marks, pinching and poking marks; certain injuries (e.g. cigarette burns) are readily identifiable
- Abdominal injury – all intra-abdominal organs can be damaged by direct impact (e.g. punches or stamps)
- Chest injury – squeezing or crushing can result in substantial injury including rib fractures, ruptured great vessels and cardiac bruising
- Skeletal injury – a range of injuries may be seen, from frank fractures, via metaphyseal fracture to subperiosteal new bone formation

---

■ Sexual abuse

There are many ways in which a child may disclose abuse; for example, it may be to a teacher, a friend or a sibling. The sexual abuse may be chronic and long term or it may be an acute or single episode. Disclosure may be delayed for many years in chronic cases, or for a few days in acute episodes, which may result in loss of forensically supportive evidence. Pubertal and pre-pubertal girls are more likely to have significant genital signs if they are examined within 7 days of the last episode of sexual abuse.

Anal signs in particular are more likely to be present in the acute phase (within the first 72 hours). Delays in proper examination should be avoided when disclosure of recent sexual contact is made. Symptoms of longer-term abuse may be general and non-specific and include sleep disturbance, enuresis and encopresis. Injuries may be acute or old and include abrasion and bruising of the genitalia, acute or healed tear of the hymen, anal bruising or lacerations.

The principles of examination and documentation of the sexually abused child are in many respects similar to those of an adult (see Chapter 12, p. 129), but with complexities added by virtue of consent issues and authority for documentation, recording and storing notes, images and other evidence such as colposcope recordings. Most jurisdictions will have specific guidelines and protocols.

In the UK, the Royal College of Paediatrics and Child Health and the Faculty of Forensic and Legal Medicine have produced guidelines related to child sexual abuse. The assessment may be undertaken by a single doctor if that doctor has the necessary knowledge, skills and experience for the case. Two doctors with complementary skills (e.g. a paediatrician and a forensic physician) will be appropriate.

It is considered essential for a permanent record of the genital or anal findings to be obtained whenever a child is examined for possible sexual abuse. A colposcope or camera may be used. The images must be of adequate quality to demonstrate the clinical findings. Further examinations may be required after initial assessments to determine whether abnormalities or features evolve or change. Examinations for acute or recent child sexual abuse are similar to those for adult sexual assault. Emphasis must be on as much detail of alleged events as possible to ensure proper consideration of body sites to be examined and forensic samples to be taken. Genito-anal examination may be particularly stressful for a child and is done at the end of the general assessment and examination. Genital examination can be done in the supine 'frog-leg' position with hips flexed and the soles of the feet touching, and if, for example, a hymenal abnormality is seen, the prone knee–chest position can additionally be used. A lateral position may be appropriate for some children, while others may be comfortable held on a carer's lap. Examiners must be aware of a potential risk that an examination may further traumatize an already traumatized child. Therapeutic needs (e.g. for genital injury) may have priority over forensic examination, but if treatment is

---

Box 13.2 Types of injury that may be seen in sexual abuse

Findings that may be noted in females:
- Genital erythema/redness/inflammation
- Oedema
- Genital bruising
- Genital abrasions
- Hymenal transections
- Hymenal clefts and notches
- Labial fusion
- Vaginal discharge in pre-pubertal girls

Anal findings in males and females may include:
- Anal/perianal erythema
- Perianal venous congestion
- Anal/perianal bruising
- Anal fissures, lacerations, scars and tags
- Reflex anal dilatation

---

required under general anaesthesia, thought should be given to forensic assessment, with appropriate consent at the time of therapeutic intervention.

The need for examination following disclosure of chronic or historic sexual abuse will need to take into account its relevance. Examination of a female alleging penetrative sexual assault pre-pubertally but disclosing in her thirties after vaginal delivery of children will provide no information. Examination of a pre-pubertal girl alleging vaginal penetration some months earlier may have value. A male alleging historic anal penetration with immediate pain and bleeding at the time may have persistent scarring.

The interpretation of physical signs found after genito-anal assessment is a very difficult and complex area. Most complainants of child sexual abuse have no genito-anal abnormalities when examined after alleged sexual abuse. It is essential that precise terminology is used in the description of abnormality and injury so that abnormal findings are clearly understood (Box 13.2). The presence of certain infections may have relevance in sexual abuse enquiries. The implications of these findings must be determined with an understanding of the context of presentation and a detailed awareness of current research findings.

■ Neglect and emotional abuse

A number of behavioural characteristics may indicate both neglect and emotional abuse, for example age-inappropriate social skills (e.g. inability to use knife and fork), bedwetting and soiling, inability to self-dress, smoking, drug and alcohol misuse, sexual precocity and absenting from school. Certain features associated with possible neglect may be evident during assessment and physical examination and include unkempt child, ill-fitting or absent items of clothes, dirty or uncut nails, local skin infections/excoriations and low centiles for weight and height. However, some of these features may be seen in normal, non-abused children. There may be a failure to thrive.

Certain groups of children are at particular risk of emotional abuse such as unplanned or unwanted children, children of the 'wrong' gender, children with behavioural issues and children in unstable or chaotic family setting. In the UK, emotional abuse is most prevalent in 5 to 15 year olds, although overall 'neglect' is the most common reason for children to be on the register.

■ Factitious disorder by proxy

Factitious Disorder by Proxy (also known as Munchausen Syndrome by Proxy or fictitious or factitious illness by proxy, fabricated illness by proxy or induced illness) is a term used to describe a setting in which a parent or carer presents a false history or appearance of illness for their child to healthcare professionals. Examples of how illness can be claimed, fabricated or induced include manipulation of required drug regimens (e.g. in diabetics), suffocation and administration of noxious substances (e.g. salt). Such approaches may result in the child presenting, or being presented repeatedly to healthcare professionals with a range of often inexplicable or puzzling symptoms. The motives behind such behaviour are unclear, but psychiatric, mental health or attention-seeking problems may be associated with such behaviour.

■ Management of child abuse

The management of child abuse will depend on the type of abuse or abuses experienced and many other factors such as their health, and where they are living. Every jurisdiction will have its own legal requirements, policies, protocols and procedures.

Every episode of child abuse that is missed has the potential for a fatal outcome. In the UK the British Medical Association published *Child Protection – a Toolkit for Doctors* in part in response to a number of high-profile cases where serious cases of child abuse had been unrecognized. The tool kit is aimed to provide an accessible guide to best practices in child protection cases, where it is believed a child may be at risk for neglect or abuse. It is emphasized that the best interests of the child must guide the decision-making process. The toolkit highlights basic principles, definitions of abuse and neglect, methods of responding to initial concerns and participation in statutory child protection procedures.

■ Further information sources

Adams JA, Girardin B, Faugno D. Adolescent sexual assault: documentation of acute injuries using photo-colposcopy. *Journal of Pediatric and Adolescent Gynecology* 2001; **14:** 175–80.

Section on Radiology, American Academy of Pediatrics. Diagnostic Imaging of child abuse. *Pediatrics* 2009; **123:** 1430–5.

American College of Radiology. *ACR Practice Guidelines for Skeletal Surveys in Children, revised 2006.* http://www. acr.org/SecondaryMainMenuCategories/quality_safety/ guidelines/pediatric/skeletal_surveys.aspx (accessed 23 November 2010).

Beh P, Payne-James JJ. Adult sexual assault. In: Gall J, Payne-James JJ (eds) *Current Practice in Forensic Medicine.* London: Wiley, 2011.

British Medical Association. *Child Protection – a Toolkit for Doctors.* May 2009. http://www.bma.org.uk/ethics/ consent_and_capacity/childprotectiontoolkit.jsp (accessed 21 July 2010).

British Society of Paediatric Radiologists. Standard Skeletal Surveys in Suspected Non-accidental Injury (Nai) in Children. http://www.bspr.org.uk/nai.htm (accessed 23 November 2010).

Children Act 1989. http://www.opsi.gov.uk/acts/acts1989/ Ukpga_19890041_en_1.htm (accessed 21 July 2010).

Children Act 2004. http://www.opsi.gov.uk/acts/acts2004/en/ ukpgaen_20040031_en_1.htm (accessed 21 July 2010).

Donald T. Children: emotional abuse. In: Payne-James JJ, Byard RW, Corey TS, Henderson C (eds). *Encyclopedia of Forensic and Legal Medicine.* London: Elsevier Academic Press, 2005.

Gallion HR, Dupree LJ, Scott TA, Arnold DH. Diagnosis of *Trichomonas vaginalis* and adolescents evaluated for possible sexual abuse: a comparison of the InPouch TV culture method and wet mount microscopy. *Journal* of Pediatric and Adolescent Gynecology 2009; **22:** 300–305.

Girardet RG, Lemme S, Biason TA, Bolton K, Lahoti S. HIV post-exposure prophylaxis in children and adolescents presenting for reported sexual assault. *Child Abuse and Neglect* 2009; **33:** 173–8.

Jenny C. Children: physical abuse. In: Payne-James JJ, Byard RW, Corey TS, Henderson C (eds). *Encyclopedia of Forensic and Legal Medicine*. London: Elsevier Academic Press, 2005.

Jenny C; Committee on Child Abuse and Neglect. Evaluating infants and young children with multiple fractures *Pediatrics* 2006; **118:** 1299–303.

Jones JG, Worthington T. Genital and anal injuries requiring surgical repair in females less than 21 years of age. *Journal of Pediatric and Adolescent Gynecology* 2008; **21,** 207–11.

Jones JS, Rossman L, Hartman M, Alexander CC. Anogenital injuries in adolescents after consensual sexual intercourse. *Academic Emergency Medicine* 2003; **10:** 1378–83.

Kavanaugh ML, Saladino RA, Gold MA. Emergency contraception services for adolescents: a National Survey of Children's Hospital Emergency Department Directors. *Journal of Pediatric and Adolescent Gynecology* 2009; **22:** 111–19.

Kellogg N, American Academy of Pediatrics Committee on Child Abuse and Neglect. The evaluation of sexual abuse in children. *Pediatrics* 2005; **116:** 506–12.

Kemp AM, Butler A, Morris S et al. Which radiological investigations should be performed to identify fractures in suspected child abuse? *Clinical Radiolology* 2006; **61:** 723–36.

Kemp AM, Dunstan F, Harrison S et al. Patterns of skeletal fractures in child abuse: systematic review. *British Medical Journal* 2008; **337:** a1518.

Kempe CH, Silverman FN, Steele BF, Droegemueller W, Silver HK. The battered-child syndrome. *Journal Of the American Medical Association* 1962; **181:** 17–24.

Maguire S, Mann MK, Sibert J, Kemp A. Are there patterns of bruising in childhood which are diagnostic or suggestive of abuse? A systematic review. *Archives of Disease in Childhood* 2005; **90:** 182–6.

Mandelstam SA, Cook D, Fitzgerald M, Ditchfield MR. Complementary use of radiological skeletal survey and bone scintigraphy in detection of bony injuries in suspected child abuse *Archives of Disease in Childhood* 2003; **88:** 387–90.

Nicoletti A. Teens and drug facilitated sexual assault. *Journal of Pediatric and Adolescent Gynecology* 2009; **22,** 187.

Palusci VJ, Cox EO, Shatz EM, Schultze JM. Urgent medical assessment after child sexual abuse. *Child Abuse and Neglect* 2006; **30:** 367–380.

Payne-James J, Rogers DJ. Drug facilitated sexual assault, 'ladettes' and alcohol. *Journal of the Royal Society of Medicine* 2002; **95:** 326–27.

Prosser I, Maguire S, Harrison SK, Mann M, Sibert JR, Kemp AM. How old is this fracture? Radiological dating of fractures in children: a systematic review. *AJR American Journal of Roentgenology* 2005; **184:** 1282–6

Royal College of Paediatrics and Child Health. *The Physical Signs of Child Sexual Abuse: an Evidence-Based Review And Guidance For Best Practice*. Lavenham, UK: Lavenham Group, 2008.

Royal College of Paediatrics and Child Health, Faculty of Forensic and Legal Medicine. *Guidelines on Paediatric Forensic Examinations in Relation to Possible Child Sexual Abuse*. Lavenham, UK: Lavenham Group, 2007; http://www.rcpch.ac.uk/doc.aspx?id_Resource=3379 (accessed 21/7/2010).

Sexual Offences Act 2003. http://www.legislation.gov.uk/ukpga/2003/42/contents (accessed 23 November 2010).

Sommers MS, Zink T, Baker RB et al. The effects of age and ethnicity on physical injury from rape. *Journal of Obstetric, Gynecologic & Neonatal Nursing* 2006; **35:** 199–207.

Watkeys, JM, Price LD, Upton PM. Maddocks A. The timing of medical examination following an allegation of sexual abuse: is this an emergency? *Archives of Disease in Childhood* 2008; **93:** 851–6.

White C, McLean I. Adolescent complainants of sexual assault: injury patterns in virgin and non-virgin groups. *Journal of Clinical Forensic Medicine* 2006; **13,** 172–80.

Wolff N, Jing S. Contextualisation of physical and sexual assault in male prisons. *Journal of Correctional Health Care* 2009; **15:** 58–77.

Young, A., Grey, M., Abbey, A., Boyd, C.J. and McCabe, S.E. (2008) Alcohol-related sexual assault victimization among adolescents: prevalence, characteristics and correlates. *Journal of Studies on Alcohol and Drugs*, **69:** 39–48.

Chapter 14

Transportation medicine

- Introduction
- Transportation law
- Transportation 'under the influence'
- Personal transport and road traffic injuries
- Railway injuries
- Aircraft fatalities
- Marine fatalities
- Further information sources

Introduction

All forms of transport (air, water or land) are associated with a risk of harm or injury. Particular environments render individuals at risk of specific types of injury. The incidence of those risks may be well established but can be increased when other factors are taken into account, including lack of experience, fatigue and the effects of drugs and alcohol.

Transportation law

Virtually every jurisdiction has laws that control the speed at which vehicles can move and the amount of alcohol and/or drugs under which an individual is lawfully deemed to be capable of controlling, or being in charge of, a means of transportation.

The basis of such laws is quite simple: the faster you are travelling, the greater the risk of loss of control and collision, and the greater the level of injury. If you are intoxicated from some substance, the more intoxicated you are, the greater

the chance of collision. Legal limits are established for acceptable levels of alcohol in blood, breath or urine. Currently in the UK, the maximum legal permissible blood alcohol concentration is 80 mg alcohol/100mL of blood, although this is hopefully going to be reduced in the future to 50 mg alcohol/100mL of blood to bring it (and the equivalent breath and urine levels) into line with the majority of Europe. The assessment of the effects of drugs and alcohol on ability to drive (in addition to a simple legal limit) is very important because of the variable individual response to the effects of alcohol and other substances. In many cases, 'driving under the influence' may be confirmed by the ability, or failure, to pass standardized tests of sobriety, or by medical examination to determine whether the ability to drive may be impaired, following preliminary impairment tests undertaken by police personnel.

Such laws apply at the personal level (e.g. the individual driving a car or a bicycle), at a management level (e.g. the individual in charge of a subway station) and at a corporate level (e.g. the senior officers in transport companies such as sea ferries). In all cases it is perceived that such individuals, or bodies, may have a duty of care to those around them, whether as private individuals (e.g. friends being given a ride to a party) or as paying clients (e.g. customers paying for transport across the sea).

In England and Wales, The Transport and Works Act 1992 defines specific offences related to the use of alcohol and drugs in transport systems, and defines the powers that police have to investigate such matters, including the power to take evidential breath, blood and urine tests.

This area of law is vast, and varies from jurisdiction to jurisdiction, but increasingly legal action is being taken at a higher corporate level such that accountability is required throughout all levels of an organization. The Corporate Manslaughter and Corporate Homicide Act 2007 came into force in 2008 and introduced a new offence, across the UK: corporate entities (companies and organizations) may now be prosecuted when there has been a gross failing, throughout the organization, in the management of health and safety where such a failure has fatal consequences.

■ Transportation 'under the influence'

In general, two types of offence are committed when 'under the influence' of alcohol or drugs. Relevant maximum permissible alcohol concentrations can be prescribed and quantified in an individual, but in many jurisdictions the effect that alcohol (or drugs) has on the ability to drive properly must also be assessed. Initial screening may be done by officers at the scene of an alleged offence or accident, using 'field impairment tests'.

Evidential 'breath alcohol machines' are used to take breath samples, and if for some reason (e.g. asthma, oral trauma) it is not possible for an individual to provide a sample, then blood or urine samples must be sought. The experience in all jurisdictions is that individuals (who might suspect they exceed the relevant legal limit) may provide a variety of reasons for not providing relevant samples (e.g. previously undiagnosed asthma, needle phobia) and, although some of those reasons may be valid, many have been tested in court and found wanting.

The medical assessment of an individual's ability to drive a motor vehicle is established by (1) undertaking a full history and examination and (2) undertaking a number of tests of coordination and reactions. The aim of the examination is to determine (1) whether the individual's ability to drive is impaired, (2) which drug/substance is causing this impairment, and (3) whether there is a medical reason for the individual's apparently impaired status (e.g. neurological disorder, psychiatric disorder). Increasingly, certain procedures that measure psychomotor function and 'divided attention tests' are used.

Divided attention tests, which assess an individual's balance and coordination, as well as the ability to follow simple instructions, include the 'walk and turn test', 'one-leg stand test', 'horizontal gaze nystagmus test' and Romberg test. If such tests are used, it is important they are reproduced and scored in identical ways. It is also important to understand that initial studies, which suggested high sensitivities and specificities in results for Drug Recognition Programs within the USA, have not been confirmed in controlled laboratory studies. The results of the few studies that have been performed suggest that the accuracy of such assessment, in general, may not be sufficiently robust for evidential purposes (in terms of determining the culpable drug/substance), but they can help corroborate other witness and toxicological evidence. Many individuals will have used a mixture of drugs and alcohol, which often renders tests for specific drugs groups inappropriate or wrong.

It is important to recognize that the results of 'field impairment tests' ('preliminary impairment tests' in the UK) do not necessarily establish impairment of driving through drugs other than alcohol, although they may be useful in screening individuals suspected of being impaired as a consequence of drug use, and provide supportive evidence of impairment. They cannot be used with certainty to confirm that drugs have been used, or the particular drug or drugs that may have consumed.

Anyone using these tests, in association with a medical examination, must be able to interpret them in the context of that medical examination, the circumstances in which field tests were undertaken, and the limitations of the evidence base on which such screening tests are established.

■ Personal transport and road traffic injuries

Those injured by collisions on the road, or off-road using personal transport can be divided into three broad groups: pedestrians, cyclists (pedal or motor) and the drivers or passengers of vehicles. Of these three broad groups, it is pedestrians who are most often injured, although the proportion of pedestrian victims in the overall road traffic-injured population varies greatly between countries depending on patterns of transport use. It is perhaps self-evident that where there is greater mingling of motor transport and pedestrians there is also a greater risk of injury to the pedestrian. Most road deaths in the world occur in developing countries.

Pedestrians

Pedestrians struck by motor vehicles suffer injuries from direct contact with the vehicle (primary injuries) or from contact with other objects, or the ground, after the primary contact with the vehicle (secondary injuries). Advances in safer vehicle design and legislation have attempted to reduce the effects of such contact but cannot eradicate them completely.

The primary injuries can often form recognizable patterns, although a variety of factors may alter the eventual constellation of injury. When an adult is hit by the front of a car, for example, the front bumper (fender) usually strikes the victim at about knee level. The exact point of contact, however, whether on the front, side or back of the leg(s), will depend on the orientation of the victim, the nature of the front of the car, and whether or not it is actively braking at the time of impact. Comparison of measurements of lower limb injuries (from the heel), with measurements of relevant parts of the car (from the ground) may assist in the reconstruction of pedestrian versus car collisions (Figure 14.1).

There are often additional primary injury sites on the thigh, hip or pelvis caused by contact with other parts of the car, such as the bonnet (the hood). At relatively low speeds (e.g. 20 kph/12 mph), the victim may be thrown off the bonnet either forwards or to one side. Between 20 and 60 kph (12–36 mph), the pedestrian may strike the bonnet (hood) and the head may strike the windscreen or

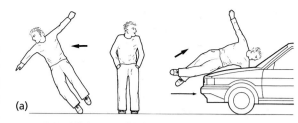

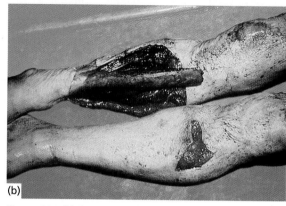

Figure 14.1 (a) A pedestrian struck by the front of a car may be projected forwards or lifted onto the vehicle; (b) 'bumper injuries' including a compound fracture of the right leg, and laceration of the left knee, probably following primary impact to this pedestrian's right leg.

the surrounding metal body work. At higher speeds (60–100 kph/36–60 mph), pedestrians may be projected up into the air; sometimes they will pass completely over the vehicle and will avoid hitting the windscreen and other points on the vehicle (Figure 14.2). Such impacts, however, will generally cause major injury, including complex fractures or traumatic amputations.

Secondary injuries are often more serious, and potentially lethal, than the primary injuries. Such secondary injuries vary from simple 'brush abrasions', caused by 'skidding' across the surface of the road, to fractures of the skull or axial skeleton, caused by direct contact with a hard surface, to hyperextension or hyperflexion fractures

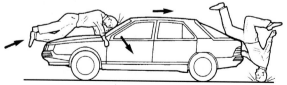

Figure 14.2 At speeds of over 23 kph (15 mph) a pedestrian can be 'scooped up' onto a car, suffering head injuries on impacting the windscreen. They may then fall off sideways or, at higher speeds, be thrown over the roof.

of the spine. It is important to remember that the external injuries are seldom lethal *per se*; it is their association with internal injuries that is important.

Even in the absence of skull fracture, traumatic brain damage, including traumatic axonal injury, is frequently observed in fatally injured pedestrians. This occurs as a consequence of the rotational, deceleration forces produced when the rapidly moving head is suddenly stopped at impact, leading to 'shearing' injuries to the brain and its coverings. Fractures of the spine, especially in the cervical and thoracic segments, may lead to cord damage. Fractures of the limbs are common but, apart from those of the legs that are associated with the primary impact sites, they are somewhat unpredictable because of random 'flailing' of the limbs following primary impact.

When an adult is struck by a larger vehicle, for example a van, a 4×4, a sport utility vehicle (SUV), truck or lorry, or when a small child is struck by any vehicle, the typical lower limb primary contact injury site described above tends to be 'higher up' (pelvis, abdomen, chest or head). It is likely that the victim will make contact with more of the front of the vehicle or be projected along the line of travel of the vehicle and 'run-over'.

'Run-over' injuries are relatively unusual and the effects are variable, depending on the area of the body involved, the weight of the vehicle and the surface area of the contact. The skull may be disrupted and the brain externalized, internal organs may be ruptured and there may be fractures of the spine. Compression of the chest may result in multiple rib fractures, causing a 'flail chest'. The rotation of the wheel may strip off

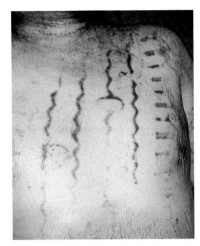

Figure 14.4 Intradermal bruising reflecting the pattern of a vehicle tyre tread. Note that the bruising is in the 'valleys' and not the 'hills' in the tread. Scaled photographic documentation of such a patterned injury will allow future comparisons to be made between it and the tread pattern of a suspect vehicle.

large areas of skin and subcutaneous tissue; this is called a 'flaying injury' (Figure 14.3). On occasion, patterned injuries are recognized on the skin surface bearing the characteristics of tyre-treads (Figure 14.4).

Car occupants

Most impacts involve the front, or the front corners, of the vehicle and approximately 80 per cent of impacts are against either another vehicle or a stationary object. This type of impact rapidly decelerates the vehicle. Less commonly, the vehicle is hit from behind, causing an 'acceleration' impact. The least common impacts are side impacts and 'roll-overs'.

Many countries now have legislation regarding the requirement to wear seatbelts, both in the front and back of moving vehicles. Unrestrained front-seat occupants in a vehicle subjected to rapid deceleration during a collision will continue to move forwards as the vehicle decelerates around them, and will impact those parts of the vehicle that are in front of them. The degree of injury sustained by the occupant is very much dependent on the vehicle's speed at the moment of impact, its deformation properties and the structure of the part (or parts) of the vehicle being impacted by the occupant (Box 14.1, Figures 14.5–14.7).

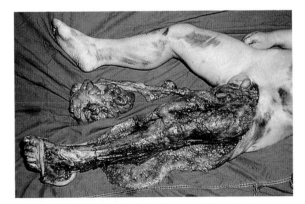

Figure 14.3 Pedestrian leg injury from a rotating wheel resulting in 'flaying' of the skin.

14 Transportation medicine

Box 14.1 Injuries that may be expected to occur in an unrestrained impact/collision

- The face and head hit the windscreen glass, frame or side-pillars, causing skull and facial fractures, injury to the brain and its coverings, and cervical spine injury.
- The chest and abdomen contact the fascia or the steering wheel, causing rib, sternal, heart and liver injuries.
- The momentum of the heart within the thorax, perhaps aided by hyperflexion, may tear the aorta at the termination of the descending part of the arch, at the point where the vessel becomes attached to the vertebral column.
- The legs of the passenger are thrown forwards and the knees may strike the parcel shelf, causing fractures.
- The legs of the driver, which are commonly braced on the brake and clutch pedals, may transmit the force of impact along the tibia and femur to the pelvis. All of these bones may be fractured or dislocated.
- On the rebound from these impacts, the heavy head may swing violently backwards and cause injury to the cervical or thoracic spine.
- The occupants of the car may be ejected out of the vehicle through the windscreen, increasing the risks of secondary injuries or being run over by another vehicle.

The unrestrained rear-seat passenger is also liable to injury through either deceleration or acceleration. The injuries, in general, may not be as severe as those caused to the front-seat occupants. In a deceleration impact, the rear-seat passengers will be thrown against the backs of the front seats and may impact the front-seat occupants. They may be projected over the front seat to hit the windscreen and even be thrown out through the windscreen. The introduction of seatbelts has dramatically reduced the number and severity of injuries to car occupants in jurisdictions where they are compulsory.

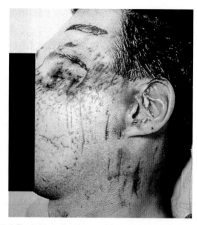

Figure 14.6 Facial injuries from shattered windscreen glass in an unrestrained driver. The toughened glass breaks into small fragments, which produce characteristic 'sparrow foot' marks. The forehead laceration was made by the windscreen rim.

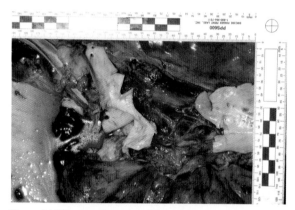

Figure 14.7 Deceleration-related thoracic aortic transection following a road traffic collision. The typical site for deceleration aortic injury is just distal to the origin of the left subclavian artery.

The function of seat belts

The mandatory use of seat belts has had a profound effect on road traffic fatality rates in the UK and other countries where similar legislation has been enacted. The combination of a horizontal lap strap and diagonal shoulder strap was introduced as a satisfactory compromise between effectiveness and social acceptability. To be effective, a seatbelt must (1) be worn and (2) worn correctly and any alteration in their fixing or structure can negate their value (Box 14.2).

The use of seatbelts can also cause injuries, the nature and severity of which is dependent on the force and nature of the impact. Any individual involved in a collision in which intrusion into the cabin has occurred, or where they have been trapped within the vehicle, should have a

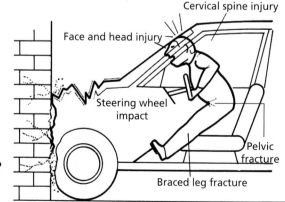

Figure 14.5 Major points of injury to an unrestrained driver of a vehicle in deceleration impact.

Cervical spine injury

Face and head injury

Steering wheel impact

Pelvic fracture

Braced leg fracture

Box 14.2 The function of seat belts

A seat belt that is correctly installed, and worn, acts in the following ways:

- It spreads the deceleration forces at impact over the whole area of contact between the straps and the body surface so that the force delivered to the body per unit area is reduced.
- It is designed to stretch during deceleration and some belts have a specific area for this to occur. This stretching slightly extends the time of deceleration and reduces the force per unit time.
- It restrains the body during deceleration, keeping it away from the windscreen, steering wheel and other obstructions at the front of the vehicle, thus reducing injury potential.
- It prevents ejection into the road through burst doors or windows, which used to be a common cause of severe injury and death.

full medical assessment, as should anyone under the influence of drugs or alcohol at the time of a collision, as such may mask significant symptoms of trauma. Such an assessment should always include, in addition to basic physiological observations, palpation and testing of range of movement of all limbs, palpation of the clavicle, lateral and anteroposterior compression of the chest, and a full abdominal examination, in order that occult fracture or internal organ injury is not missed.

Air bags

Air bags were developed in an attempt to aid the protection of all car occupants following a collision by rapidly deploying a 'soft method of restraint' that is only present when required. Most modern cars now have sophisticated air-bag systems, many providing protection not only from front impacts but also from the sides or corners of the vehicle.

The deployment of an air bag relies upon the explosive production of gas, usually from the detonation of a pellet commonly made of sodium azide. For the deployment to be timed correctly, the deceleration of the vehicle following impact needs to be sensed and the detonation of the pellet completed in microseconds so that the bag is correctly inflated at the time the occupant of the car is beginning to move towards the framework of the vehicle.

Air bags are designed to provide protection to the 'average-sized adult' in the front of the car and this protection depends upon the occupant responding to the impact in an 'average' fashion. Air bags can cause injuries, most frequently abrasions or burns, and guidelines exist as to the minimum size

that a person should be when sitting in an air-bag protected seat. Most cars have the option of disabling air bags if those of short stature (generally children) are occupying such seats. Air bags, in general, should never be used in the presence of baby seats. At particular risk are babies who are placed on the front passenger seat in a rear-facing baby seat that is held in place by the seat belt. The back of the baby seat may lie within the range of the bag when it is maximally expanded, and fatalities have been recorded following relatively minor vehicle impacts when the air bag has struck the back of the baby seat.

Motorcycle and pedal cycle injuries

Most injuries to motorcyclists are caused by falling from the machine onto the roadway. Many of the injuries can be reduced or prevented by the wearing of suitable protective clothing and a crash helmet. Abrasions caused by contact with the road surface are almost universal following an accident at speed, and injuries to the limbs and to the chest and spine occur very commonly because of contact with other objects or vehicles, entanglement with the motor bike or direct contact with the road (Figure 14.8). Despite the introduction of the mandatory wearing of crash helmets in the UK, head injuries are still a common cause of morbidity and mortality. In countries where there is no mandatory requirement for motorcycle helmets, the incidence is substantially increased. A more unique injury occurs from 'tail-gating', where the motorcyclist drives under the rear of a truck, causing severe head injuries or even decapitation. This injury has been reduced by

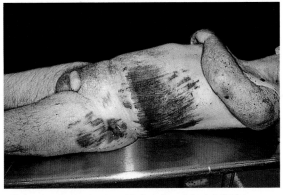

Figure 14.8 Extensive 'brush' abrasion of the left flank in a motor cyclist thrown across a rough surface.

147

the presence of bars at the sides and rear of trucks to prevent both bikes and cars passing under the vehicle.

Injuries associated with pedal cycles are very common because of the large numbers of cycles in use. Most injuries associated with cycles tend to be of mild or moderate severity because of their low speeds. However, impact by vehicles can result in severe and fatal injuries. Secondary injuries, especially to the head and chest, are common when cyclists fall from their relatively high riding position on such an inherently unstable machine.

Other transportation methods (e.g. the Segway Personal Transporter) may also have their own types and range of risk of injury or fatality.

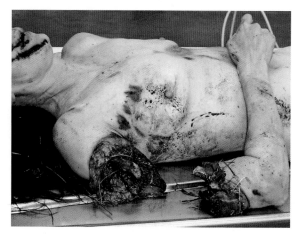
Figure 14.9 Amputation of the right arm and bruising of the face and chest in a pedestrian struck by a passing train.

■ Railway injuries

These are most common in countries with a large railway network, such as India and China, and in countries where rail crossings are unprotected or unmanned. Although mass disasters, such as the derailment of a train, occasionally lead to large numbers of casualties, most deaths and injuries occur as an aggregation of numerous individual incidents, most of which are accidents, such as at level crossings or as a result of children playing on the line. Railway lines are a common site for suicide attempts.

Medically, there is nothing specific about railway injuries except the frequency of very severe mutilation. The body may be severed into many pieces and soiled by axle grease and dirt from the wheels and track. Where passengers fall from a train at speed, multiple injuries caused by repeated impacts and rolling may be seen, often with multiple abrasions from contact with the coarse gravel of the line ballast.

Suicides on railways fall into two main groups: those that lie on the track (sometimes placing their neck across a rail so that they are beheaded) and those that jump in front of a moving train from a platform, bridge or other structure near to the track. Jumping from a moving train is much less common. The injuries present will depend on the exact events, but they are usually extensive and severe when there has been contact with a moving train, although they may be localized with black soiling at the crushed decapitation or amputation site if the individual has lain across the track (Figure 14.9).

There is a risk of secondary injury if survival occurs where other factors such as electrified lines are present. On electrified lines, an additional cause of suicidal or accidental injury or death is present in the form of electric shock from either a live rail or overhead power lines. The voltage in these circuits is high, often in region of 600 V. Death is rapid and often associated with severe burns at the points of contact or earthing.

A careful search for unusual injuries inconsistent with the setting, and examination for a vital response to the severe blunt force injuries, should be made, as homicides may be concealed by staging the scene, with the deceased being placed on the rail track in an attempt to conceal the true cause of death.

Railway workers may be injured or killed by falling under, or by being struck by, moving rolling stock or by being trapped between the buffers of two trucks while uncoupling or coupling the rolling stock. The injuries associated with the squeezing between rolling stock are often those of a flail chest, with or without evidence of traumatic asphyxia.

■ Aircraft fatalities

Aviation incidents can be divided into two main groups: those that involve the crew and the large numbers of passengers of a modern, commercial aircraft, and those that involve the occupants of small, relatively slow, light aircraft.

Large aircraft are pressurized and, if the integrity of the cabin is breached, there can be rapid decompression and the passengers may suffer barotrauma. If the defect in the cabin is large enough, victims may exit through the defect and fall to their death. When an aircraft hits the ground, the results will depend on the rapidity of transfer of the forces, and this is dependent on the speed of the aircraft and the angle of impact. If the forces are very severe, all passengers may be killed by deceleration injuries and by multiple trauma owing to loss of integrity of the fuselage.

In lesser impacts, the results may be similar to those of motor vehicle crashes, although the forces are usually greater and the injuries sustained are proportionately more severe. The usual lap-strap seat belt offers little protection in anything but the most minor accident. Fire is one of the greatest hazards in air crashes and accounts for many deaths.

In light aircraft crashes, the velocity, and hence the forces, may be less than in large commercial aircraft, but they are still often fatal. The investigation of air accidents is a task for specialist medical personnel, who are often available from the national air force or from a civil authority. There should always be a full autopsy on the pilot or suspected pilot, with full microscopic and toxicological examination to exclude natural disease, drugs and alcohol.

■ Marine fatalities

Fatalities in the marine setting embrace a range of marine-specific and general injury types. The range of activities include commercial diving, recreational diving, use of powered water sport bikes, sailing, motor cruising and commercial marine transport (e.g. oil tankers, container ships, passenger vessels). The likelihood of dying in a marine environment is enhanced by not wearing appropriate safety gear. In the recreational setting, fatalities occur when individuals fall from vessels and drown, or succumb to hypothermia, or cannot be recovered back on board.

Physical injuries in recreational sailing are widespread and examples include those of suffering direct trauma (e.g. head or neck following uncontrolled gybe; Figure 14.10), loss of digits or limbs when caught up in winches or anchor cable, limb fractures or skull fractures from direct impact from flailing blocks and burn injury from uncontrolled rope movement. Drowning may occur from being trapped after inversion of the vessel.

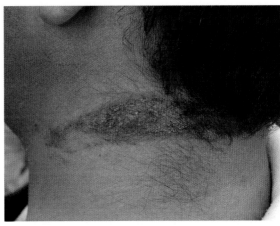

Figure 14.10 Abrasion of neck caused by mainsheet during uncontrolled gybe.

Motor-powered vessels may cause injury from explosion or fire, or those in the water may sustain injury from rotating propellers.

Commercial vessels may cause their own specific problems, such as asphyxiation in storage tanks or falls from heights. Most of these scenarios are of an industrial/occupational nature and may involve potential breaches of health and safety legislation. In the UK The Marine Accident Investigation Branch (MAIB) examines and investigates all types of marine accidents to, or on board, UK ships worldwide, and other ships in UK territorial waters.

■ Further information sources

Aghayev E, Thali M, Jackowski C et al. Virtopsy – Fatal motor vehicle accident with head injury. *Journal of Forensic Sciences* 2004; **49**: 809–13.

Bhatti JA, Razzak JA. Railway associated injuries in Pakistan. *International Journal of Injury Control and Safety Promotion* 2010; **17**: 41–4.

Boniface K, McKay MP, Lucas R, Shaffer A, Sikka N. Serious injuries related to the Segway® personal transporter: a case series. *Annals of Emergency Medicine* 2010; [Epub ahead of print].

Chao T-C, Lau G, Eng-Swee Teo C. Falls from a height: the pathology of trauma from vertical deceleration, Chapter 20 In: Mason JK, Purdue BN (eds). *The Pathology of Trauma*, 3rd edn. London: Arnold, 2000; p. 313–26.

Clark JC, Milroy CM (2000). Injuries and deaths of pedestrians, Chapter 2. In: Mason JK, Purdue BN (eds). *The Pathology of Trauma*, 3rd edn. London: Arnold, 2000; p. 17–29.

Conroy C, Hoyt DB, Eastman AB *et al*. Motor vehicle-related cardiac and aortic injuries differ from other thoracic injuries. *Journal of Trauma* 2007; **62:** 1462–7.

Corporate Manslaughter and Corporate Homicide Act 2007. http://www.legislation.gov.uk/ukpga/ 2007/19/contents (accessed 23 November 2010).

Cullen SA, Drysdale HC. Aviation accidents, Chapter 19. In: Mason JK, Purdue BN (eds) *The Pathology of Trauma*, 3rd edn. London: Arnold, 2000; p. 300–12.

Deaner RM, Fitchett VH. Motorcycle trauma. *Journal of Trauma* 1975; **15:** 678–81.

Graham JW. Fatal motorcycle accidents. *Journal of Forensic Sciences* 1969; **14:** 79–86.

Goonewardene SS, Baloch K, Porter K, Sargeant I, Punchihewa G. Road traffic collisions-case fatality rate, crash injury rate, and number of motor vehicles: time trends between a developed and developing country. *American Surgeon* 2010; **76:** 977–81.

Hitusugi M, Takatsu A, Shigeta A. Injuries of motorcyclists and bicyclists examined at autopsy. *The American Journal of Forensic Medicine and Pathology* 1999; **20:** 251–5.

Karger B, Tiege K, Bühren W, DuChesne A. Relationship between impact velocity and injuries in fatal pedestrian–car collisions. *International Journal of Legal Medicine* 2000; **113:** 84–8.

Liu BC, Ivers R, Norton R, Boufous S, Blows S, Lo SK. Helmets for preventing injury in motorcycle riders. *Cochrane Database Systematic Reviews* 2008; **1:** CD004333.

Milroy CM, Clark JC. Injuries and deaths in vehicle occupants, Chapter 1. In: Mason JK, Purdue BN (eds) *The Pathology of Trauma*, 3rd edn. London: Arnold, 2000; p. 1–16.

Murphy GK. Death on the railway. *Journal of Forensic Sciences* 1976; **21:** 218–26.

National Highway Traffic Safety Administration. Recent trends in motorcycle fatalities. *Annals of Emergency Medicine* 2002; **39:** 195–7.

Nikolic S, Atanasijevic T, Mihailovic Z *et al*. Mechanisms of aortic blunt rupture in fatally injured front-seat passengers in frontal car collisions: an autopsy study. *American Journal of Forensic Medicine and Pathology* 2006; **27:** 292–5.

Obafunwa JO, Bulgin S, Busuttil A. Medico-legal considerations of deaths from watersports among Caribbean tourists. *Journal of Clinical Forensic Medicine* 1997; **4:** 65–71.

Oström M, Eriksson A. Natural death while driving. *Journal of Forensic Sciences* 1987; **32:** 988–8.

Penttilä A, Lunetta P. Transportation medicine, Chapter 35. In: Payne-James J, Busuttil A, Smock W (eds). *Forensic Medicine – Clinical and Pathological Aspects*. London: Greenwich Medical Media, 2003; p. 525–41.

Rosenkrantz KM, Sheridan RL. Trauma to adult bicyclists: a growing problem in the urban environment. *Injury* 2003; **34:** 825–9.

Sato Y, Oshima T, Kondo T. Airbag injuries: a literature review in consideration of demands in forensic autopsies. *Forensic Science International* 2002; **128:** 162–7.

Saukko P, Knight B. Transportation injuries, Chapter 9. In: Saukko P, Knight B (eds) *Knight's Forensic Pathology*, 3rd edn. London: Arnold, 2004; p. 281–300.

Schmidt P, Haarhoff K, Bonte W. Sudden natural death at the wheel – a particular problem of the elderly? *Forensic Science International* 1990; **48:** 155–62.

Sevitt S. The mechanisms of traumatic rupture of the thoracic aorta. *British Journal of Surgery* 1977; **64:** 166–73.

Shkrum MJ, McClafferty KJ, Green RN *et al*. Mechanisms of aortic injury in fatalities occurring in motor vehicle collisions. *Journal of Forensic Sciences* 1999; **44:** 44–56.

Shkrum MJ, McClafferty KJ, Nowak ES, German A. Driver and front seat passenger fatalities associated with air bag deployment. Part 2: a review of injury patterns and investigative issues. *Journal of Forensic Sciences* 2002; **47:** 1035–40.

Siegel JH, Smith JA, Tenebaum N *et al*. Deceleration energy and change in velocity on impact: key factors in fatal versus potentially survivable motor vehicle crash (mvc) and aortic injuries (AI): the role of associated injuries as determinants of outcome. *Annual Proceedings of the Association for the Advancement of Automotive Medicine* 2002; **46:** 315–38.

Smith TG 3rd, Wessells HB, Mack CD, Kaufman R, Bulger EM, Voelzke BB. Examination of the impact of airbags on renal injury using a national database. *Journal of the American College of Surgeons* 2010; **211:** 355–60.

Swan KG, Swan BC, Swan KG. Deceleration thoracic injury. *Journal of Trauma* 2001; **51:** 970–4.

Thali MJ, Braun M, Bruschweiler W, Dirnhofer R. Matching tire tracks on the head using forensic photogrammetry. *Forensic Science International* 2000; **113:** 281–7.

Thali MJ, Braun M, Aghayev E *et al*. Virtopsy – scientific documentation, reconstruction and animation in forensic: individual and real 3D data based geo-metric approach including optical body/object surface and radiological CT/MRI scanning. *Journal of Forensic Sciences* 2005; **50:** 428–42.

Töro K, Hubay M, Sótonyi P, Keller E. Fatal traffic injuries among pedestrians, bicyclists and motor vehicle occupants. *Forensic Science International* 2005; **151:** 151–6.

Transport and Works Act 1992. http://www.legislation.gov.uk/ukpga/1992/42/contents (accessed 23 November 2010).

Zettas JP, Zettas P, Thanasophon B. Injury patterns in motorcycle accidents. *Journal of Trauma* 1979; **19:** 833–6.

Zivot U, Di Maio VJ. Motor vehicle–pedestrian accidents in adults: relationship between impact speed, injuries and distance thrown. *American Journal of Forensic Medicine and Pathology* 1993; **14:** 185–6.

14 Transportation medicine

Chapter

15

Asphyxia

- Introduction
- Classification of asphyxia
- Phases and signs of 'asphyxia'
- Types of mechanical asphyxial mechanisms
- Further information sources

Introduction

The literal translation of the word 'asphyxia' from the Greek means 'absence or lack of pulsation'; quite how this word has came to denote the effects of 'the lack of oxygen' is not clear, but it is now a word commonly used to describe a range of conditions for which the lack of oxygen, whether it is partial (hypoxia) or complete (anoxia), is considered to be the cause (Table 15.1).

In forensic medicine, asphyxia often describes a situation where there has been a physical obstruction between the mouth and nose to the alveoli, although other 'asphyxial mechanisms' exist, in which there is an inability to utilize oxygen at the cellular level without there being a physical airway obstruction. The term asphyxia is not a term frequently used in clinical medicine and, given the incomplete understanding of the pathophysiology of many deaths occurring following the application of pressure to the chest and neck, for example, its use as a useful descriptive term in such scenarios is perhaps questionable.

Table 15.1 Examples of 'asphyxial' conditions

Underlying cause of death	Name
Lack of oxygen in the inspired air	Suffocation
Blockage of the external orifices	Suffocation/smothering
Blockage of the internal airways by obstruction	Gagging/choking
Blockage of the internal airways by external pressure	Strangulation/hanging
Restriction of chest movement	Traumatic asphyxia
Failure of oxygen transportation	(For example carbon monoxide poisoning)
Failure of oxygen utilization	(For example cyanide poisoning)

■ Classification of asphyxia

Although there are currently moves to develop an internationally agreed classification for asphyxia, for the purposes of exploring what is generally currently broadly agreed in the forensic community as 'asphyxia', a simple classification of 'asphyxial mechanisms' is described below:

- ■ Mechanical (Figure 15.1)
  - strangulation (pressure applied to the neck by means of a ligature, or by hands etc.)
  - hanging (pressure applied to the neck by means of a ligature combined with the weight of the body)
  - choking (physical obstruction within the airways)
  - compression asphyxia (pressure applied to the chest or abdomen, resulting in a physical interference with the ability to breathe effectively)
  - smothering (physical obstruction of the mouth/ nose preventing effective breathing).
- ■ Non-mechanical
  - carbon monoxide poisoning (chemical interference with respiration at a cellular level – see Chapter 22, p. 212)
  - cyanide poisoning (as above).
- ■ Miscellaneous
  - drowning (physical interference with effective respiration; see Chapter 16, p. 164).

Asphyxial insults are not necessarily fatal, the outcome being largely dependent on the nature of the insult, its degree, and its length of time. It is possible for some survivors to suffer no significant adverse long-term health effects, although others may 'survive' in a vegetative state following irreversible hypoxic–ischaemic brain injury, depending on the length of time inadequate oxygenation was experienced. In the living, appropriate examination, documentation and investigations will optimize the recovery of forensically useful evidence in order to assist subsequent legal proceedings and, if such an individual presents to hospital, it is appropriate for such an examination to be made by a suitably experienced forensic physician at the earliest opportunity. Where the insult has resulted in death, examination by a forensic pathologist is recommended in order to identify potentially subtle evidence of assault.

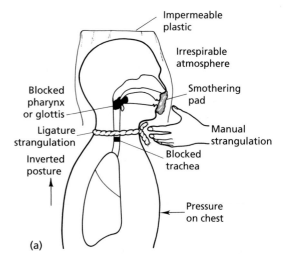

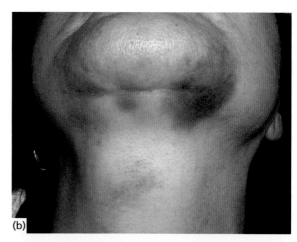

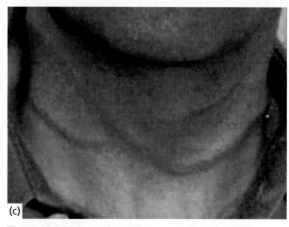

Figure 15.1 **(a)** Examples of the causes of mechanical asphyxia. **(b)** Grip marks to the neck and jaw following attempted manual strangulation. **(c)** Ligature mark after attempted garrotting - note congestion ('tide mark') above double ligature.

■ Phases and signs of 'asphyxia'

The general sequence of events currently described in most 'asphyxial episodes' is: the dyspnoea phase, convulsive phase, pre-terminal respiratory phase, then gasping for breath followed by the terminal phase (see Box 15.1).

> **Box 15.1** Sequence of events that may be seen in asphyxial episodes
>
> - **Dyspnoea phase** – expiratory dyspnoea with raised respiratory rate, cyanosis and tachycardia (may last for a minute or more)
> - **Convulsive phase** – loss of consciousness, reduced respiratory movements, facial congestion, bradycardia, hypertension, fits (may last for a couple of minutes)
> - **Pre-terminal respiratory phase** – no respiratory action, failure of respiratory and circulatory centres, tachycardia, hypertension (may last a couple of minutes)
> - **Gasping for breath** – respiratory reflexes
> - **Terminal** – loss of movement, areflexial, pupillary dilatation

Research into the pathophysiology of 'asphyxia' is ongoing, including attempts to analyse the sequence of events depicted in recordings made by individuals who hang themselves. It remains to be seen whether such a sequence of events is 'asphyxial mechanism specific', and whether there is reliable, objective, evidence for a non-fatal outcome at any (or all) of the pre-terminal phases described above.

Traditionally, the 'classic signs of asphyxia' were described as:

- petechial haemorrhages in the skin of the face and in the lining of the eyelids;
- congestion and oedema of the face;
- cyanosis (blue discoloration) of the skin of the face;
- right heart congestion and abnormal fluidity of the blood.

None of these 'classic signs' is, however, specific for 'asphyxia', and they are commonly seen, for example, in those dying from congestive cardiac deaths. Raised intravascular pressure in blood vessels in the head/neck explains the first three signs, while right heart congestion and fluidity of blood can be considered irrelevant to ascribing death to 'asphyxia'. Of these 'classic signs', the finding of petechiae in the face/neck is of most importance to the forensic pathologist; it is a finding that requires an explanation, and a careful search for any evidence capable of supporting a diagnosis of 'pressure having been applied to the neck or chest' (Figure 15.2). Additional non-specific findings in 'asphyxial deaths' include congestion of the viscera and petechiae (Tardieu spots) (Figure 15.3).

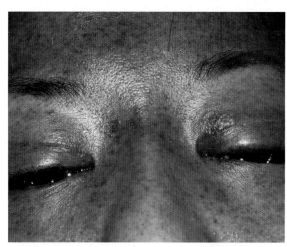

Figure 15.2 Petechial (and more confluent) haemorrhages in the facial skin and conjunctivae following manual strangulation.

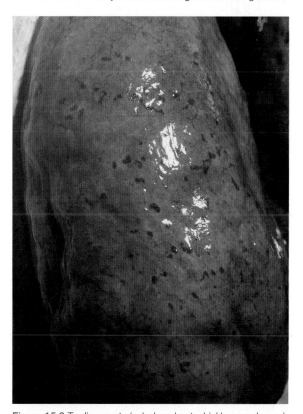

Figure 15.3 Tardieu spots (subpleural petechial haemorrhages) following manual strangulation. These are no longer considered to be specific for asphyxia.

In survivors of an 'asphyxial episode', careful clinical examination may show:

- pain and tenderness around the neck and structures within the neck;
- damage to the larynx and associated cartilages;
- damage to the hyoid bone;
- dried saliva around the mouth;
- cyanosis (particularly if the survivor is found immediately after the attack);
- congestion and oedema of the structures above any level of compression;
- petechiae (see Chapter 8, p. 80) above the level of the compressive force that has caused the asphyxia;
- haemorrhage from the mouth, nose and ears, presumably as a consequence of raised intravascular pressure; incontinence of faeces and urine.

■ Types of mechanical asphyxial mechanisms

Pressure to the neck

Three forms of the application of direct pressure to the neck are of importance in forensic medicine, namely manual strangulation, ligature strangulation and hanging. In each of these it is not possible to predict how rapidly death will occur; in some cases, death will be relatively 'slow', allowing time for the development of the 'classic signs of asphyxia' (although such signs may be evident following the application of pressure to the neck for a matter of seconds), while in other cases such signs will be entirely absent.

The application of pressure to the neck may lead to any of the following, the precise nature of which is dependent upon the type, site and extent of the pressure applied:

- obstruction of the jugular veins, causing impaired venous return of blood from the head to the heart (leading to cyanosis, congestion, petechiae);
- obstruction of the carotid arteries which, if severe, causes cerebral hypoxia;
- stimulation of carotid sinus baroreceptors at the bifurcation of the common carotid arteries resulting in a neurologically mediated cardiac arrest;

- elevation of the larynx and tongue, closing the airway at the level of the pharynx (unless extreme pressure is applied to the neck, the cartilaginous trachea is more resistant to compression).

Following mechanical pressure to the neck, loss of consciousness can occur rapidly; traditionally, loss of consciousness following hanging was thought to occur within 10 seconds, and such a time-frame would generally seem to be confirmed by analysis of filmed hangings. The time taken to produce a fatal outcome, however, has not been satisfactorily established, although filmed hanging analysis suggests a lack of recognizable respiratory movements after 2 minutes and a lack of muscle movements after 7.5 minutes. Experimental occlusion of dog tracheas indicated the potential for their survival up to 14 minutes following obstructive asphyxiation.

'Vagal inhibition' or reflex cardiac arrest

It has been recognized for some time that the mechanical stimulation of the carotid sinus baroreceptors in the neck can result in an unpredictable, and sometimes fatal, outcome. Fatalities have been described, for example, following apparently minimal pressure being applied to the neck, and such events have been attributed to vagal inhibition or reflex cardiac arrest (Figure 15.4). Therapeutic carotid sinus pressure is carried out on individuals with an arrhythmia, while being closely monitored, and is considered to be generally safe. The clinical response, however, has also been described as being unpredictable, and deaths have occurred because of ventricular arrhythmias/asystole.

Stimulation of the carotid sinus baroreceptors results in impulses being transmitted via the carotid sinus nerve (a branch of the glossopharyngeal nerve) to the nucleus of the tractus solitarius, and vagal nuclei, in the medulla. Parasympathetic impulses descend to the heart via the vagus nerve leading to a profound bradycardia and potentially asystole.

Death may supervene at any time following the application of pressure to the neck, and it is thought that such 'vagal inhibition' may explain why so many individuals found hanging show none of the classic signs of asphyxia.

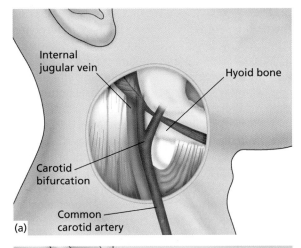

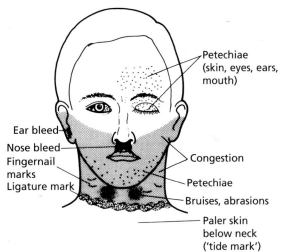

Figure 15.5 Possible features of strangulation when cardiac arrest is delayed.

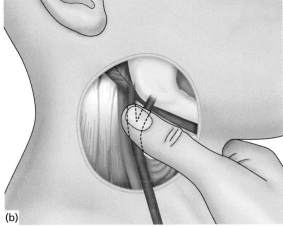

Figure 15.4 The carotid sinus baroreceptor and pressure to the neck: **(a)** the location of the carotid sinus at the bifurcation of the common carotid artery in the neck, and **(b)** pressure to the neck causing compression of the carotid sinus.

The length of time that pressure to the neck/chest must be maintained to produce congestion and petechiae in a living victim is a matter of continued controversy, but it is generally accepted that a minimum of 10–30 seconds is required. In the absence of petechiae, it follows that if death resulted from the application of pressure to the neck, death must have supervened within that length of time, a factor that may be of legal relevance when considering a defendant's actions.

Strangulation

Manual strangulation is used to describe the application of pressure to the neck using the hands, and is a relatively common mode of homicide, particularly where there is disparity between the sizes of the assailant and victim. The external signs of manual strangulation (Figure 15.5) can include bruises and abrasions on the front and sides of the neck, and the lower jaw; the pattern of skin surface injuries is often difficult to interpret because of the dynamic nature of an assault, and the possibility of the repeated reapplication of pressure during strangulation. Bruises caused by fingertip pressure (rounded or oval-shaped bruises up to approximately 2 cm in size) and fingernail scratches (linear or crescent-shaped abrasions, imprints or skin breaches) may be seen, the latter being made either by the assailant or the victim (Figure 15.6).

When pressure to the neck is sustained, additional features of manual strangulation can include the 'classic asphyxial signs', including facial petechiae. In the living victim, clinical evaluation may reveal pain on swallowing, hoarseness, stridor, neck, head or back pain.

Ligature strangulation may be homicidal, suicidal or accidental and involves the application of pressure to the neck by an item capable of constricting the neck, such as a scarf, neck-tie, stocking or telephone cable etc. (Figure 15.7). There is frequently a clear demarcation of congestion, cyanosis and petechiae above the level of the constricting ligature, and there is usually a 'ligature mark' on the neck at the site of constriction. This mark is probably formed by a combination of compression and abrasion of the skin, and may reflect the nature of the ligature itself, replicating the pattern of a plaited ligature, for example. Careful documentation of any pattern visible within a

155

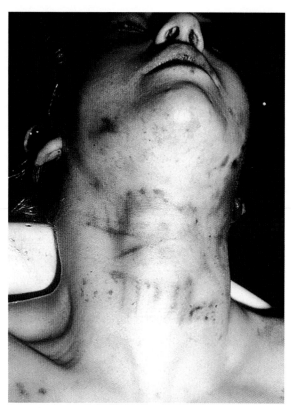

Figure 15.6 Surface injuries on the neck and jaw in manual strangulation. Note multiple bruises and abrasions; some of these injuries are caused by the victim trying to release the grip of the assailant.

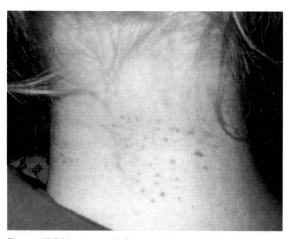

Figure 15.7 Ligature mark from a nylon scarf. Although the fabric was broad, tight stretching of the fabric resulted in a well-defined linear 'band' that could be mistaken for that made by a cord or wire.

ligature mark, with scaled photographs, may enable comparison to be made with an item suspected of being used as a ligature in that case at a future date. Soft and broad-surface ligatures, however, may leave very little evidence of compression on the skin of the neck, or even injury to underlying structures.

Marks on the neck in ligature strangulation may encircle the neck horizontally, although clothing, or hair, may be interposed between the ligature and skin, resulting in discontinuities in the mark. There may be marks suggestive of crossover of the ligature, or knots, but there will be no pattern suggestive of a suspension point, distinguishing ligature strangulation from hanging, in which the individual's body weight against a ligature leads to pressure being exerted on the neck. At post-mortem examination, ligature marks are frequently seen as brown parchmented bands, reflecting post-mortem drying of the abraded skin. While accidental and suicidal ligature strangulation does occur, it is recommended that such cases are treated with great caution until homicide can be excluded by thorough investigation.

Pressure can be applied to the neck by means other than the hands or a ligature; restraint techniques may involve the use of 'arm-locks' or 'choke-holds', and investigations into deaths following police/security service contact frequently involve the evaluation of potential effects of restraint techniques used prior to death. Such techniques may or may not result in the production of asphyxial signs or neck injury.

The extent of injury to soft tissues, muscles and the skeleton of the neck (hyoid bone and thyroid cartilage) varies depending upon the nature of the pressure applied to the neck. Post-mortem dissection of neck structures should always be carried out following 'drainage' of the vasculature of the neck, which can be achieved by carrying out the dissection after removal of the brain and heart. Such a technique avoids the production of artefactual haemorrhage at the back of the larynx (Figure 15.8). There may be bruising within the 'strap muscles' in the neck and injury to the superior horns of the thyroid cartilage, which are particularly vulnerable to compressive injury (Figure 15.9). Suspected fractures should be confirmed under the microscope as triticeous cartilage mobility at the tips of the horns may simulate fractures. The greater horns of the hyoid bone may also be injured, albeit less frequently than the thyroid cartilage. Calcification and ossification of the hyoid bone and thyroid cartilage occurs with increasing age, and such change is associated with less flexible structures that are more prone to injury following neck compression. Internal neck injuries are commonly less extensive in ligature strangulation, with haemorrhage often being more localized to the site of ligature application.

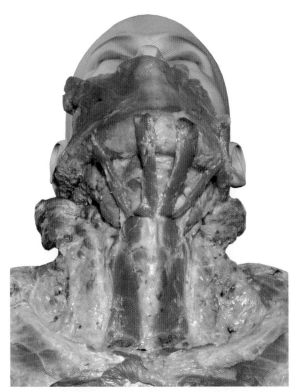

Figure 15.8 Layered *in situ* dissection of the anterior neck structures is essential in order to evaluate injuries following pressure to the neck. Such dissection must be carried out following 'drainage' or 'decompression' of the blood vessels in the neck to avoid artefactual haemorrhage.

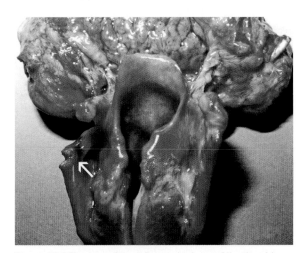

Figure 15.9 Fracture of the left superior horn of the thyroid cartilage following strangulation.

Hanging

Hanging describes suspension of the body by the neck. Any material capable of forming a ligature can be used for hanging. The pressure of the ligature on the neck is produced by the weight of the body; it is not necessary for the body to be completely suspended, with the feet off the ground and the body hanging free under gravity, as death may result from hanging where the body is slumped in a sitting, kneeling or half-lying position, with the point of suspension occurring at the level of, for example, a door-handle. As with ligature strangulation, a ligature mark is commonly present – often accompanied by a deep indentation or furrow in the skin – but discontinuous at some point around the neck. This discontinuity reflects the suspension point, which may be at the sides or back of the neck, or even at the front of the neck. If the ligature mark is seen to rise at the sides of the neck, for example, to form an inverted V-shaped mark at the back of the head, the suspension point was at the back of the head (Figures 15.10 and 15.11).

The precise mechanism of death in hanging is incompletely understood, although research is ongoing. In the absence of classical signs of asphyxia, even in hangings in which there is complete suspension, the inference must be that death has occurred more rapidly than it takes for such signs to appear, raising the possibility that carotid sinus pressure and neurogenic cardiac arrest has played an important role.

Hanging by judicial execution involves a 'drop', for example through a trapdoor, calculated to result in cervical spinal cord injury and fracture-dislocation of the cervical spine, but without decapitation. However, excluding judicial execution hangings, internal injury

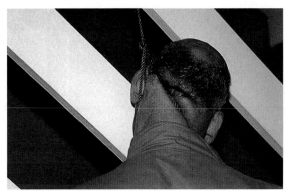

Figure 15.10 Suicidal hanging: the rope rises to a point, leaving a gap in the ligature mark – the suspension point – on the neck.

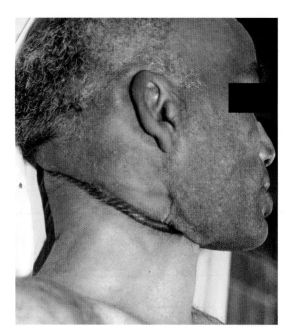

Figure 15.11 A deep furrowed ligature mark under the chin, and rising to the back of the neck, in hanging. Note the spiral weave pattern visible in the parchmented mark.

to neck structures in hangings is frequently inconspicuous, and may be entirely absent.

Non-judicial hanging is mostly a suicidal act of males. Some cases are accidental and entanglement with cords and ropes can occur, for example with restraint harnesses or window-blind cords in children. Occasionally, a homicide is staged to resemble a suicidal hanging, and the pathologist must be alert to the presence of injuries not capable of being explained by hanging. Post-mortem toxicological analysis should be performed in all hangings in order to determine whether the individual was capable of self-suspension.

In survivors of accidental or suicidal hanging there may be no adverse sequelae. For some there may be residual hypoxic brain damage that may be profound, or only detectable by neuropsychological assessment. Others have motor and/sensory loss as a result of brain damage.

Choking

Accidental ingestion of objects or food can cause choking, the internal obstruction of the upper air passages by an object or substance impacted in the pharynx or larynx. Choking is, most commonly, accidental and common causes include misplaced dentures in adults and inhaled objects such as small toys, balls, etc., in children. In medical practice there are risks associated with individuals who are sedated or anaesthetized, when objects such as extracted teeth or blood from dental or ear, nose and throat (ENT) operations may occlude the airway without provoking the normal protective reflex of coughing. Obstruction commonly leads to respiratory distress with congestion and cyanosis of the head and face.

Café coronary

One of the commonest causes of choking is the entry of food into the air passages. If food enters the larynx during swallowing, it usually causes gross choking symptoms of coughing, distress and cyanosis, which can be fatal unless the obstruction is cleared by coughing or some rapid treatment is offered. However, if the piece of food is large enough to occlude the larynx completely, it will prevent not only breathing but also speech and coughing. The individual may die silently and quickly, the cause of death remaining hidden until the autopsy. This is the so-called café coronary (Figure 15.12).

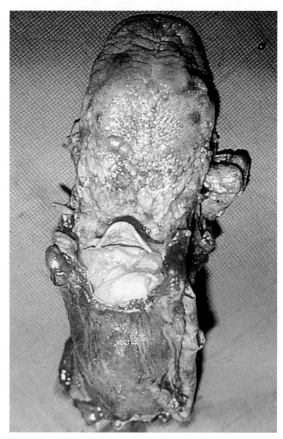

Figure 15.12 Impaction of food in the larynx – café coronary.

Compressional and positional asphyxia

Pressure on the trunk (chest and/or abdomen) can result in an inability to breathe effectively and result in death. Workmen trapped in collapsed earth trenches, or buried in grain silos, for example, can find that they are unable to expand their chests, leading to marked 'asphyxial signs'. Similarly, individuals trapped under heavy machinery experience an inability to breathe effectively. Occasionally, individuals are crushed by the weight of many other people fleeing danger, such as during a fire in a sports stadium. These examples of 'compression asphyxia' are commonly referred to as traumatic or crush asphyxia (Figure 15.13).

A less dramatic presentation of asphyxial signs is commonly seen in individuals who find themselves in such an awkward body position that they too are unable to breathe effectively. They may, for example, attempt to squeeze through small gaps in railings, or small open windows, and become wedged preventing expansion of the chest (Figure 15.14). Others may find themselves hanging head first over the side of a bed, with their head flexed into their chest, restricting air entry. Such a scenario is termed positional or postural asphyxia, and those involved are usually unable to extricate themselves from the position in which they find themselves because of impaired cognition or consciousness as a result of intoxication.

Individuals with impaired neurological function owing to neurological disease may also succumb to positional asphyxia, for example by attempting to get out of a hospital bed with 'cot sides', and becoming wedged between the bed and a wall.

Controversy exists in the forensic community regarding the potential role of restraint techniques by police, in particular where arms are being secured behind the back and the subject is being

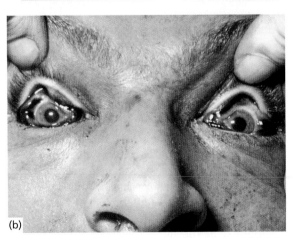

(a)

(b)

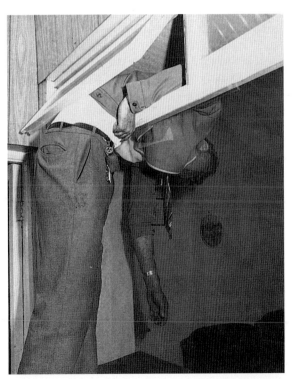

Figure 15.13 Traumatic asphyxiation in the workplace: **(a)** there is gross congestion of the head and face, with petechiae following burial, up to the axillae, in an avalanche of iron ore, and **(b)** gross conjunctival haemorrhages following chest compression by ash.

Figure 15.14 Postural asphyxiation. This intoxicated individual slipped and fell from a window sill while trying to climb through a fanlight window. He became wedged and could not make sufficient respiratory movements. Facial (and left arm) congestion and hypostasis is present.

placed in a face-down position. Deaths in such a scenario rarely involve restraint in isolation but occur on a background of intense exertion, substance misuse and mental health problems; it is likely that such deaths represent the culmination of a number of adverse physiological factors. Nevertheless, restraint techniques used by police/security forces and others must minimize the risk of positional asphyxia.

Suffocation and smothering

Suffocation is a term usually used to describe a fatal reduction of the concentration of oxygen in the respired atmosphere, and often incorporates 'smothering'. A reduction in atmospheric oxygen can occur, for example, in a decompressed aircraft cabin, or in a grain silo. Mechanical obstruction of the upper airways can lead to suffocation, as is seen when plastic bags are accidentally, homicidally, or suicidally placed over the head (Figure 15.15). Post-mortem examination in such cases rarely reveals any of the 'classic asphyxial signs'.

Similarly, smothering – the physical occlusion of the nose and mouth – may leave no 'asphyxial signs' in survivors or the deceased. If the individuals are unable to struggle, owing to extremes of age or intoxication, for example, they may have no evidence of injury, including around the mouth or nose. Occasionally, examination will reveal intraoral injury (including bruising or laceration of the insides of the lips or bruising of the gums in an edentulous individual) and soft tissue dissection

of the face may reveal subcutaneous bruising around the mouth and nose. Smothering may therefore be impossible to diagnose at post-mortem examination.

Retention of items/objects alleged to have been used to smother individuals that survive, for example, may have evidential value. Saliva, for example, may be identified on a pillow used in an attack and DNA matching may corroborate the account given.

Autoerotic asphyxia

Autoerotic asphyxia is the term used to describe those fatalities occurring during some form of solitary sexual activity. Many other terms have been used to describe deaths such as these including sexual asphyxia, sex hanging, asphyxiophilia, Kotzwarrism, autoasphyxiophilia and hypoxyphilia. The recurrent feature tends to be the use of a device, appliance or restraint that causes neck compression, leading to cerebral hypoxia, with the aim of heightening the sexual response. Such deaths, which usually involve men, occur predominantly as a result of failure of safety devices.

The presence of the following features should be considered when 'diagnosing' autoerotic asphyxiation:

- evidence of solo sexual activity;
- private or secure location;
- evidence of previous similar activity in the past;
- no apparent suicidal intent;
- unusual props including ligatures, clothing, and pornography;
- failure of a device or set-up integral to the activity causing death.

Death results from the application of pressure to the neck, and as with other ligature-related deaths, the presence of classic asphyxial signs is variable. The presence of gags or other means of occluding the airways may lead to a death more akin to upper airway occlusion than pressure to the neck, and the addition of an asphyxiant substance (such as nitrous oxide gas) within coverings over the head may lead to suffocation. The presence of injuries suggestive of assault must be looked for carefully, and the possibility of third-party involvement must always be considered in such cases.

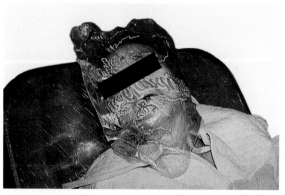

Figure 15.15 Suicidal plastic bag asphyxia. Suffocation by plastic bag often leaves no autopsy asphyxial signs, and removal of the bag by another individual prior to autopsy would cause significant interpretation problems.

■ Further information sources

Adelson LA. *The Pathology of Homicide. A Vade Mecum for Pathologist, Prosecutor and Defense Counsel.* Springfield, IL: Charles C Thomas, 1974.

Adjutantis G, Coutselinis A, Dritsas C. Suicidal strangulation. *Forensic Science* 1974; **3:** 283–4.

Alexander S, Ping WC. Fatal ventricular fibrillation during carotid sinus stimulation. *American Journal of Cardiology* 1966; **18:** 289–91.

Bell MD, Rao VJ, Wetli CV, Rodriquez RN. Positional asphyxiation in adults. A series of 30 cases from the Dade and Broward County Florida Medical Examiner Offices from 1982 to 1990. *American Journal of Forensic Medicine and Pathology* 1992; **13:** 101–7.

Boghossian E, Clement R, Redpath M, Sauvageau A. Respiratory, circulatory, and neurological responses to hanging: a review of animal models. *Journal of Forensic Sciences* 2010; **55:** 1272–7.

Busuttil A. Asphyxial deaths in children. Chapter 16. In: Busuttil A, Keeling JW (eds) *Paediatric Forensic Medicine and Pathology.* London: Hodder Arnold, 2008; p. 329–35.

Byard RW. Autoerotic death. In: Payne-James JJ, Byard RW, Corey TS, Henderson C (eds) *Encyclopaedia of Forensic and Legal Medicine.* Volume 1. Oxford: Elsevier Science, 2005; p. 157–65.

Byard RW, Bramwell NH. Autoerotic death. A definition. *American Journal of Forensic Medicine and Pathology* 1991; **12:** 74–6.

Byard RW, Cohle SD. Accidents. In: Byard RW (ed.) *Sudden Death in Infancy and Childhood and Adolescence*, 2nd edn. Cambridge: Cambridge University Press, 2004; p. 11–73.

Byard RW, Wilson GW. Death scene gas analysis in suspected methane asphyxia. *American Journal of Forensic Medicine and Pathology* 1992; **13:** 69–71.

Byard RW, Gilbert JD, Klitte A, Felgate P. Gasoline exposure in motor vehicle accident fatalities. *American Journal of Forensic Medicine and Pathology* 2002; **23:** 42–4.

Clement R, Redpath M, Sauvageau A. Mechanism of death in hanging: a historical review of the evolution of pathophysiological hypotheses. *Journal of Forensic Sciences* 2010; 55: 1268–71.

Cohen MV. Ventricular fibrillation precipitated by carotid sinus pressure: case report and review of the literature. *American Heart Journal* 1972; **84:** 681–6.

Daly MD, Angell-James JE, Elsner R. Role of carotid-body chemoreceptors and their reflex interactions in bradycardia and cardiac arrest. *Lancet* 1979; **1:** 764–7.

Di Maio DJ, Di Maio VJM. *Forensic Pathology.* Boca Raton, FL: CRC Press, 1993.

Duband S, Timoshenko AP, Morrison AL, Prades JM, Debout M, Peoc'h M. Ear bleeding: A sign not to be underestimated in cases of strangulation. *American Journal of Forensic Medicine and Pathology* 2009; **30:** 175–6.

Ely SF, Hirsch CS. Asphyxial deaths and petechiae: a review. *Journal of Forensic Sciences* 2000; **45:** 1274–7.

Gill JR, Ely SF, Hua Z. Environmental gas displacement: three accidental deaths in the work place. *American Journal of Forensic Medicine and Pathology* 2002; **23:** 26–30.

Gilson T, Parks BO, Porterfield CM. Suicide with inert gases. *American Journal of Forensic Medicine and Pathology* 2003; **24:** 306–8.

Greenwood RJ, Dupler DA. Death following carotid sinus pressure. *Journal of the American Medical Association* 1962; **181:** 605–9.

Härm T, Rajs J. Types of injuries and interrelated conditions of victims and assailants in attempted and homicidal strangulation. *Forensic Science International* 1981; **18:** 101–3.

Hood I, Ryan D, Spitz WU. Resuscitation and petechiae. *American Journal of Forensic Medicine and Pathology* 1988; **9:** 35–7.

Humble JG. The mechanism of petechial haemorrhage formation. *Blood* 1949; **4:** 69–75.

Khokhlov VD. Pressure on the neck calculated for any point along the ligature. *Forensic Science International* 2001; **123:** 178–81.

Lasczkowski G, Risse M, Gamerdinger U, Weiler G. Pathogenesis of conjunctival petechiae. *Forensic Science International* 2005; **147:** 25–9.

Maxeiner H, Brockholdt B. Homicidal and suicidal ligature strangulation – a comparison of the post-mortem findings. *Forensic Science International* 2003; **137:** 60–6.

Plattner T, Bollinger S, Zollinger U. Forensic assessment of survived strangulation. *Forensic Science International* 2005; **153:** 202–7.

Pollanen MS. Subtle fatal manual neck compression. *Medicine, Science, and the Law* 2001; **41:** 135–40.

Prinsloo I, Gordon I. Post-mortem dissection artefacts of the neck; their differentiation from ante-mortem bruises. *South African Medical Journal* 1951; **25:** 358–61.

Purdue BN. Asphyxial and related deaths, Chapter 15. In: Mason BN, Purdue BN (eds) *The Pathology of Trauma*, 3rd edn. London: Arnold, 2000; p. 230–52.

Puschel K, Türk E, Lach H. Asphyxia-related deaths. *Forensic Science International* 2004; **144:** 211–14.

Rao VJ, Wetli CV. The forensic significance of conjunctival petechiae. *American Journal of Forensic Medicine and Pathology* 1988; **9:** 32–4.

Reay DT, Eisele JW. Death from law enforcement neck holds. *American Journal of Forensic Medicine and Pathology* 1982; **3:** 253–8.

Rossen R, Kabat H, Anderson JP. Acute arrest of cerebral circulation in man. *Archives of Neurology and Psychiatry* 1943; **50:** 510–28.

Saukko P, Knight B. *Knight's Forensic Pathology*, 3rd edn. London: Arnold Publishing, 2004.

Sauvageau A, LaHarpe R, Geberth VJ; Working Group on Human Asphyxia. Agonal sequences in eight filmed hangings: analysis of respiratory and movement responses to asphyxia by hanging. *Journal of Forensic Sciences* 2010; **55:** 1278–81.

Schmunk GA, Kaplan JA. Asphyxial deaths caused by automobile exhaust inhalation not attributable to carbon monoxide toxicity: study of 2 cases. *American Journal of Forensic Medicine and Pathology* 2002; **23:** 123–6.

Sep D, Thies KC. Strangulation injuries in children. *Resuscitation* 2007; **74:** 386–91.

Simpson K. Deaths from vagal inhibition. *Lancet* 1949; **1:** 558–60.

Swann HG, Brucer M. The cardiorespiratory and biochemical events during rapid anoxic death; obstructive asphyxia. *Texas Reports on Biology and Medicine* 1949; **7:** 593–3.

Verma SK. Pediatric and adolescent strangulation deaths. *Journal of Forensic and Legal Medicine* 2007; **14:** 61–4.

Walker A, Milroy CM, Payne-James JJ. Asphyxia. In: Payne-James JJ, Byard RW, Corey TS, Henderson C (eds) *Encylopedia of Forensic and Legal Medicine*. Oxford: Elsevier, 2005.

Wright RK, Davis J. Homicidal hanging masquerading as sexual asphyxia. *Journal of Forensic Sciences* 1976; **21:** 387–9.

Chapter 16

Immersion and drowning

■ Introduction

The presence of a body in water does not necessarily indicate drowning. Most bodies found in water are there as a result of accident or suicide. However, certain clues when a body is recovered (e.g. ligatures to hands and feet) may suggest a criminal act. Drowning can occur in only a few inches of water, and when investigating a possible drowning death as much knowledge as possible of the circumstances and locus is needed to make a proper and accurate determination of the cause of death. Jumping or diving into water may result in limb or head injuries that render a person incapable of swimming. Bodies are frequently retrieved from water; this process in itself may require the expertise of marine recovery units as there may be considerable hazard in ensuring the body is returned to dry land. The process of recovery may hamper investigation and contaminate a potential crime scene.

The pathological investigation of deaths following the recovery of a body from water is difficult, given that a wide range of potential explanations

for death exist; some examples are given in Box 16.1. The pathologist must attempt to address all of these potential explanations for death and determine if there is any pathological evidence capable of supporting a diagnosis of drowning. The death investigation must also address other questions such as how did the individual get into the water and what prevented survival?

Box 16.1 Examples of reasons for death in a body recovered from water

- Died of natural causes before entering the water (e.g. a myocardial infarction)
- Died of natural causes while in the water, having entered the water either voluntarily or accidentally (e.g. micturating into a canal and losing balance)
- Died from exposure and hypothermia in the water (particularly in the thin, the young and the elderly)
- Died of injuries or other unnatural cause before entering the water (e.g. an assault)
- Died of injuries after entering the water (e.g. being hit by a boat or jet ski)
- Died from submersion, but not drowning
- Died from true drowning as a result of aspiration of water into the lungs

■ Evidence of immersion

A number of changes appear on the skin and body surface after a body has been in water for enough time. The changes described later appear at very variable times, as there are many factors that may influence how these changes appear. Relevant factors that may influence the condition of a body include whether the water is salt or fresh, whether the water source is tidal or non-tidal, the presence of possible predators, water temperature, clothing worn on the body and type of surface at the base of the water.

Generally, if left in water for long enough, the skin of the hands and feet will become wrinkled and macerated. The fingertips become opaque and wrinkled ('washerwoman's fingers'; Figure 16.1) within a few hours of immersion in cold water (and a shorter time in warm water). As immersion time increases, macerated skin begins to separate, leading to skin peeling and 'degloving' of the skin of the hands and feet (Figure 16.2). Loss of pigment layers may be apparent, causing colour change in skin, which can sometimes mislead as to the ethnic origin of the deceased.

Estimating the post-mortem interval from signs of immersion, and decomposition, in a body recovered from water is completely unreliable and entirely temperature dependent. Once again there is an oft-quoted (but not evidence-based) 'rule of thumb' recognizing that decomposition in water in temperate climates occurs at roughly half the rate of a body left in air.

Bloating of the body (face, abdomen and genitals) owing to gas formation in soft tissues and body cavities is often evident after approximately

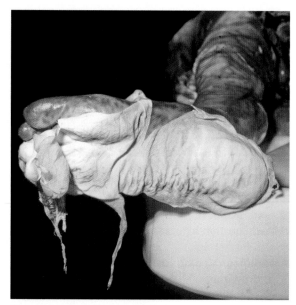

Figure 16.2 Peeling of the epidermis from the foot (degloving) following a few weeks of immersion.

a few days' immersion in temperate conditions, after which skin and hair loosening leads to their detachment. However, the skin and hair can remain *in situ* for weeks at a time.

Gaseous decomposition and bloating often causes the body to 'float to the surface' of the water in which it is submerged, leading to its discovery. If the body has a lot of fat it may sink for only a short period, even in the absence of bloating.

■ Post-mortem artefact and immersion

Bodies moved by the flow of water may come into contact with sand/silt, rocks, piers and other underwater obstructions, all of which can injure the skin and deeper structures (Figure 16.3) Contact of a body with propeller blades classically leads to deep 'chop' wounds and/ or lacerations. Post-mortem injuries produced in such circumstances must be differentiated from ante-mortem injuries suggestive of assault.

Other artefactual injuries characterized by immersion include damage to the body by marine life (for example, fish, crustaceans, molluscs and larger animals; Figure 16.4) and as the post-mortem interval increases, fragments/limbs may become detached and lost.

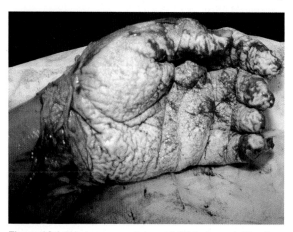

Figure 16.1 'Washer woman's hands'. Waterlogged skin after 1 week of immersion in a cold climate.

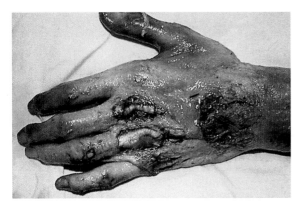

Figure 16.3 Post-mortem injuries to the back of the hand in a body recovered from a shallow river. Such injuries are likely to have been caused by contact against the river bed.

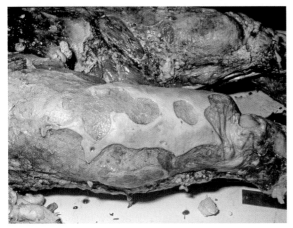

Figure 16.4 Post-mortem injuries caused by marine creature predation. This body was recovered from the sea and the circular skin defects are likely to have been caused by crustaceans such as crabs.

■ Pathological diagnosis of drowning

Pathophysiology of drowning

Regardless of the composition of water/fluid, drowning – the process of experiencing respiratory impairment from submersion in a liquid – may result in pulmonary surfactant insufficiency/damage, pulmonary oedema, alveolitis, hypoxaemia and metabolic acidosis.

As time in cold water continues, so does the likelihood of hypothermia (core body temperature 35°C). As hypothermia develops, cognitive function becomes impaired increasing the risks of (1) wrong decisions and (2) aspiration of water.

Drowning is a mixture of both mechanical presence of water within the respiratory system (causing a mechanical asphyxia) and fluid and electrolyte changes which vary according to the medium (sea water versus fresh water) in which immersion has occurred.

Fresh water is hypotonic compared with plasma and, when inhaled, is rapidly absorbed into the bloodstream, causing transient (but clinically irrelevant) electrolyte dilution and hypervolaemia. It causes alveolar collapse/atelectasis because of alteration of surface tension properties of pulmonary surfactant, resulting in intrapulmonary (left to right) shunts.

Sea water is hypertonic compared with plasma and, when inhaled, results in fluid shifts into alveoli, plasma electrolyte hyperconcentration and hypovolaemia. Sea water inhalation causes surfactant loss.

Aspiration of fresh or sea water leads to systemic hypoxaemia causing myocardial depression, reflex pulmonary vasoconstriction and altered pulmonary capillary permeability, contributing to pulmonary oedema. There is an inverse relationship between survival and the volume of aspirated fluid (sea water being twice as 'lethal' as fresh water), but even small quantities (i.e. as little as 30 mL) cause arterial hypoxaemia.

Signs of drowning

Autopsy findings ascribed to drowning reflect the pathophysiology of submersion and aspiration of the drowning medium (Box 16.2). However, none of these findings are diagnostic of drowning or present in all verified drownings, and so the autopsy diagnosis of drowning is one that can cause considerable difficulty.

■ Alternative mechanisms of death in immersion

Attempts to explain death in individuals recovered from water without autopsy signs of aspiration of water led to the concept of 'dry drowning', although alternative explanations for such deaths include trauma, the effects of intoxication, arrhythmia, laryngospasm or some other neurologically mediated mechanism.

Stimulation of trigeminal nerve receptors by immersing the face (and pharyngeal/laryngeal

Box 16.2 Findings that may be associated with drowning

- **External foam/froth and frothy fluid in the airways** reflects an admixture of bronchial secretion/mucus, proteinaceous material and pulmonary surfactant with aspirated fluid (Figure 16.5). This froth/foam has been likened to 'whisked egg white' in texture and consistency, with a different quality to that seen in, for example, cardiac failure.
- **Emphysema aquosum/heavy lungs** describes hyperexpanded and 'water-logged' lungs, whose medial margins meet in the midline and which do not collapse on removal from the body. There may be rib imprints on the surface of the lungs, and copious frothy fluid may exude from their cut surfaces. Combined lung weights of over 1 kg has been said to indicate fresh-water drowning (Figure 16.6).
- **Pleural fluid accumulation** has been associated with drowning, the volume of which controversially being said to reflect the post-mortem interval.
- **Subpleural haemorrhages (Paultauf's spots)** probably reflect haemolysis within intra-alveolar haemorrhages, and have been described in 5–60% of drownings.
- **Miscellaneous signs** including middle ear congestion/haemorrhage, bloody/watery fluid in the intracranial sinuses, engorgement of solid organs, reduced weight of the spleen and muscular haemorrhages in the neck and back have all been proposed as additional physical signs of drowning.
- **Microscopy of the lungs** revealing alveolar distension, haemorrhage and rupture, and narrowed capillaries, has been proposed as a sign of drowning but remains open to debate.

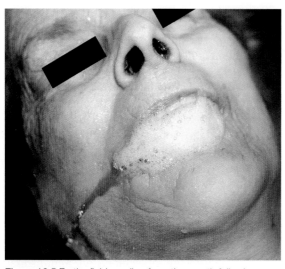

Figure 16.5 Frothy fluid exuding from the mouth following drowning.

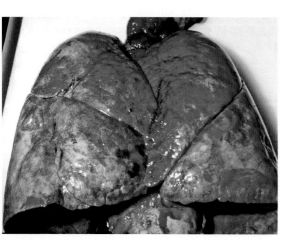

Figure 16.6 Emphysema aquosum following drowning. The lungs are hyperinflated, crossing the midline and obscuring the pericardial sac. There are subpleural haemorrhages in the right lung middle lobe (Paultauf's spots).

mucosa) in water has been shown to elicit reflex apnoea, bradycardia and peripheral vasoconstriction in humans – the 'diving response' – which is augmented by anxiety/fear, a water temperature of less than 20°C and possibly alcohol, increasing the likelihood of the development of a fatal arrhythmia. Cardiac arrest has also been documented following entry of water into the nose.

The cold shock response, which is initiated by peripheral subcutaneous receptors, causes respiratory effects (inspiratory gasp and uncontrolled hyperventilation, respiratory alkalosis and cerebral hypoxia) and cardiovascular effects (tachycardia, increased cardiac output, hypertension and 'heart strain' potentially leading to cardiac irritability and ventricular fibrillation), which appear temperature dependent.

Co-stimulation of both diving and cold shock responses may precipitate supraventricular arrhythmias.

■ The role of alcohol in drowning

Alcohol is frequently found in the blood of adult drowning victims but a causative role has not been proven. The strongest association between the two is in relation to 'fall-related' cases; concussive head injuries may be exacerbated by alcohol, with immersion/submersion contributing to a fatal outcome. Vasodilation from alcohol intake may hasten hypothermia. If a person is heavily intoxicated through alcohol (or other drugs) his ability to respond appropriately to save himself may be hampered by confusion, ataxia and incoordination as a direct result of the alcohol.

■ Other investigations in bodies recovered from water

Post-mortem blood chloride and specific gravity analyses used to be performed in some centres in order to differentiate fresh and sea water drowning; such tests are of no utility in the diagnosis of drowning. Blood strontium analysis has been proposed as a marker of drowning, but this test has not found widespread acceptance.

Diatoms

Diatoms are microscopic organisms present in sea and fresh water, and have a siliceous capsule that survives acid digestion in the laboratory (Figure 16.7). The presence of diatoms in organs (kidneys and brain) and the bone marrow has been taken to imply that an individual found in the water drowned in that water, where diatoms found in their body 'match' those found in the water (see also Chapter 24, p. 236). However, the interpretation of diatom testing remains controversial, as diatoms have been found to be ubiquitous in food and the environment, have been found in non-drowning deaths and have been absent in 'known' cases of drowning. The use of diatomology in the forensic diagnosis of drowning must be used with caution and in the context of other available evidence, but may be useful in corroboration of findings.

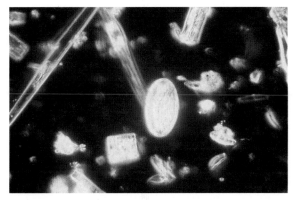

Figure 16.7 Diatoms from lake water.

■ Further information sources

Azaparren JE, Vallejo G, Reyes E et al. Study of the diagnostic value of strontium, chloride, haemoglobin and diatoms in immersion cases. Forensic Science International 1998; **91:** 123–32.

Copeland AR. An assessment of lung weights in drowning cases – the Metro Dade County experience from 1978 to 1982. American Journal of Forensic Medicine and Pathology 1985; **6:** 301–4.

De Burgh Daly M, Angell-James JE, Elsner R. Role of carotid-body chemoreceptors and their reflex interactions in bradycardia and cardiac arrest. Lancet 1979; **1:** 764–7.

Datta A, Tipton MJ. Respiratory responses to cold water immersion: neural pathways, interactions, and clinical consequences awake and asleep. Journal of Applied Physiology 2006; **100:** 2057–64.

Foged N. Diatoms and drowning – once more. Forensic Science International 1983; **21:** 153–9.

Golden FS, Tipton MJ, Scott RC. Immersion, near drowning and drowning. British Journal of Anaesthesia 1997; **79:** 214–25.

Hendy NI. The diagnostic value of diatoms in cases of drowning. Medicine, Science and the Law 1973; **13:** 23–34.

Lunetta P, Penttila A, Sajantila A. Circumstances and macropathologic findings in 1590 consecutive cases of bodies found in water. American Journal of Forensic Medicine and Pathology 2002; **23:** 371–6.

Lunetta P, Smith GS, Penttilä A, Sajantila A. Unintentional drowning in Finland 1970–2000: a population-based study. International Journal of Epidemiology 2004; **33:** 1053–63.

Lunetta P, Modell JH. Macroscopical, microscopical, and laboratory findings in drowning victims – A comprehensive review. Chapter 1. In: Tsokos M (ed.) Forensic Pathology Reviews – Volume 3. Totowa, NJ: Humana Press, 2005; p. 3–77.

Milovanovic AV, Di Maio VJM. Death due to concussion and alcohol. American Journal of Forensic Medicine and Pathology 1999; **20:** 6–9.

Modell JH. Drowning. New England Journal of Medicine 1993; **328:** 253–6.

Modell JH, Davis JH. Electrolyte changes in human drowning victims. Anesthesiology 1969; **30:** 414–20.

Modell JH, Moya F. Effects of volume of aspirated fluid during chlorinated fresh water drowning. Anesthesiology 1966; **27:** 662–72.

Modell JH, Gaub M, Moya F et al. Physiological effects of near drowning with chlorinated fresh water, distilled water and isotonic saline. Anesthesiology 1966; **27:** 33–41.

Modell JH, Moya F, Newby EJ et al. The effects of fluid volume in seawater drowning. Annals of Internal Medicine 1967; **67:** 68–80.

Modell JH, Bellefleur M, Davis JH. Drowning without aspiration: is this an appropriate diagnosis? *Journal of Forensic Sciences* 1999; **44:** 1119–23.

Morild I. Pleural effusion in drowning. *American Journal of Forensic Medicine and Pathology* 1995; **16:** 253–6.

Orlowski JP. Drowning, near-drowning, and ice-water submersions. *Pediatric Clinics of North America* 1987; **34:** 75–92.

Peabody AJ. Diatoms and drowning – a review. *Medicine, Science and the Law* 1980; **20:** 254–61.

Pearn J. Pathophysiology of drowning. *Medical Journal of Australia* 1985; **142:** 586–8.

Pounder DJ. Drowning. In: Payne-James JJ, Byard RW, Corey TS, Henderson C (eds) *Encylopedia of Forensic and Legal Medicine*. Volume 1. Oxford: Elsevier, Academic Press, 2005; p. 227–32.

Saukko P, Knight B. Immersion deaths, Chapter 16. In: *Knight's Forensic Pathology*, 3rd edn. London: Arnold, 2004; p. 395–411.

Suzuki T. Suffocation and related problems. *Forensic Science International* 1996; **80:** 71–8.

Tipton MJ. The initial responses to cold-water immersion in man. *Clinical Science* 1989; **77:** 581–8.

van Beeck EF, Branche CM, Szpilman D *et al.* A new definition of drowning: towards documentation and prevention of a global public health problem. *Bulletin of the World Health Organization* 2005; **83:** 853–6.

16 Immersion and drowning

Chapter 17

Heat, cold and electrical trauma

- Introduction
- Injury caused by heat
- Cold injury (hypothermia)
- Electrical injury
- Further information sources

Introduction

Heat, cold and electricity are some of the 'physical agents' that can cause non-kinetic injuries to the body.

Injury caused by heat

Burns are caused by the transfer of energy from a physical or chemical source into living tissues, which causes disruption of their normal metabolic processes and commonly leads to irreversible changes that end in tissue death. Exposure of living tissue to high temperatures can cause damage to cells, the extent of which is a function of the temperature to which the tissues are exposed, and the length of time of that exposure. Complete epidermal necrosis can occur at 44°C if exposed for 6 hours, while such necrosis occurs within 5 seconds at 60°C and less than 1 second at 70°C.

The heat source may be dry or wet; where the heat is dry, the resultant injury is called a 'burn', whereas with moist heat from hot water, steam and other hot liquids it is generally known as 'scalding'. Certain settings, such as war zones or terrorist attacks result in particular types of thermal injury, from improvised explosive devices, which may be associated with all other features of blast injury, posing particular management problems.

Burns

Dry burns may be conveniently classified by their severity (degree of burn injury and depth of tissue burned) and extent (burn area).

Severity of burn

Several systems of classification of burn severity exist, which can sometimes lead to confusion as there may be some overlap of terms (Figure 17.1). Perhaps the most widely used historically is:

- first degree – erythema and blistering (vesiculation);
- second degree – burning of the full-thickness of the epidermis and exposure of the dermis;
- third degree – destruction down to subdermal tissues, sometimes with carbonization and exposure of muscle and bone.

In recent years another classification has been used to reflect potential treatment options and this describes three main categories of burn as 'full thickness' (destroying the full thickness of skin) and 'partial thickness', which is divided into 'superficial' and 'deep'.

> ## Box 17.1 A classification of burns related to extent of tissue damage
>
> - Very superficial burns – for example those caused by sunburn – may simply cause reddening with mild blistering that may occur after 12–18 hours. After 5–10 days the damaged layers of cells peel off without residual scarring
> - Partial-thickness burns destroy the whole of the epidermis and possibly part of the next cellular layer – the dermis
> - Superficial partial-thickness burns result in fluid production which lifts off the dead epidermis forming blisters and subsequently scabs. Sensory nerves are damaged and the burn is very painful. New epithelium grows quickly and the burn heals in 10–14 days with little or no scarring
> - Deep partial-thickness burns are often less painful as nerve endings are destroyed and scarring is likely to be marked if the wound is allowed to heal spontaneously without skin grafting
> - Full-thickness burns destroy all skin elements and may require substantial reconstructive surgery because of the potential for incapacitating scarring (Figure 17.1)

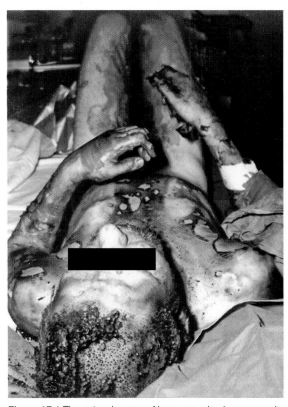

Figure 17.1 The extensiveness of burns on a body recovered from a fire may be varied. This individual had second and third degree burns after dousing himself with petrol before setting himself on fire (self-immolation). Note the molten and singed hair.

Extent of burn

The size of the area of burning may be more important in the assessment of the dangers of the burn than the depth. Mapping the area of skin burned on body charts (for example the Lund and Browder chart) may be helpful, although body surface area affected by burns may be conveniently expressed as a percentage of the total body surface area using the 'Rule of Nines' (Figure 17.2).

Factors influencing mortality risk include burn area, increasing age and the presence of inhalation airway injury; the presence of multiple risk factors substantially increases the risk of death from burns. There is considerable individual variation and the speed and extent of emergency treatment will play a significant part in the morbidity and mortality from burns. In dry burns, any clothing can offer some protection against heat, unless it ignites. Scars or burns from such injury may reflect the pattern or style of clothing warn at the time of burn (Figure 17.3).

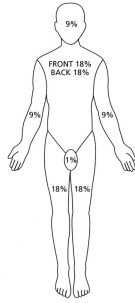

Figure 17.2 The 'Rule of Nines'.

Scalds

The general features of scalds are similar to those of burns, with erythema and blistering, but charring of the skin is only found when the liquid is extremely hot, such as with molten metal. The pattern of scalding will depend upon the way in which the body has

Figure 17.3 row

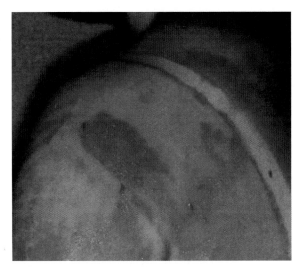

Figure 17.3

This may have great relevance when two different accounts of how the injury was sustained are given.

If only small quantities of hot liquid hit the skin, cooling will be rapid, which will reduce the amount of damage done to the skin. However, if clothing is soaked by hot fluid, the underlying skin may be badly affected, as the fabric will retain the hot liquid against the skin surface. Scalding is seen in industrial accidents where steam pipes or boilers burst and it is also seen in children who pull kettles and cooking pots down upon themselves.

Scalds are also seen in child physical abuse and are the most common intentional thermal injury in children. A recent systematic review of the literature identified features most commonly associated with accidental and intentional scalds when a child is placed in a tub or bath of hot water. Accidental scalds (from hot beverages/liquids being pulled of a table top, etc.) are predominantly 'spill' injuries from 'flowing liquid', characterized by scalds with irregular margins and burn depth, and lacking a 'glove and stocking' distribution. Intentional scalds are predominantly those caused by forced immersion in hot water, giving rise to symmetrical 'glove and

been exposed to the fluid: immersion into hot liquid results in an upper 'fluid level', whereas splashed or scattered droplets of liquid result in scattered punctate areas of scalding. Runs or dribbles of hot fluid will leave characteristic areas of scalding. These runs or dribbles will generally flow under the influence of gravity and this can provide a marker to the orientation or position of the victim at the time the fluid was moving (Figure 17.4). Children pulling saucepans with hot liquid off a cooker can result in this type of injury.

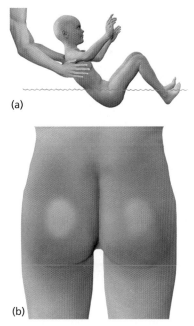

Figure 17.5 Pattern of scalding from forced immersion in a hot bath. Note the clear demarcation between scalded and uninjured skin representing the fluid level of the bath. Sparing of skin on the buttocks reflects firm contact between those parts and the base of the bath.

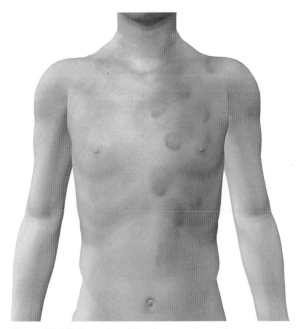

Figure 17.4 Pattern of scalding from running water.

stocking' injuries to the limbs, sparing skin folds (and buttocks in those forced to sit in hot water), which are of uniform depth (Figure 17.5). Other injuries or marks suggestive of non-accidental injury may accompany intentional scalds (see Chapter 13, p. 137).

Pathophysiological consequences of thermal injury

Burned/scalded tissue elicits an acute inflammatory response, leading to increased capillary permeability at the injured site; tissue fluid loss associated with thermal injury can be severe enough to cause de-hydration, electrolyte disturbance and hypovolaemic shock and, if the burn area exceeds 20% of the total body surface area, the release of systemic inflammatory mediators which may lead to acute lung injury and multiple organ dysfunction/failure. Burned skin provides no protection against infection, increasing the risk of sepsis in survivors.

Exposure to heat/hyperthermia

Hyperthermia – a condition where the core body temperature is greater than 40°C (100°F) – occurs when heat is no longer effectively dissipated, lead-ing to excessive heat retention. Its development is more likely in those who have taken substances (e.g. drugs, including cocaine and amphetamine) that elevate metabolic rate/heat production or re-duce sweating, or in those with medical conditions (e.g. hyperthyroidism). Autopsy findings in 'heat ill-ness', including 'heat stroke', are non-specific but can include pulmonary and/or cerebral oedema, visceral surface petechiae and features in keeping with 'shock' and multiple organ failure in those who survive for a short period.

Pathological investigation of bodies recovered from fires

When a fire results in a fatality, there should be a low threshold for treating the death with caution, in view of the potential for there to have been an attempt made to conceal a homicide by 'burning the evidence'. The need for safety of investiga-tors after events such as gas explosions, is a very important consideration in the examination of fire scenes.

The fire scene must be examined by special-ist investigators with expertise in the interpreta-tion of the causes and 'point of origin' or 'seat' of fires, and the use of accelerants, such as petrol (see Chapter 23, p. 232). Attendance at the scene by a pathologist is important and assists subse-quent interpretation of post-mortem findings (Figures 17.6 and 17.7). The position of the body when discovered is important because sometimes, when flames or smoke are advancing, the vic-tim will retreat into a corner, a cupboard or other

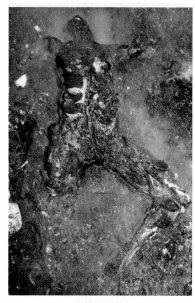

Figure 17.6 Charred body at the scene of a fire showing the 'pugilist attitude' and post-mortem skin splits on the chest. Extreme care must be taken to preserve the teeth in such cases, in order to assist identification of the deceased.

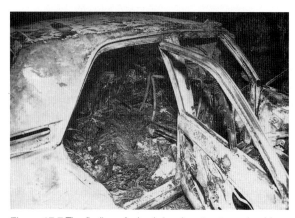

Figure 17.7 The finding of a body in a burnt-out car should always be treated with suspicion. Carboxyhaemoglobin levels may be low in rapid flash petrol fires leading to difficulties in assessing vitality at the time of the fire.

hiding place, or they may simply move to a place furthest away from the fire or to a doorway or window, all of which may indicate that the victim was probably still alive and capable of movement for some time after the start of the fire.

The pathological investigation of bodies recovered from fires should attempt to:

- confirm the identity of the deceased;
- determine whether the deceased was alive at some time during the fire (or was dead before it started);
- determine why the deceased was in the fire (and why they could not get out of it);
- determine the cause of death; and
- determine (or give an opinion as to) the manner of death.

Visual identification from facial features may be possible if there has been limited fire damage to the body, but heat damage can cause major distortion of such features even in the absence of direct burns.

Personal effects may assist identification, as will unique medical features and factors such as the presence of scars and tattoos, but where there is severe charring of the body more robust means of identification must be relied on such as dental examination and comparison of the dentition with available ante-mortem records or DNA analysis.

Post-mortem radiography should usually be performed before dissection, with particular emphasis on radiographs to assist identification (dentition, surgical prostheses, etc.), to identify fractures (including healing fractures with callus) and to exclude projectiles such as bullets and shrapnel (Figure 17.8).

Determination of 'vitality' (the fact that someone was alive) during the fire at post-mortem examination may be possible by the finding of soot in the airways, oesophagus and/or stomach – the implication that respiration was required to inhale the soot. The presence of soot below the level of the vocal cords, often accompanied by thermal injury of the epithelial lining of the airways, is particularly useful, and may be confirmed under the microscope (Figures 17.9–17.11). Blood samples can be taken for a rapid assessment of carboxyhaemoglobin, as a convenient marker of the inhalation of the combustion products of fire i.e. the inhalation of carbon monoxide, a product of incomplete combustion.

While carboxyhaemoglobin levels are commonly elevated in fire deaths (a level of over 50 per cent

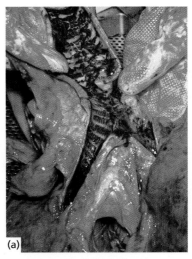
(a)

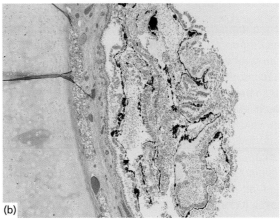
(b)

Figure 17.9 Pathological evidence of vitality at the time of the fire. Soot staining following inhalation of the combustion products of fire is clearly visible to the 'naked eye' in this trachea **(a)**, and such a finding can be confirmed under the microscope **(b)**.

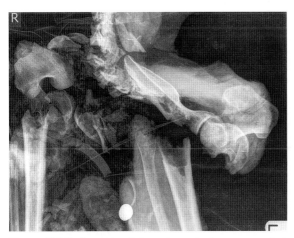

Figure 17.8 Radiography of charred remains is recommended in order to look for projectiles. These fragmented burnt remains include part of a disposable lighter.

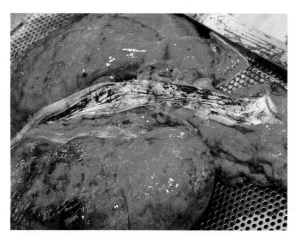

Figure 17.10 Soot staining can be seen in the oesophagus in this body recovered from a house fire. Such staining indicates that the deceased was alive – and able to swallow – at the time of the fire.

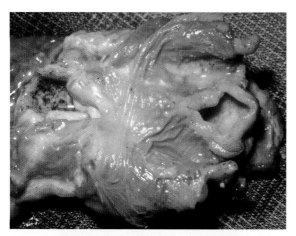

Figure 17.11 Thermal injury to the back of the throat provides evidence of the inhalation of hot gases during a fire, and provides a useful sign of vitality at the time of a fire.

often being considered good evidence of death having occurred as a consequence of breathing in the combustion products of fire), lower levels do not necessarily mean that the deceased was not alive at some time during the fire. In some circumstances, such as flash-over fires and petrol conflagrations in vehicles, for example, it is not uncommon to find low post-mortem carboxyhaemoglobin levels. Other factors may raise carboxyhaemoglobin levels. Cigarette smokers, for example, may 'tolerate' an elevated background carboxyhaemoglobin level (which may be as high as 20 per cent in heavy cigar smokers), whereas individuals with chronic heart and/or lung disease may not tolerate even very low levels before succumbing in a fire (Box 17.2).

Box 17.2 Examples of reasons for failure to escape from a fire

- Deceased was already dead before the start of the fire
- Deceased was intoxicated (alcohol and/or drugs)
- Deceased was elderly and/or disabled
- Deceased was immobile
- Deceased was rapidly overcome by fumes/smoke because of 'poor physiological reserve' (e.g. ischaemic heart disease or chronic obstructive airways disease)
- Deceased had insufficient time to escape the fire owing to the nature of the fire itself (an explosion or 'flash fire')
- There was panic/confusion
- Escape routes were obstructed (deliberately or accidentally)
- Deceased was in an unfamiliar environment (and did not know where the escape route was)

Deaths occurring during a fire

The majority of burnt bodies recovered from fires will not have died from the direct effect of burns, but from exposure to the products of combustion (smoke, carbon monoxide, cyanide and a cocktail of toxic combustion by-products) and/or the inhalation of hot air/gases (Box 17.3).

Box 17.3 Examples of mechanisms of death in fires

- Interference with respiration (owing to a reduction in environmental oxygen and/or the production of carbon monoxide and other toxic substances)
- Inhalation heat injury leading to laryngospasm, bronchospasm and so-called 'vagal inhibition' and cardiac arrest
- Exposure to extreme heat and shock
- Trauma
- Exacerbation of pre-existing natural disease or burns

Deaths occurring after a fire may occur because of the large variety of potential complications of thermal injury such as hypovolaemic shock following fluid loss, overwhelming infection, the inhalation of combustion products (causing acute lung injury), renal failure or blood-clotting abnormalities.

While the determination of 'manner of death' usually rests with the appropriate medico-legal authority, an opinion from the forensic pathologist is frequently sought. The interpretation of injury in bodies recovered from fire is complicated by arte-facts related to exposure to fire:

■ the so-called 'pugilist attitude' of the body reflects differential heat-related contraction of muscle, leading to flexion of the forearms, hands and thighs (Figure 17.12);

- post-mortem splitting of fragile burnt skin (Figure 17.13);
- fire- and heat-related fractures; and
- heat-related 'extradural haemorrhage', caused when severe heat has been applied to the scalp, resulting in expansion of the blood in the skull diplöe and the intracranial venous sinuses, which rupture, resulting in the formation of a collection of brown and spongy blood outside the meninges (Figure 17.14).

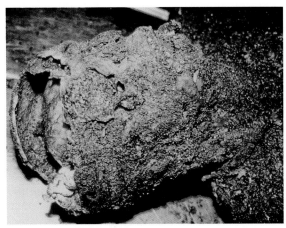

Figure 17.14 Post-mortem fire-related skull fractures in a severely charred body. There is a reddish-brown heat haematoma/extradural haemorrhage on the inner surface of the carbonized cranial vault.

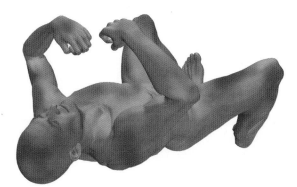

Figure 17.12 Appearance of 'pugilistic attitude' as a respose to heat effect more on flexor than extensor muscle grasp.

Such artefacts often cause concern to police and/or fire officers attending the scene, and may be misinterpreted as representing the effects of ante mortem violence.

Careful consideration of all apparently traumatic lesions must be made in order to determine the true nature of such post mortem lesions; the lack of naked eye or microscopic evidence of vitality (such as erythema, blistering, tissue swelling, bruising or an acute inflammatory reaction) will frequently distinguish artefact from trauma inflicted before death, unless they were inflicted at, or around, the time of death. In cases where there is doubt, an evaluation of the overall pattern and distribution of such lesions may assist in the interpretation of artefact versus ante-mortem trauma.

The manner of death may be homicide (following arson or where death was caused by violence before the fire being set), accident (e.g. an intoxicated individual attempting to cook, or from a discarded cigarette) or, rarely, suicide (self immolation).

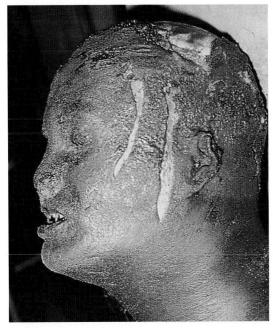

Figure 17.13 Post-mortem artefactual skin splitting in charred skin. No haemorrhage can be seen in the depths of the splits and they should not be confused with ante-mortem injuries.

Cold injury (hypothermia)

Cold injury (hypothermia) has both clinical and forensic aspects, as many people suffer from and die of hypothermia even in temperate climates in winter. In marine disasters, hypothermia may be as common a cause of death as drowning. In the very cold waters of seas, and lakes in high latitudes, death from immersion may occur within a few minutes from sheer heat loss and before true drowning can occur.

Deaths from exposure occur through heat loss from radiation, convection, conduction, respiration and evaporation. Environmental temperatures below 10°C are probably sufficient to cause harmful hypothermia in vulnerable individuals.

Hypothermia occurs when a person's normal body temperature of around 37°C (98.6°F) drops below 35°C (95°F). It is usually caused by being in a cold environment. It can be triggered by a combination of factors, including prolonged exposure to cold (such as staying outdoors in cold conditions or in a poorly heated room for a long time), rain, wind, sweat, inactivity or being in cold water.

It is usually healthy individuals who succumb to death from hypothermia caused by a cold environment. If a body gets cold, the normal response is to warm up by becoming more active, putting on more clothing layers or moving indoors. If exposure to the cold continues, other physiological processes will attempt to prevent any further heat loss. These processes include shivering (which keeps the major organs at normal temperature), restricting blood flow to the skin and releasing hormones to generate heat. After prolonged exposure to the cold, these responses are not enough to maintain body temperature. At this point, shivering stops and heart rate decreases. This can happen quickly. Alcohol consumption worsens hypothermia as it causes vascular dilatation and increased heat radiation. Wind and rainfall exacerbate the drop in body temperature. The body may rapidly lose temperature when immersed in cold water, as water has a cooling effect that is 20–30 times that of dry air. Hypothermia may confer a protective effect on survival following cold water immersion, but survival may be accompanied by severe hypoxic brain injury.

In many patients there may be an underlying medical cause (such as thyroid or pituitary dysfunction), or it may be associated with immobile or demented patients or conditions such as pneumonia. It is characterized by depression (poor functioning) of the cardiovascular and nervous systems.

Generally, the elderly, children and trauma patients are susceptible to hypothermia. Hypothermia can be classified into *mild* (core temperature 32–35°C compared with a normal of 37.5°C), *moderate* (30–32°C), or *severe* (<30°C). Below a core temperature of 32°C, shivering ceases and thus this extra muscle activity will no longer generate heat,

worsening the situation. Unconsciousness may occur between core temperatures of 27°C and 30°C, while ventricular fibrillation and apnoea occur at core temperatures below 27°C. Those who may be prone to developing hypothermia are those in extreme weather conditions (e.g. climbers, walkers, skiers, sailors), homeless people who are unable to find shelter, heavy drug and/or alcohol users (collapsing in the open) and those who have been immersed in cold water.

Hypothermia is usually diagnosed on the basis of typical symptoms and environment, and can be divided into mild, moderate and severe cases (Box 17.4). When unconscious, a person will not appear to have a pulse or be breathing. Treatment of severe hypothermia may not be successful. The key to treatment is a controlled rewarming that must be under medical supervision, and may require intervention such as dialysis.

Box 17.4 Features of mild, moderate and severe hypothermia

- **Mild cases**
  - shivering
  - feeling cold
  - lethargy
  - cold, pale skin
- **Moderate cases**
  - violent, uncontrollable shivering
  - cognitive impairment
  - confusion
  - loss of judgment and reasoning
  - loss of coordination, including difficulty moving around or stumbling
  - memory loss
  - drowsiness
  - slurred speech
  - apathy
  - slow, shallow breathing
  - weak pulse
- **Severe cases**
  - loss of control of hands, feet and limbs
  - uncontrollable shivering that suddenly stops
  - unconsciousness
  - shallow or no breathing, weak
  - irregular or no pulse
  - stiff muscles
  - dilated pupils

It is important to remember that the weather does not have to be unusually cold for hypothermia to develop and, even in moderately cold winter weather, many elderly individuals will become hypothermic.

Children have a high body surface-to-weight ratio and lose heat rapidly. In some cases of deliberate neglect or careless family circumstances, infants may be left in unheated rooms in winter and suffer hypothermia.

In an unrefrigerated body, the finding of indistinct red or purple skin discoloration over large joints, such as the elbows, hips or knees (and in areas of skin in which such discoloration cannot be hypostasis) raises the possibility of hypothermia and is found in approximately 50 per cent of presumed hypothermia deaths (Figure 17.15). The nature of such discoloration ('frost erythema') is not completely understood, but may reflect capillary damage and plasma leakage; microscopy reveals no red blood cell extravasation, distinguishing it from bruising.

Classically, haemorrhagic gastric lesions (Wischnewsky spots) may be seen in hypothermia

deaths; these lesions represent mucosal necrosis with haematin formation (Figure 17.16). However, their presence is not specific to hypothermia as they are identical to those lesions seen in some deaths following sepsis and shock, as well as in cases of alcohol misuse. They are thought to be caused by a disturbance of gastric microcirculation and exposure of haemoglobin to gastric acid.

Other gastrointestinal lesions sometimes found in deaths caused by hypothermia include haemorrhagic erosions and infarction in the small bowel (because of red blood cell 'sludging' and submucosal thrombosis), and haemorrhagic pancreatitis with fat necrosis.

Cold injury to the extremities may be severe enough to cause frost bite, which reflects tissue injury that varies in severity from erythema to infarction and necrosis following microvascular injury and thrombosis (Figure 17.17).

Hypothermia may cause behavioural abnormalities that can lead to death-scene findings that appear suspicious. Paradoxical undressing is a phenomenon that describes the finding of partially clothed – or naked – individuals in a setting of lethal hypothermia. The pathophysiology of this is uncertain but it may reflect confusion and abnormal processing of peripheral cutaneous stimuli in a cold environment, leading the individual to perceive warmth and thus to shed clothing.

The phenomenon of 'hide and die syndrome' describes the finding of a body that appears to be hidden, for example under furniture or in the corner of a room, etc., often surrounded by disturbed furniture, clothes or other artefacts. It is thought that this phenomenon reflects a terminal primitive 'self-protective' behaviour and may be more commonly

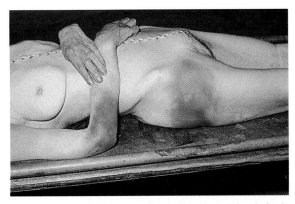

Figure 17.15 Pinkish discoloration over the large joints in fatal hypothermia.

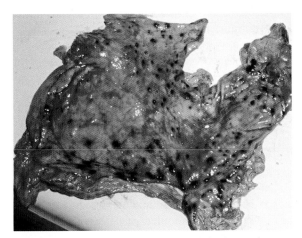

Figure 17.16 Numerous superficial haemorrhagic gastric erosions of the lining of the stomach in hypothermia. These are often called 'Wischnewsky' spots.

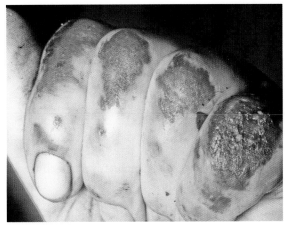

Figure 17.17 Frostbite of the knuckles.

observed where there is a slow decrease in core body temperature.

■ Electrical injury

Injury and death from the passage of an electric current through the body is common in both industrial and domestic circumstances. The essential factor in causing harm is the current (i.e. an electron flow) which is measured in milliamperes (mA). This in turn is determined by the resistance of the tissues in ohms (Ω) and the voltage of the power supply in volts (V). According to Ohm's Law, to increase the current (and hence the damage), either the resistance must fall or the voltage must increase, or both.

Almost all cases of electrocution, fatal or otherwise, originate from the public power supply, which is delivered throughout the world at either 110 V or 240 V. It is rare for death to occur at less than 100 V. The current needed to produce death varies according to the time during which it passes and the part of the body across which it flows. Usually, the entry point is a hand that touches an electrical appliance or live conductor, and the exit is to earth (or 'ground'), often via the other hand or the feet. In either case, the current will cross the thorax, which is the most dangerous area for a shock because of the risks of cardiac arrest or respiratory paralysis.

When a live metal conductor is gripped by the hand, pain and muscle twitching will occur if the current reaches about 10 mA. If the current in the arm exceeds about 30 mA, the muscles will go into spasm, which cannot be voluntarily released because the flexor muscles are stronger than the extensors: the result is for the hand to grip or to hold on. This 'hold-on' effect is very dangerous as it may allow the circuit to be maintained for long enough to cause cardiac arrhythmia, whereas the normal response would have been to let go so as to stop the pain.

If the current across the chest is 50 mA or more, even for only a few seconds, fatal ventricular fibrillation is likely to occur, and alternating current (AC, common in domestic supplies) is much more dangerous than direct current (DC) at precipitating cardiac arrhythmias.

The tissue resistance is important. Thick dry skin, such as the palm of the hand or sole of the foot, may have a resistance of 1 million ohms, but when wet, this may fall to a few hundred ohms and the current, given a fixed supply voltage, will be markedly increased. This is relevant in wet conditions such as bathrooms, exterior building sites or when sweating.

The mode of death in most cases of electrocution is ventricular fibrillation caused by the direct effects of the current on the myocardium and cardiac conducting system. These changes can be reversed when the current ceases, which may explain some of the remarkable recoveries following prolonged cardiac massage after receipt of an electric shock. The victims of such an arrhythmia will be pale, whereas those who die as a result of peripheral respiratory paralysis are usually cyanosed. Even rarer are the instances in which the current has entered the head and caused primary brain-stemparalysis, which has resulted in failure of respiration. This may occur when workers on overhead power supply lines or electric railway wires touch their heads against high-tension conductors, usually 660 V.

The scene of a suspected electrical death should be reviewed to try and identify causative agents and ensure that no risk persists. Health and safety legislation may require that an electrical death (e.g. in the work setting) should be fully reviewed to prevent further electrical exposure.

The electrical lesion

Unless the circumstances are accurately known, it can be difficult to know whether a dead victim has been in contact with electricity. When high voltages or prolonged contact have occurred, extensive and severe burns can be seen, but a few seconds of contact with a faulty appliance may leave minimal signs. Where the skin is wet or where the body is immersed, as in a bath, there may be no signs at all, as the entrance and exit of the current may be spread over such a wide area that no focal lesion exists.

Usually, however, there is a discrete focal point of entry and, as the electrical current is concentrated at that point, enough energy can be released to cause a thermal lesion. The entry points may be multiple and obvious, or they may be single and very inconspicuous. As the most commonplace is on the hands, these should always be examined with particular care (Figures 17.18 and 17.19).

The focal electrical lesion is usually a blister, which occurs when the conductor is in firm contact with the skin and which usually collapses soon after infliction, forming a raised rim with a concave centre. Characteristically, the skin is pale, often white, and there is an areola of pallor (owing to

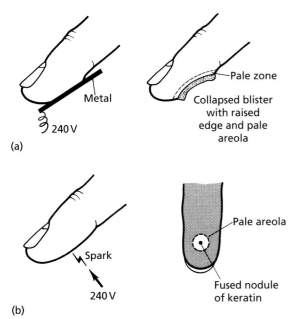

(a)

(b)

Figure 17.18 Electrical mark on the skin: collapsed blister formation following firm contact (a) and a 'spark burn' across an air gap.

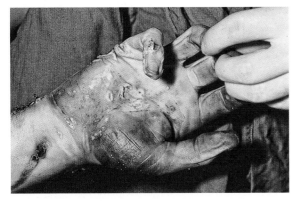

Figure 17.19 Multiple electrical marks/burns on the hand, associated with scorching and blistering.

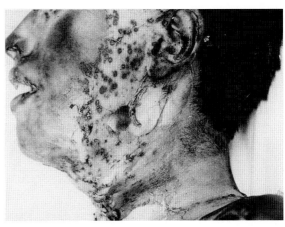

Figure 17.20 Multiple burns from high-voltage (multi-kilovolt) electrical supply lines. The 'crocodile skin' is caused by arcing of the current over a considerable distance.

Internally, there are no characteristic findings in fatal electrocution. The skin lesions are mainly thermal in nature, but opinions vary as to whether histological appearances are specific to electricity. It has been said that the cell nuclei line up in parallel rows because of the electric field, but similar appearances can occur in purely thermal burns. There are specific intracellular lesions on electron microscopy, but the gross pathological diagnosis relies upon the external appearances.

Death from lightning

Hundreds of deaths occur each year from atmospheric lightning, especially in tropical countries. A lightning strike from cloud to earth may involve property, animals or humans. Huge electrical forces are involved, producing millions of amperes and phenomenal voltages. Some of the lesions caused to those who are struck directly or simply caught close to the lightning strike are electrical, but other will be from burns and yet others result from the 'explosive effects' of a compression wave of heated air leading to 'burst eardrums', pulmonary blast injury and muscle necrosis/myoglobinuria. All kinds of bizarre appearances may be found, especially the partial or complete stripping of clothing from the victim, which may arouse suspicions of foul play. Severe burns, fractures and gross lacerations can occur, along with the well-known magnetization or even fusion of metallic objects in the clothing. The usual textbook description is of 'fern or branch-like' patterns on the skin – the so-called Lichtenberg

local vasoconstriction), sometimes accompanied by a hyperaemic rim. The blister may vary from a few millimetres to several centimetres. The skin often peels off the large blisters leaving a red base. The other type of electrical mark is a 'spark burn', where there is an air gap between metal and skin. Here, a central nodule of fused keratin, brown or yellow in colour, is surrounded by the typical areola of pale skin. Both types of lesion often lie adjacent to each other. In high-voltage burns, multiple sparks may crackle onto the victim and cause large areas of damage, sometimes called 'crocodile skin' because of its appearance (Figure 17.20).

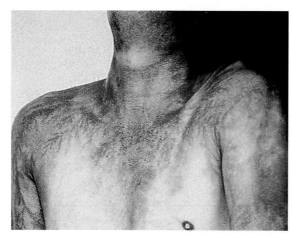

Figure 17.21 The 'Lichtenberg figure' and lightening fatalities. Note the fern-like branching pattern of skin discoloration on the chest.

figure (Figure 17.21) – but others claim that such marks are not seen. Red streaks following skin creases or sweat-damped tracks are more likely, although many bodies are completely unmarked.

■ Further information sources

Arturson MG. The pathophysiology of severe thermal injury. *Journal of Burn Care and Rehabilitation* 1985; **6:** 129–46.

Ayoub C, Pfeifer D. Burns as a manifestation of child abuse and neglect. *American Journal of Diseases in Children* 1979; **133:** 910–14.

Busche MN, Gohritz A, Seifert S *et al.* Trauma mechanisms, patterns of injury, and outcomes in a retrospective study of 71 burns from civil gas explosions. *Journal of Trauma* 2010; **69:** 928–33.

Celik A, Ergün O, Ozok G. Pediatric electrical injuries: a review of 38 consecutive patients. *Journal of Pediatric Surgery* 2004; **39:** 1233–7.

Cherrington M, Olson S, Yarnell PR. Lightning and Lichtenberg figures. *Injury* 2003; **34:** 367–71.

D'Souza AL, Nelson NG, McKenzie LB Pediatric burn injuries treated in US emergency departments between 1990 and 2006. *Pediatrics* 2009; **124:** 1424–30.

Hussmann J, Kucan JO, Russell RC, Bradley T, Zamboni WA. Electrical injuries – morbidity, outcome and treatment rationale. *Burns* 1995; **21:** 530–5.

Kauvar DS, Wolf SE, Wade CE, Cancio LC, Renz EM, Holcomb JB Burns sustained in combat explosions in Operations Iraqi and Enduring Freedom (OIF/OEF explosion burns). *Burns* 2006; **32:** 853–7.

Lund CC, Browder NC. The estimation of areas of burns. *Surgery, Gynaecology, Obstetrics* 1944; **79:** 352–358.

Madea B, Tsokos M, Preuß J. Death due to hypothermia, Chapter 1. In: Tsokos M (ed.) *Forensic Pathology Reviews*, Volume 5. Totowa, NJ: Humana Press, 2008; p. 3–21.

Maquire S, Moynihan S, Mann M *et al.* A systematic review of the features that indicate intentional scalds in children. *Burns* 2008; **34:** 1072–81.

McCance KL, Huether SE. *Pathophysiology. The Biologic Basis For Disease in Adults and Children*, 6th edn. St Louis, MO: Mosby Inc., 2009.

Moritz AR, Henriques FC. Studies of thermal injury II. The relative importance of time and surface temperature in the causation of cutaneous burns. *American Journal of Pathology* 1947; **23:** 695–720.

Nixdorf-Miller A, Hunsaker DM, Hunsaker JC 3rd. Hypothermia and hyperthermia medico-legal investigation of morbidity and mortality from exposure to environmental temperature extremes. *Archives of Pathology and Laboratory Medicine* 2006; **130:** 1297–304.

Roeder RA, Schulman CI. An overview of war-related thermal injuries. *Journal of Craniofacial Surgery* 2010; **21:** 971–5.

Rothschild MA. Lethal hypothermia. Paradoxical undressing and hide-and-die syndrome can produce very obscure death scenes, Chapter 11. In: Tsokos M (ed.) *Forensic Pathology Reviews*, Volume 1. Totowa, NJ: Humana Press, 2004; p. 263–72.

Ryan CM, Schoenfeld DA, Thorpe WP *et al.* Objective estimates of probability of death from burn injuries. *New England Journal of Medicine* 1998; **338:** 362–6.

Selvaggi G, Monstrey S, Van Landuyt K, Hamdi M, Blondeel P. Rehabilitation of burn injured patients following lightning and electrical trauma. *NeuroRehabilitation* 2005; **20:** 35–42.

Shkrum MJ, Ramsay DA. *Forensic Pathology of Trauma: Common Problems for the Pathologist*. Totowa, NJ: Humana Press, 2007.

Suominen PK, Vallila NH, Hartikainen LM, Sairanen HI, Korpela RE. Outcome of drowned hypothermic children with cardiac arrest treated with cardiopulmonary bypass. *Acta Anaesthesiologica Scandinavica* 2010; **54:** 1276–81.

Vege A. Extremes of temperature. In: Payne-James JJ, Corey T, Henderson C, Byard R (eds). *Encyclopedia of Forensic and Legal Medicine*, Volume 2 Oxford: Elsevier Academic Press, 2005; pp. 300–3.

Wick R, Gilbert JD, Simpson E, Byard RW. Fatal electrocution in adults – a 30-year study. *Medicine, Science, and the Law* 2006; **46:** 166–72.

Chapter

18

Principles of toxicology

■ Introduction

Drugs and alcohol influence lives in many ways. The heroin- and crack-dependent addict arrested for robbery, the recreational cocaine user suspended following drug screening at work, the student arrested for driving under the influence of drugs and alcohol, and the chronic alcoholic dying in police custody because of unrecognized alcohol withdrawal are all examples of how drug abuse can have huge impacts on individuals. However, this impact may well be low compared with the number of cancer patients dying in pain because they have been treated with inadequate doses of pain relievers as a result of their physicians fearing legal proceedings against them. Doctors treating patients dying of severe pain risk being accused of illegal prescribing or, even more tragically, being charged with euthanasia because post-mortem drug testing demonstrates blood concentrations said to exceed the 'therapeutic range' (although what a therapeutic range in a cadaver might constitute is hard to say).

One of the key tasks faced by forensic practitioners is to determine the role that a specific drug (or drugs) plays in instances of impairment and death. This task is made complicated by a series of issues, many of which arise simply because physicians,

toxicologists and lawmakers fail to understand the basic issues of forensic science, and the way these issues may interplay in complex legal, clinical and pathological matters. As a consequence, the interpretation of forensic evidence is often based more on anecdote and intuition than controlled scientific studies. Inadequate or bad science, or the misinterpretation of established sciences can lead to wrong legal decisions. Faulty and unjust conclusion can only be avoided if the limitations of the science are understood.

Stories of exotic poisonings give rise to plots that fascinate television viewers but which, more often than not, can pose vexing problems for forensic scientists. Fortunately, they are uncommon. Detailed knowledge of exotic poisons is a skill not much in demand today. What is required is the ability to recognize (and manage) the common complications of commonly abused drugs, such as stimulants, opiates, cannabinoids, hallucinogens, solvents, some anaesthetics and some prescription medications. With each edition of this book the molecular mechanisms of addiction and drug abuse have become clearer. At the same time, our ability to measure drug concentrations in any tissue has become ever more precise. The problem is to determine what those measurements signify.

■ Principles

The term 'toxic' can be applied in different ways. Some use the term synonymously with 'poisonous', meaning to imply that ingestion of a particular substance will cause death. Others mean only to imply that some sort of illness will result if the substance is ingested. The definition of 'lethal dose' is more precise, but now that the molecular mechanisms of many poisons are known, the relevance of this concept is not as important as it once was. Drug sensitivity and resistance vary from individual to individual (if for no reason other than their size). Thus 'lethal dose' is said to represent the dose of that drug at which all subjects given the drug will die, and that dosage will be expressed in grams, micrograms or milligrams per kilogram.

The abbreviation LD_{50} specifies the dose at which 50% of those who take a particular dose will die. The LD_{50} depends partly on the mode of drug administration, because the route of ingestion determines exactly how much drug is ultimately absorbed into the system. Put another way, the route of ingestion determines bioavailability. A drug injected intravenously is 100% bioavailable because the entire dose of drug enters the circulation. The amount absorbed after oral ingestion is variable. A 10 mg dose of morphine given intravenously would be expected to result in a peak plasma concentration of between 100 and 200 nanograms per millilitre. But if that same amount were given by mouth the peak plasma concentration would be only a fraction of that seen after intravenous injection. Because of anatomic and metabolic differences, the LD_{50} for any particular drug varies from experimental animal to experimental animal, and in no case can results obtained from the study of experimental animals be directly extrapolated to humans. The process of extrapolation from animals to humans is so unreliable that courts in many different countries have held that animal studies alone do not suffice to prove causation in humans.

The issue of receptor physiology is extremely important. Drugs exert their effects by binding with receptors. How well a particular drug will bind to a receptor determines how effectively it will act (or how toxic it will be). It does not help much to know that opiates bind to the mu (μ) receptor. What matters is how effectively any particular opiate binds to the receptor, and receptor-binding ability is altered by many factors. On a weight for weight basis, oxycodone is many times more powerful than morphine, simply because it is a better fit for the binding site on the μ receptor than is morphine. Receptors are subject to mutation. More than 140 different mutations have been identified within the μ receptor itself. Mutations cause receptors to change shape. Structural distortions of the receptor make some drugs fit better while others fit worse. The actual result cannot be predicted without knowledge of the mutation and the structure of the receptor, but this knowledge is never available to Coroners or forensic toxicologists as they have neither the facilities nor the budget to study receptor or enzyme genetic composition. How may this be important in clinical practice? An example could be the patient who asks for a 'stronger' pain medication not because he or she is a drug seeker, but because they carry a mutation that prevents the current pain reliever from binding normally to the μ receptor.

■ Definitions

Drug tolerance

Tolerance occurs after chronic exposure to a specific drug. An individual is said to be tolerant when increasingly large doses of the drug produce less and less effect. One might suppose that the classic mechanisms of receptor down-regulation and desensitization explain these phenomena, but they do not, and the reason why tolerance occurs is not really understood. Extraordinary degrees of tolerance can be attained. During the course of drug administration, the effective dose of any particular drug can increase 100- to 1000-fold, and the process may occur very rapidly: for example, cocaine tolerance begins to emerge after the first dose of drug is administered.

Drug dependence

Dependence is said to exist when an individual cannot function normally in the absence of a specific drug. Dependence goes hand in hand with tolerance as it too is controlled, at least partly, by receptor distribution, density and genetic make-up. The current Diagnostic and Statistical Manual of Mental Disorders (DSM-IV) defines substance dependence as:

When an individual persists in use of alcohol or other drugs despite problems related to use of the substance, substance dependence may be diagnosed. Compulsive and repetitive use may result in tolerance to the effect of the drug and withdrawal symptoms when use is reduced or stopped. This, along with Substance Abuse are considered Substance Use Disorders.... .

Substance dependence can be diagnosed with or without concomitant physiological dependence, evidence of tolerance, or even evidence of withdrawal (see Box 18.1).

Box 18.1 DSM-IV recognizes the following substance dependencies

- 303.90 Alcohol
- 304.40 Amphetamine (or amphetamine-like)
- 304.30 Cannabis
- 304.20 Cocaine
- 304.50 Hallucinogen
- 304.60 Inhalant
- 305.10 Nicotine
- 304.00 Opioid
- 304.90 Phencyclidine (or phencyclidine-like)
- 304.10 Sedative, hypnotic, or anxiolytic
- 304.80 Polysubstance dependence
- 304.90 Other (or unknown) substance

Drug withdrawal

Withdrawal refers to the development of symptoms when a drug is abruptly discontinued. Only individuals who are already dependent on a drug can experience withdrawal symptoms. For drug withdrawal to occur a substance must be taken in large quantities for a long time. In simple withdrawal syndrome, such as seen after long-term cocaine abuse, or even heroin addiction, individuals feel increasingly ill and may require sedation but after a certain number of days have passed, recovery begins and the symptoms dissipate. However, withdrawal from certain other drugs, especially benzodiazepines, can provoke uncontrollable seizures and may prove fatal.

Drug idiosyncrasies

This term is used to describe unanticipated drug reactions. For the most part these reactions are allergic in nature. They fall into the category of hypersensitivity reaction, where an inappropriate and excessive reaction to an allergen (such as pollen, dust, animal hair or certain foods) causes symptoms. These symptoms may range in severity from those of a mild allergic reaction to anaphylactic shock. Pathologists have been debating for more than half a century whether the pulmonary oedema associated with heroin abuse might be a type of hypersensitivity reaction, although this hypothesis has never been convincingly proven.

Drug interactions

This term describes unanticipated symptoms and signs that result after two or more different drugs have been given. Interactions may be good or bad, depending on which types of drugs are involved. Many permutations are possible: a drug could interact with other drugs, endogenous chemical agents, dietary components, or chemicals used in, or resulting from, diagnostic tests (such as a contrast medium used for angiography).

In recent years the term drug interaction has come to take on a completely new meaning for clinicians and forensic scientists. If two drugs are both metabolized by the same enzyme system, one may interfere with the metabolism of the other. For example, two different P450 hepatic enzymes (CYP3A and CYP2B6) metabolize methadone. Methadone induces production of CYP3A, so that abnormally low concentrations of carbamazepine, which is also metabolized by that enzyme, might unexpectedly result. However if methadone is taken with a drug that inhibits CYP3A, such as diltiazem (also metabolized by CYP3A), methadone will not be metabolized and concentrations will be unexpectedly high.

Until fairly recently, it was not generally recognized that drugs could interact with the channels that control electrical conduction in the myocardium. The shape of the cardiac action potential is determined by the sequential opening and closing of dedicated channels within the cell membrane of cardiomyocytes. These channels conduct potassium, sodium and calcium. There are several varieties of each channel, as well as many genetic variations (genetic polymorphism). Some polymorphisms are harmless but others are not. If the channel is sufficiently altered it may not function properly, preventing normal ion conductance. The channel responsible for most unexpected drug reactions (arrhythmias and sudden death) is the one that conducts potassium back into the cell after depolarization (known as hERG, or 'slow repolarizing potassium conductance channel'). Drugs that combine with this channel can disrupt the normal cycle of cardiac repolarization, causing fatal cardiac arrhythmias. Recently it was discovered that arsenic is an hERG channel poison, and it may well be that an arsenic–hERG interaction was responsible for the death of Emperor Napoleon. Unanticipated drug–hERG interactions are the main reason for drug recalls in the United States and Europe.

■ Testing matrices

General principles

Drugs can reliably be detected and quantitated in any tissue of the body. It is the interpretation of those quantities that is critical. Interpeting the significance of any drug found is the major issue facing forensic practitioners on a daily basis. Detection proves that ingestion or at least exposure has taken place, but the mere presence of a drug, even in seemingly large quantities, says nothing about toxicity and even less about intention or motivation. Does it really matter whether urinary cocaine metabolite concentrations exceed some specified range? It does not, unless the individual's state of hydration is known, as well as the specific gravity and acidity of their urine, and usually this information is rarely available in the forensic setting. No matter how many decimal points are added to the results, specific measurements have inherent limitations.

The effect of media stories regarding techniques for forensic measurement and analysis (what can be termed the 'CSI effect') can be pernicious. Many practitioners believe (wrongly) that precise laboratory measurements can supply information that could not have been gathered by accurate history and scene investigation alone. Each investigative modality has its contribution to make to a forensic investigation. There are a number of misunderstandings concerning toxicology, and failure to consider them can lead to needless effort and expense, not to mention an incorrect conclusion.

Suppose a left-handed heroin user is found dead with a needle mark in his left antecubital fossa. Some might take that as proof that another person administered the injection, which would be likely. It would be an unnecessary waste of laboratory resources to measure drug concentrations in the skin adjacent to an injection site because, once a drug is injected into the blood stream, it circulates throughout the body. Skin measurement of drug concentrations would have meaning only if concentration measurements were made of skin taken from both sides of the body, and were found to be different. The same might be said for the value of vaginal, rectal or nasal swabs. Route of administration cannot be determined by measuring the drug concentration in those areas. The recovery of cocaine from the vagina does not necessarily mean it was absorbed via that route. It just means that the circulation persisted for some time after drug use. That being the case, distribution of drug to nasal, rectal and vaginal mucosa would be anticipated.

Analysis of drug paraphernalia may also be a poor use of resources; unless the decedent was participating in a needle-exchange programme, they may have reused the syringe many times. Drugs will, no doubt, be detected in the syringe, but whether their presence has anything to do with the death being investigated is an open question.

It is not generally appreciated that the site where the blood sample is collected at autopsy may well determine the final analytical result. After death, concentrations of weakly basic drugs (such as cocaine) are higher on the left side of the heart than on the right, and concentrations in the heart are higher than those in the leg. Drug concentrations in blood collected from any tissue taken at autopsy may, or may not, bear a reliable relationship to concentrations that existed in life.

Regardless of whether the specimen is from the heart or the leg, there is ample proof that post-mortem drug concentrations almost always exceed those measured in the immediate ante-mortem period. It follows that autopsy blood measurements, taken in isolation, cannot implicate any drug as a cause of death. Quantification can only prove exposure or ingestion. The concept of 'normal' or 'therapeutic' drug concentration measurements made in the living does not have any relevance to the dead. It makes no sense to discuss therapeutic drug concentration in cadavers: blood is a living tissue and cadavers cannot be said to have blood, only reddish clumped liquid that was once living blood.

Whether or not an individual dies from taking a drug often depends on the phenomenon of tolerance (decreasing effect with increasing dose), but for all intents and purposes, there is no effective way to measure tolerance after death. Thus, a laboratory result that might seem to indicate a massive drug overdose, could merely be an incidental finding. The highest blood cocaine level ever reported in a human was measured in a man (> 35 000 ng/mL) who had no physical complaint other than the 45-calibre bullet that traversed his brain!

Often, it is sufficient just to demonstrate that a drug is present. For example, was the rape complainant really a victim of drug-facilitated assault, or was he/she a promiscuous chronic drug abuser? Was the individual with an unconfirmed urine test positive for opiates really a drug abuser, or was he/she taking a cough medication containing codeine? A simple way to help answer the question is to take a hair sample. Drugs are stable in hair for perpetuity. Prior drug use in an alleged rape victim is easy enough to establish, simply by hair testing. In the instance of the individual with the urine test positive for opiates, the presence of other components of cough syrup in their hair would probably yield a correct interpretation of the findings. There is not always a need to test hair, but there is often a reason to collect and store a sample, even if it is never analysed.

Specific testing matrices

Blood and urine

Blood is still the preferred testing matrix for drug detection. It is always collected into a sodium fluoride-containing tube (which prevents further drug degradation). There are differences between pre- and post-mortem blood specimens. When blood is drawn in the hospital, either for therapeutic drug monitoring or drug detection, only the plasma is analysed. In death, concentrations in whole blood are measured. Drug concentrations, especially the concentration of alcohol, are different in plasma and whole blood. Serum and plasma contain 10–15% more water than whole blood. It follows that plasma ethanol concentrations are 10–15% higher than corresponding whole-blood concentrations. The difference may seem small, but it is more than enough to convict or exonerate a driver accused of driving under the influence.

Urine was once the preferred specimen for post-mortem drug screening but, increasingly, cardiac blood samples are considered a better testing matrix. Advances in technology have substantially reduced the costs of gas chromatography/mass spectrometry (GC/MS), and screening whole-blood involves not much more expense than the cost of screening urine, but provides greatly enhanced sensitivity. After death, drug concentrations tend to increase faster in cardiac blood than elsewhere in the body, making such samples more sensitive indicators of drug use, although they are less specific. The routine screening of cardiac blood also helps avoid another problem: at autopsy, there is often no urine in the bladder. Some centres have dispensed with urine testing entirely; they first screen cardiac blood with GC/MS and then confirm their findings in a peripheral blood sample.

Vitreous humour

In the USA many forensic pathologists also collect vitreous humour, although that is often not the case in the UK. Vitreous humour is a useful testing medium, especially for the diagnosis of electrolyte disorders, renal failure, hyperglycaemia and ethyl alcohol ingestion. The vitreous humour is, in many ways, protected from the external environment, and it may be the only reliable testing matrix available when individuals have drowned or when bodies are found after an extended period of environmental exposure. Measurement of alcohol concentrations in the vitreous humour may even help distinguish between post-mortem alcohol formation and ante-mortem ingestion. There is an emerging tendency to also measure the concentrations of abused drugs in the vitreous humour, although for the present, too few measurements have been reported to allow accurate extrapolation from vitreous humour concentrations to concentrations in other tissues.

Hair testing

Measurement of abused drug concentrations in hair can yield valuable information about drug exposure and drug compliance, and sometimes hair testing can reveal the presence of drugs that were completely unexpected. Once deposited in hair, drugs and their metabolites are stable indefinitely. It requires very little effort to collect hair at autopsy, place it in a sealed envelope and file the sample. For reasons that are not entirely clear, the parent drug is often found in higher concentrations within the hair than is the metabolite. Should questions about drug use arise some time in the distant future, they will be easily answered if a hair sample has been retained.

Liver

Liver analysis can be especially valuable in cases where the drug sought (such as a tricyclic antidepressant) is highly bound to protein. Liver analysis is also valuable if the drug undergoes enterohepatic circulation. Some drugs, such as morphine, may be detectable in the liver long after they have been cleared from the blood, only because they remain in the enterohepatic circulation for so long. There is, however, one important caveat: most drugs readily diffuse from the stomach into the right lobe of the liver so, as a rule, only the left lobe of the liver should be used for analytical testing.

Stomach

The testing of stomach contents is only worthwhile if (1) the volume of the gastric contents is recorded, (2) a homogeneous specimen is analysed and (3) the total drug content within the stomach is computed. It does no good to know the drug concentration in gastric fluid if the total volume of the gastric contents is not also known. It may also be possible to identify small pill fragments by microscopic examination of the gastric fluid. Very little should be made of low-level drug concentrations found in stomach, as ion trapping may cause small amounts of some charged drugs, such as cocaine and morphine, to appear in the gastric contents, even if the drug has been injected intravenously. However, the detection of high concentrations of some drugs in the stomach (such as morphine) does not necessarily prove oral ingestion; it may just be an artefact produced by enterohepatic circulation.

■ Interpretation

Post-mortem drug concentration measurements cannot be interpreted in isolation, if for no other reasons than that tolerance eventually emerges to most abused drugs. A living heroin addict may very well have a higher morphine concentration than an occasional heroin user lying in the morgue, but both might have much lower morphine concentrations than a hospice patient treated with a diamorphine syringe driver. Tolerance is not the only issue.

Drugs taken previously are likely to be stored in deep body compartments, only to be released as the body decomposes (a process that begins immediately after death). Drug measurements made under these circumstances might give the false impression that the drugs were, in fact, circulating in the blood at the time of death. This phenomenon was strikingly illustrated in a recent study of post-mortem blood fentanyl concentrations. Fentanyl concentrations were measured in post-mortem specimens collected in 20 medical examiner cases from femoral blood, heart blood, heart tissue, liver tissue and skeletal muscle. In a subset of seven cases femoral blood was obtained shortly after death and then again at autopsy. The mean collection times of between the two post-mortem samples were 4.0 hours and 21.6 hours, respectively. In four of the cases fentanyl concentrations rose from 'none detectable' in the samples taken shortly after death, to concentration as high as 52.5 μg/L. If only the toxicology results were considered in isolation, a pathologist confronted with a case of unexpected sudden death might very well make the mistake of classifying fentanyl as the cause of death, even though none was present in the blood at the time of death.

Finally, there is the issue of genetic polymorphism. Not only does post-mortem redistribution (Figure 18.1) ensure that concentration measured at autopsy will

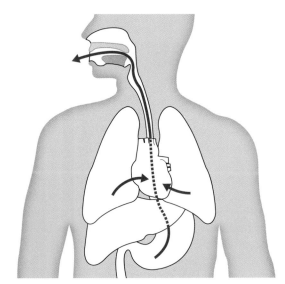

Figure 18.1 Post-mortem redistribution. Blood values measured after death have little or no relationship between levels that existed in life. Aspiration of stomach contents into the lungs often occurs at the time of death, and drugs that were in the lungs diffuse into the heart. Blood from the illiofemoral vessels is generally considered preferable for testing.

be higher than in life, there is always the possibility that high drug concentrations, even those measured in life, do not always reflect drug overdose: the individual simply may not have been able to metabolize the correct dose of drug they had been given. This possibility was only realized a few years ago when a newborn died of morphine poisoning that originated in the mother's breast milk. As is often the case, she had been prescribed codeine for post-labour pain. When the infant died unexpectedly it was discovered that the mother was an ultra-rapid metabolizer of cytochrome P450 2D6, causing her to produce much more morphine when taking codeine than would normally be expected. Individuals with a normal genetic compliment convert roughly 10% of codeine into morphine, accounting for codeine's modest pain-relieving effects, but because of the mother's genetic make-up, much higher concentrations of morphine were found in the infant than would normally be predicted, even though the mother was not taking excessive doses of codeine.

■ Further information sources

American Psychiatric Association. *Diagnostic and Statistical Manual of Mental Disorders (DSM-IV)*. Arlington, VA: American Psychiatric Association.

Drummer OH. Forensic toxicology. *EXS* 2010; **100:** 579–603.

Ferner RE. Post-mortem clinical pharmacology. *British Journal of Clinical Pharmacology*, 2008; **66:** 430–43.

Jung BF, Reidenberg MM. Interpretation of opioid levels: comparison of levels during chronic pain therapy to levels from forensic autopsies. *Clinical Pharmacology and Therapeutics* 2005; **77:** 324–34.

Karch SB, Stephens BG, Ho CH. Methamphetamine-related deaths in San Francisco: demographic, pathologic, and toxicologic profiles. *Journal of Forensic Sciences* 1999; **44:** 359–68.

Karch S (ed.). *Drug Abuse Handbook*, 2nd edn. Boca Raton, FL: CRC Press, 2007.

Karch S. *Karch's Pathology of Drug Abuse*, 4th edn. Boca Raton, FL: CRC Press, 2008.

Kintz P, Villain M, Cirimele V. Hair analysis for drug detection. *Therapeutic Drug Monitoring* 2006; **28:** 442–6.

Koren G, Cairns J, Chitayat D *et al*. Pharmacogenetics of morphine poisoning in a breastfed neonate of a codeine-prescribed mother. *Lancet* 2006; **368:** 704.

LeBeau M, Moyazani A. *Drug-Facilitated Sexual Assault, A Forensic Handbook*. London: Academic Press, 2001.

Levine B. *Principles of Forensic Toxicology*, 3rd edn, Washington, DC: American Association for Clinical Chemistry, 2010.

Moriya F, Hashimoto Y. Redistribution of basic drugs into cardiac blood from surrounding tissues during early-stages postmortem. *Journal of Forensic Sciences* 1999; **44:** 10–16.

Olson KN, Luckenbill K, Thompson J *et al*. Postmortem redistribution of fentanyl in blood. *American Journal of Clinical Pathology* 2010; **133:** 447–53.

Pélissier-Alicot AL, Gaulier JM, Champsaur P, Marquet P. Mechanisms underlying postmortem redistribution of drugs: a review. *Journal of Analytical Toxicology* 2003; **27:** 533–44.

Pounder DJ. The nightmare of postmortem drug changes. *Legal Medicine* 1993: 163–91.

Chapter 19

Alcohol

- ■ Ethanol sources and concentrations
- ■ Ethanol absorption
- ■ Elimination of alcohol
- ■ Ethanol measurement
- ■ Clinical effects of alcohol
- ■ Post-mortem considerations
- ■ Further information sources

■ Ethanol sources and concentrations

Alcohol (ethanol) may be ingested or it may be present by virtue of bacterial action occurring after death. Depending on local practice, blood alcohol concentrations can be expressed in many different units and notations, but they are all interchangeable in their meaning. The definition of what constitutes a standard drink of alcohol also varies from country to country. In the USA it is 14 g (17.74 mL) ethanol, but in the UK it is 7.9 g (10.00 mL) of ethanol. In most countries there are tables listing the alcohol content of common beverages by brand name, and there are standard formulae (such as the Widmark Formula, see Appendix 2, p. 243) for calculating the amount of alcohol ingested and the time of ingestion. As an alternative to the complex equations used by toxicologists, many forensic practitioners find it easier to remember a simple formula first introduced by American toxicologist Charles Winnek (Box 19.1). It must always be remembered that Winnek's formula is intended only to provide a rough working estimate. If a trial is to ensue, the Widmark formulae must be employed.

> ### Box 19.1 Winnek's formula
>
> Winnek's formula is based on the simple observation that, on average, a 150-pound (68 kg) man will have a blood alcohol concentration (BAC) of 0.025% after drinking 1 ounce (29.5 mL) of 100-proof (50%) alcohol. It follows that:
>
> BAC = (150/body weight in pounds) (% ethanol/50) (ounces consumed) (0.025)
>
> Thus, if a 200-pound (90.7 kg) man drank five 12-ounce (354.9 mL) cans of beer, and the beer contained 4% ethanol, then the BAC would be approximately:
>
> BAC = (150/200) (4/50) (60) (0.025) = 0.090% (90 mg%)

■ Ethanol absorption

Alcohol is absorbed from the stomach and small intestine by diffusion, with most of the absorption occurring in the small intestine. The rate of absorption varies with the emptying time of the stomach but, as a rule, the higher the alcohol concentration of the beverage, the faster the rate of absorption. Gastric absorption accounts for 30 per cent and 10 per cent of ethanol administered with food and water, respectively, and only a small percentage of the ethanol undergoes first-pass metabolism in the liver. The more rapid absorption of ethanol administered with water compared with food leads to higher blood ethanol levels. The maximum absorption rate occurs after consuming an alcoholic beverage containing approximately 20–25% (by volume or v/v) alcohol solution on an empty stomach. The absorption rate may be less when alcohol is consumed with food or when a 40% (v/v) alcohol solution is consumed on an empty stomach. The rate may also slow when high fluid volume/low alcohol content beverages, such as beer, have been consumed.

Elimination of alcohol

The human body converts ethanol into acetaldehyde via the actions of alcohol dehydrogenase, leading to the production of acetic acid and then acetaldehyde. Acetaldehyde is responsible for most of the clinical side-effects produced by alcohol. Ultimately, the measured alcohol concentration depends on both weight and sex because these two factors determine the total volume of body water and consequently the blood alcohol concentration (BAC). As a rule, the more a person weighs, the larger the volume of water his or her body will contain. It follows that, after consuming equal amounts of alcohol, someone who is obese or has a greater proportion of body fat will have a lower BAC than a thin person. Women have more fat tissue than men of the same weight and, therefore, a smaller volume of body water. As a result, BAC will be slightly higher in women than in men after consuming an equal amount of alcohol.

Alcohol elimination occurs at a constant rate in each individual. The median rate of decrease in BAC is generally accepted as around 15 mg per cent (mg%) per hour, but the actual range is 10–20 mg% per hour, although the extremes are rarely encountered except in chronic alcoholics. The elimination rate in the vast majority of individuals is between 13 and 18 mg% per hour, with the majority of values lying at the higher end of the curve. Very few people eliminate alcohol at a rate as low as 10 mg% per hour.

Ethanol measurement

Breath testing is used by most enforcement agencies in most countries with respect to road traffic (driving) offences. Many different devices are available for measuring the ethanol content of expired air, and these mostly work in a similar fashion: ethanol contained in the sample is oxidized with an electrochemical sensor. If done correctly, the value measured is directly proportional to the concentration of the ethanol present in the body. 'Breathalyser' type devices have repeatedly been proven accurate and reliable, and they do not react with acetone, which might be present in a poorly controlled diabetic. Quality control and standardization of such evidential machines is important to ensure accurate analysis. In the presence of factors such as use of alcohol-containing mouthwash or regurgitation of stomach contents, different jurisdictions may apply different protocols, to overcome risks of false elevations, by repeating evidential breath tests after a period of time or replacement by either blood or urine analysis.

Clinical effects of alcohol

Ethanol is a potent central nervous system depressant, and the degree of apparent intoxication correlates well with the amount consumed. As blood concentrations rise, initial feelings of relaxation and cheerfulness give way to blurred vision, loss of coordination and behavioural issues. After excessive drinking, unconsciousness can occur. Extreme levels of consumption can lead to alcohol poisoning and death, although tolerance may allow the consumption of massive amounts of alcohol and result in blood alcohol concentrations that would surely lead to death in the alcohol naive. Thus blood alcohol concentrations have very little meaning when taken in isolation except that, of course, a large amount of alcohol has been consumed. A blood alcohol concentration exceeding 0.40 per cent (400 mg%) may be lethal in a non-drinker but might produce few, if any, symptoms in a chronic alcoholic. If an individual is severely intoxicated, aspiration of vomit may lead to asphyxiation and death. Chronic alcoholism is associated with a host of medical conditions, but these are not within the scope of this book. The Forensic Science Service within the UK has produced a leaflet *Blood Alcohol Concentration and General Effects* (Figure 19.1) but the majority of clinicians would be uncomfortable classifying the effects (even in general terms) within quite narrow specific quantified ranges, as in this publication, because of the huge variability in response to consuming alcoholic drinks.

It is also important to understand that there are substantial risks for those who are dependent on alcohol and suffer alcohol withdrawal. Untreated alcohol

Blood Alcohol Concentrations and General Effects

The table below is for guidance only and may not apply to any specific individual. Although categorised for ease of reference, the symptoms can overlap considerably and gradually increase in severity with increasing concentrations. Whilst the effects described could apply to a social drinker, they depend on the person's degree of habituation. A heavy drinker would be expected to show less-noticeable effects and a person unaccustomed to alcohol more pronounced symptoms. Therefore the effects of any given blood alcohol level cannot be obtained simply from the table. Tolerance should be considered, together with other information such as evidence from other witnesses and the findings of any medical/psychiatric examination. Because of the number of factors involved, it is not possible to determine a particular level of alcohol that could cause memory loss in a specific individual, or render an individual unable to form an intent, or to give informed consent to, for example, sexual activity.

10 – 50 mgs%	Little outward effects, feelings of relaxation and well-being, increased sociability
50 – 100 mgs%	Increased self-confidence and talkativeness, mild euphoria, reduced co-ordination and slightly slowed reactions. Legal limit for driving is 80 mgs%
100 – 150 mgs%	Impaired balance, thickened speech, clumsiness, reduced alertness, lowered social reserve, increased garrulousness and volubility
150 – 200 mgs%	Drunkenness, slurred speech, glazed eyes, flushed complexion, staggered gait, drowsiness, exaggerated emotional responses, impaired co-ordination, reduced inhibitions, dizziness, nausea, disorientation
200 – 250 mgs%	Marked or heavy drunkenness, confusion, grossly impaired co-ordination, vomiting, reduced awareness, short-term memory may be impaired
250 – 300 mgs%	Extreme drunkenness, stupor, impaired consciousness, reduced reflexes, depressed respiration, incontinence
300 – 400 mgs%	Unconsciousness, absence of reflexes, coma
Around 400 mgs% and above	Possible death by respiratory depression or cardiac arrest.

References
1. H.J.Walls and A.R.Brownlie: Drink, Drugs and Driving, 2nd Edition (1985)
2. Simpson's Forensic Medicine, Ed. B Knight, 11th Edition (1997)
3. W.E.Cooper, T.G.Schwar and L.S.Smith: Alcohol, Drugs and Road Traffic (1979)
4. K.M.Dubowski: Am J Clin Pathol 74:749 (1980)
5. M.J.Ellenhorn, D.G.Barceloux: Medical Toxicology, Diagnosis & Treatment of Human Poisoning (1988)
6. R.Baselt: Disposition of Toxic Drugs and Chemicals in Man, 7th Edition (2004).

© Forensic Science Service Ltd. (2007). All rights reserved.

Figure 19.1 Blood alcohol concentrations and general effects.

withdrawal can be fatal and those involved in clinical assessment and management must understand how to diagnose and treat such individuals. The degree of alcohol withdrawal can be quantified using the Clinical Withdrawal Assessment of Alcohol Scale (Figure 19.2).

■ Post-mortem considerations

The situation is much more complicated after death. Bacterial enzymes (predominantly alcohol dehydrogenase and acetaldehyde dehydrogenase) act upon carbohydrates within the cadaver. Glycogen or lactate is converted to pyruvate and then ethanol. The amount of alcohol produced depends on the amount of glycogen or substrate available. Accordingly, post-mortem ethanol production will be greater in some tissues than in others. For example, the glycogen content of liver is 8 g/100 g wet tissue weight, whereas that of vitreous humour is only 90 mg/100 g.

Other factors also help determine how much alcohol will be produced. Terminal hyperthermia, such as might be seen in a patient with sepsis, or storage of the body at high ambient temperatures, will accelerate alcohol production, as will bowel trauma or disruption of the bowel owing to surgery or malignancy. Aircraft accidents or other causes of severe body disruption almost always cause the production of ethanol in large quantities.

Whether any alcohol detected was formed before or after death is fairly easy to determine. The easiest way is to compare the ethanol content of urine (UAC) which, unless the decedent was diabetic, contains no carbohydrates, and vitreous humour (which only contains very small amounts of carbohydrate) with the amount measured in blood. If the ethanol was definitely consumed and not formed post mortem, then determination of the ratio between vitreous humour and blood ethanol concentrations can be very useful. If the UAC:BAC ratio is less than 1:2, this is generally considered confirmation that ethanol concentrations were rising at time of death. A ratio of greater than 1:3 suggests that the decedent was in the post-absorptive stage. Ratios much greater than 1:3 indicate heavy consumption over a long period of time.

Clinical Institute Withdrawal Assessment of Alcohol Scale, Revised (CIWA-Ar)

Patient: _____ Date: _____ Time: _____ (24 hour clock, midnight = 00:00)

Pulse or heart rate, taken for one minute: _____ Blood pressure: _____

NAUSEA AND VOMITING — Ask "Do you feel sick to your stomach? Have you vomited?" Observation.
0 no nausea and no vomiting
1 mild nausea with no vomiting
2
3
4 intermittent nausea with dry heaves
5
6
7 constant nausea, frequent dry heaves and vomiting

TACTILE DISTURBANCES — Ask "Have you any itching, pins and needles sensations, any burning, any numbness, or do you feel bugs crawling on or under your skin?" Observation.
0 none
1 very mild itching, pins and needles, burning or numbness
2 mild itching, pins and needles, burning or numbness
3 moderate itching, pins and needles, burning or numbness
4 moderately severe hallucinations
5 severe hallucinations
6 extremely severe hallucinations
7 continuous hallucinations

TREMOR — Arms extended and fingers spread apart. Observation.
0 no tremor
1 not visible, but can be felt fingertip to fingertip
2
3
4 moderate, with patient's arms extended
5
6
7 severe, even with arms not extended

AUDITORY DISTURBANCES — Ask "Are you more aware of sounds around you? Are they harsh? Do they frighten you? Are you hearing anything that is disturbing to you? Are you hearing things you know are not there?" Observation.
0 not present
1 very mild harshness or ability to frighten
2 mild harshness or ability to frighten
3 moderate harshness or ability to frighten
4 moderately severe hallucinations
5 severe hallucinations
6 extremely severe hallucinations
7 continuous hallucinations

PAROXYSMAL SWEATS — Observation.
0 no sweat visible
1 barely perceptible sweating, palms moist
2
3
4 beads of sweat obvious on forehead
5
6
7 drenching sweats

VISUAL DISTURBANCES — Ask "Does the light appear to be too bright? Is its color different? Does it hurt your eyes? Are you seeing anything that is disturbing to you? Are you seeing things you know are not there?" Observation.
0 not present
1 very mild sensitivity
2 mild sensitivity
3 moderate sensitivity
4 moderately severe hallucinations
5 severe hallucinations
6 extremely severe hallucinations
7 continuous hallucinations

ANXIETY — Ask "Do you feel nervous?" Observation.
0 no anxiety, at ease
1 mild anxious
2
3
4 moderately anxious, or guarded, so anxiety is inferred
5
6
7 equivalent to acute panic states as seen in severe delirium or acute schizophrenic reactions

HEADACHE, FULLNESS IN HEAD — Ask "Does your head feel different? Does it feel like there is a band around your head?" Do not rate for dizziness or lightheadedness. Otherwise, rate severity.
0 not present
1 very mild
2 mild
3 moderate
4 moderately severe
5 severe
6 very severe
7 extremely severe

AGITATION — Observation.
0 normal activity
1 somewhat more than normal activity
2
3
4 moderately fidgety and restless
5
6
7 paces back and forth during most of the interview, or constantly thrashes about

ORIENTATION AND CLOUDING OF SENSORIUM — Ask "What day is this? Where are you? Who am I?"
0 oriented and can do serial additions
1 cannot do serial additions or is uncertain about date
2 disoriented for date by no more than 2 calendar days
3 disoriented for date by more than 2 calendar days
4 disoriented for place/or person

Total CIWA-Ar Score _____

Rater's Initials _____
Maximum Possible Score 67

This assessment for monitoring withdrawal symptoms requires approximately 5 minutes to administer. The maximum score is 67 (see instrument). Patients scoring less than 10 do not usually need additional medication for withdrawal.

Figure 19.2 Assessment of alcohol withdrawal. Reproduced from Sullivan, JT Sykora, K, Schneiderman, J, Naranjo, CA, and Sellers, EM. Assessment of alcohol withdrawal: The revised Clinical Institute Withdrawal Assessment for Alcohol scale (**CIWA-Ar**). *British Journal of Addiction* 1989; **84:** 1353–1357.

The **CIWA-Ar** is not copyrighted and may be reproduced freely.

■ Further information sources

Ahmed, S., M.A. Leo, C.S. Lieber, Interactions between alcohol and beta-carotene in patients with alcoholic liver disease. *American Journal of Clinical Nutrition* 1994; **60:** 430–6.

Alkana RL, Finn DA, Jones BL *et al*. Genetically determined differences in the antagonistic effect of pressure on ethanol-induced loss of righting reflex in mice. *Alcoholism, Clinical and Experimental Research* 1992; **16:** 17–22.

Baraona E, Gentry RT, Lieber CS. Blood alcohol levels after prolonged use of histamine-2-receptor antagonists. *Annals of Internal Medicine* 1994; **121:** 73–4.

Baraona E, Gentry RT, Lieber CS. Bioavailability of alcohol: role of gastric metabolism and its interaction with other drugs. *Digestive Diseases* 1994; **12:** 351–67.

Caplan YH, Levine B. Vitreous humor in the evaluation of postmortem blood ethanol concentrations. *Journal of Analytical Toxicology* 1990; **14:** 305–7.

Carpenter EB, Seitz DG. Intramuscular alcohol as an aid in management of spastic cerebral palsy. *Developmental Medicine and Child Neurology* 1980; **22:** 497–501.

Droenner P, Schmitt G, Aderjan R, Zimmer H. A kinetic model describing the pharmacokinetics of ethyl glucuronide in humans. *Forensic Science International* 2002; **126:** 24–9.

Dubowski KM. Alcohol determination in the clinical laboratory. *American Journal of Clinical Pathology* 1980; **74:** 747–50.

Dubowski KM. National Safety Council's Committee on Alcohol and Drugs. *American Journal of Forensic Medicine And Pathology* 1986; **7:** 266.

Erwin VG, Radcliffe RA, Jones BC Chronic ethanol consumption produces genotype-dependent tolerance to ethanol in LS/Ibg and SS/Ibg mice. *Pharmacology, Biochemistry and Behavior* 1992; **41:** 275–81.

Flanagan RJ. Guidelines for the interpretation of analytical toxicology results and unit of measurement conversion factors. *Annals of Clinical Biochemistry* 1998; **35:** 261–7.

Forensic Science Service. *Blood alcohol concentration and general effects*. London: Forensic Science Services, 2007.

Frezza M, di Padova C, Pozzato G *et al*. High blood alcohol levels in women. The role of decreased gastric alcohol dehydrogenase activity and first-pass metabolism. *New England Journal of Medicine* 1990; **322:** 95–9.

Hahn RG, Jones AW, Norberg A. Abnormal blood-ethanol profile associated with stress. *Clinical Chemistry* 1992; **38:** 1193–4.

Helander A, Beck O, Jones AW. Urinary 5HTOL/ 5HIAA as biochemical marker of postmortem ethanol synthesis. *Lancet* 1992; **340:** 1159.

Jones AW. Ethanol distribution ratios between urine and capillary blood in controlled experiments and in apprehended drinking drivers. *Journal of Forensic Science* 1992; **37:** 21–34.

Jones AW, Andersson L. Influence of age, gender, and blood-alcohol concentration on the disappearance rate of alcohol from blood in drinking drivers. *Journal of Forensic Science* 1996; **41:** 922–6.

Jones AW, Beylich KM, Bjørneboe A *et al*. Measuring ethanol in blood and breath for legal purposes: variability between laboratories and between breath-test instruments. *Clinical Chemistry* 1992; **38:** 743–7.

Jones AW, Hahn RG, Stalberg HP. Pharmacokinetics of ethanol in plasma and whole blood: estimation of total body water by the dilution principle. *European Journal of Clinical Pharmacology* 1992; **42:** 445–8.

Jones AW, Holmgren P. Urine/blood ratios of ethanol in deaths attributed to acute alcohol poisoning and chronic alcoholism. *Forensic Science International* 2003; **135:** 206–12.

Lieber CS. Alcohol and the liver: 1994 update. *Gastroenterology* 1994; **106:** 1085–105.

Moriya F, Ishizu H. Can microorganisms produce alcohol in body cavities of a living person?: a case report. *Journal of Forensic Science* 1994; **39:** 883–8.

Pounder DJ, Smith DR. Postmortem diffusion of alcohol from the stomach. *American Journal Of Forensic Medicine and Pathology* 1995; **16:** 89–96.

Stark MM, Payne-James JJ. *Symptoms and Signs of Substance Misuse*, 2nd edn. London: Greenwich Medical Media, 2003.

Sturner WQ, Coumbis RJ. The quantitation of ethyl alcohol in vitreous humor and blood by gas chromatography. *American Journal of Clinical Pathology* 1966; **46:** 349–51.

Sullivan JT, Sykora K, Schneiderman J, Naranjo CA, Sellers EM. Assessment of alcohol withdrawal: the revised Clinical Institute Withdrawal Assessment for Alcohol Scale (CIWA-Ar). *British Journal of Addiction* 1989; **84:** 1353–7.

Widmark EMP. *Principles and Applications of medicolegal Alcohol Determination*. Davis, CA: Biomedical Publications, 1981. http://www.seattle-duiattorney.com/dui/widmark-equation.php.

Winek CL, Carfagna M. Comparison of plasma, serum, whole blood ethanol concentrations. *Journal of Analytical Toxicology* 1987; **11:** 267–8.

Chapter

20

■ Harm reduction
■ Legal status of drugs
■ Commonly misused drugs
■ Drug facilitated sexual assault
■ Further information sources

Licit and illicit drugs

■ Harm reduction

When considering the use of licit or illicit (legal or illegal drugs) it is important to recognize that an essential part of the treatment of substance misuse is the principle of harm reduction. Harm reduction (or harm minimization) refers to a range of public health policies designed to reduce the harmful consequences associated with drug use and other high-risk activities, This may embrace a number of areas, but perhaps the area where complications of substance misuse (of which there are many) have been substantially reduced is with regard to intravenous drug misusers. Skin infections from unsafe injection practices are the most common, even when free needle exchanges are available. Some countries (including the UK) proactively encourage needle exchange even within prisons to reduce the physical and infective risks.

Stigmata of intravenous drug use are commonly seen in association with injection site ulcer, abscess, deep vein thrombosis, venous ulcer and post-phlebitic limb (Figures 20.1–20.4). Severe complications requiring hospitalization, such as necrotizing fasciitis, may occur. Injectors may be very adept at gaining vascular access for the administration of drugs, and any clinician should be aware of the wide variety of sites that may be used for injection (Figure 20.5). Infectious systemic complications occur less often,

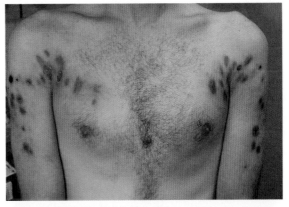

Figure 20.1 Multiple drug injection sites.

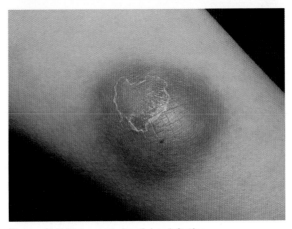

Figure 20.2 Abscess at site of drug infection.

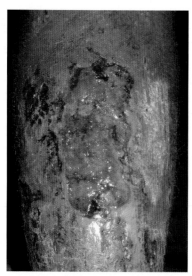

Figure 20.3 Venous ulcer following deep vein thrombosis secondary to intravenous drug administered into femoral vein.

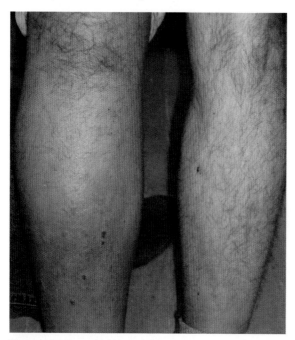

Figure 20.4 Post-phlebitic limb following repeated injection into femoral vein.

such as transmission of human immunodeficiency virus (HIV) and hepatitis, but in some areas of the world essentially all injection drug users are infected with the hepatitis C virus. In the case of anthrax the source of infection is believed by some to be the animal skins used to transport the heroin into Europe, but person-to-person spread occurs via the exchange of saliva or blood. Valvular infection, secondary to the injection of non-sterile material, can lead to valve

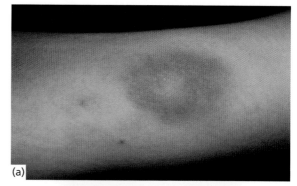

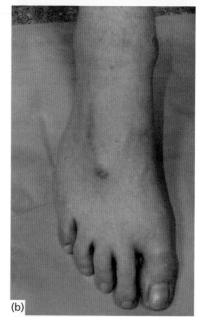

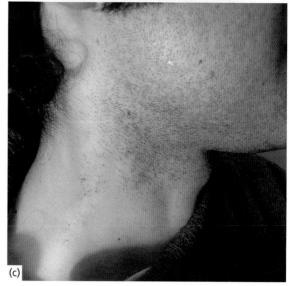

Figure 20.5 Sites of intravenous (IV) injection. **(a)** Forearm; **(b)** foot; **(c)** neck.

destruction and some confusing medical symptoms, as when bacterial vegetations separate from the valve and circulate through the body. At the same time that the incidence of this complication seems to be decreasing, the rate for valvular infection with mixed organisms, many drug resistant, seems to be increasing. Other complications are so rare as to merit little attention, but occasionally, as with the anthrax outbreak amongst injecting drug users in Scotland in 2009, even rare complications can become clinically significant.

■ Legal status of drugs

The legal status of drugs varies widely around the world and different jurisdictions have different ways of classifying drugs in relation to their perceived harm to society. The penalties associated with crimes such as possession, possession with intent to supply, and importation may reflect the political, religious, cultural or social environment of the country in question. Re-classification of drugs may occur, perhaps as a political response to concerns of the general public. Drugs are available throughout the world and their cost and availability is influenced by demand and effect. Increasingly 'legal highs' are being developed; these are often synthetic drugs that mimic the effects of some illegal drugs, and which may then be sold via the Internet. Governments and authorities face an uphill struggle as ways to develop substances that avoid legal sanction are used to get round the inevitable clamp down as some legal highs become fashionable. Some governments deal with the issue by determining that any drugs with similar structures to those already classified as unlawful, that are developed in the future will automatically be considered unlawful.

■ Commonly misused drugs

There are many different types of drugs of misuse. The use of any particular drug varies, depending on geography, social setting, fashion, availability, cost, legal status, and effects. Seemingly disparate agents may exert their effects via similar final common pathways (for example, khat and methamphetamine). Drugs can be classified into eight main groups according to their mode of action (Table 20.1).

Stimulants

All drugs in this group act by increasing concentrations of a neurotransmitter called dopamine. Dopamine is located within certain vital areas of the hind-brain. Dopamine has many different actions, but perhaps the best known involves mediating the sense of pleasure. Some drugs, such as cocaine (Figure 20.6), simply prevent the reuptake of dopamine, allowing it to accumulate in the space between nerve endings (synaptic cleft), while others, such as the amphetamines (khat has nearly the same structure as amphetamine, as does the drug called fenethylline or Captagon in the Middle East), have a similar action to cocaine but, in addition, cause presynaptic neurons to release additional dopamine stored within their endings. The net result is that even more dopamine accumulates within the synapses leading, in turn, to enhanced dopamine effect. However, like many of the newer antidepressants, cocaine also blocks the reuptake of serotonin (sometimes causing a disorder known as serotonin syndrome) and blocks the reuptake of all catecholamines, especially norepinephrine. It is this last action that explains most of the vascular disease associated with stimulant abuse. Excessive

Table 20.1 Drugs classified into eight main groups according to their mode of action

Drug group	Examples
Stimulants	Amphetamines, Captagon, cocaine, ephedra, khat
Opiates and opioids	Naturally occurring opiates, synthetic opioids
Sedative hypnotics	Zolpidem
Hallucinogens	LSD (lysergic acid diethylamide), mescaline
Dissociative anaesthetics	GHB (γ-hydroxybutyrate), PCP (phencyclidine), *Salvia divinorum*
Cannabinoids	'Spice', THC (tetrahydrocannabinol)
Solvents	Toluene, glue, lighter fuel
New synthetic agents	Piperazines

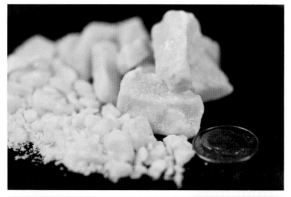

Figure 20.6 Cocaine.

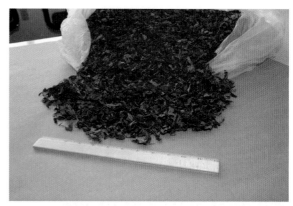

Figure 20.9 Khat.

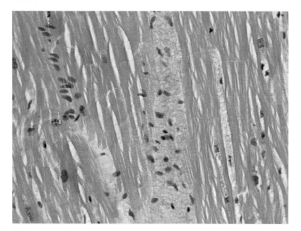

Figure 20.7 Fibrosis of the heart secondary to stimulant abuse.

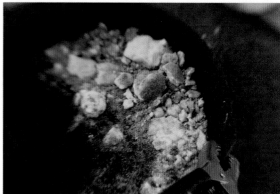

Figure 20.10 Crystal meth.

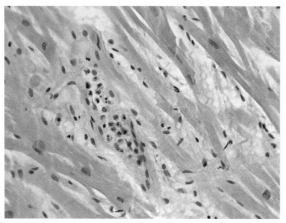

Figure 20.8 Zone of micro-infarction in the heart secondary to stimulant abuse.

concentrations of catecholamines within the heart cause scarring (Figure 20.7) or even micro-infarction of the myocardium (Figure 20.8). This process disrupts the normal electrical flow of the heart, causing an irregular heartbeat. The result can be fatal.

When moderate doses of stimulants are ingested, the main effect is a profound state of euphoria, which rapidly dissipates in the case of cocaine, which has a half–life of 1 hour, but persists for much longer in the case of other drugs, such as methamphetamine, which has a half–life closer to 12 hours. The half-lives of other amphetamines and khat fall somewhere in between. All stimulants, except for khat, can be injected, insufflated (snorted) or smoked. Khat (Figure 20.9) is chewed. The onset of effects after smoking or injecting occurs much more rapidly than when the drug is taken orally because drug reaches the brain more quickly. Rapid onset usually implies that a drug's effects will be more rapidly terminated. Blood levels after smoking cocaine free-base are comparable to those seen after cocaine injected intravenously. The term 'crystal meth' (Figure 20.10) is reserved for methamphetamine that has been allowed to crystallize slowly – the less volatile the solvent, the larger the crystals that form – but it is also smoked, resulting quickly in high plasma concentrations. Chemically crystal meth and methamphetamine are identical: both can be dissolved, injected, insufflated or smoked. Large crystals are highly prized by methamphetamine smokers, but the effects produced are no different than with uncrystallized methamphetamine.

Physical effects of stimulant use generally include dilation of pupils, increased heart rates and raised blood pressure. The problem for a clinician involved in attempting to assess or determine the type of drug used in an intoxicated individual is that few users (either dependent on, or using drugs recreationally) use a single drug, and thus drugs from different groups may produce a wide variety of clinical states. Heavy cocaine users may occasionally manifest paranoid symptoms but this is an uncommon event. When frank psychosis does occur, it is often in the form of Magnun syndrome, where users believe that 'bugs' are crawling out of their skin (called formication). Extreme forms of this syndrome are manifest by self-injury. Methamphetamine abusers not infrequently manifest symptoms of florid paranoid psychosis. The unique feature of methamphetamine psychosis is that it may reoccur years after drug usage has been discontinued. Its occurrence seems to be related to methamphetamine-induced damage to cortical white matter. These pathological changes are quite easily visualized with magnetic resonance imaging (MRI) scanning. This ability is not shared by cocaine or other stimulants.

The most feared consequence of any type of stimulant abuse is the syndrome referred to as 'excited delirium'. Although not recognized as a specific International Classification of Diseases entity, the existence of this disorder is accepted by forensic pathologists, forensic physicians. forensic toxicologists and by many authoritative bodies, including the American Medical Association and the American Academy of Emergency Physicians, The syndrome, often lethal, is notable for the acute onset of hyperthermia and agitated violent behaviour that often culminates in a sudden unexplained death. The contribution of restraint, struggle and the use of conducted energy devices (CEDs) to the cause of death in these cases is the object of considerable controversy (see Chapter 11, p. 126); there is good evidence that a central nervous system (CNS) dysfunction of dopamine signalling underlies the delirium and produces fatal autonomic dysfunction.

The vascular complications of stimulant abuse are numerous. Mostly, but not entirely, they relate to catecholamine excess. Excessive amounts of norepinephrine (noradrenaline) damage the walls of blood vessels, and can cause dissection, stroke and coronary artery spasm. The presence of excess norepinephrine also accelerates the onset of coronary artery disease, induces cardiac enlargement and produces scarring (referred to as interstitial fibrosis (see Figure 20.7) of the myocardium. The combination of myocardial fibrosis and cardiac enlargement is referred to as myocardial remodelling. Remodelling greatly favours the occurrence of sudden cardiac death. Both cocaine and methamphetamine interact with the ion pores controlling the normal electrical cycling of the heart (the action potential) but react with different channels. Cocaine blocks the sodium channel (a property shared by all local anaesthetics) and the hERG potassium channel. Methamphetamine does not share either of those properties, but does interact with L-type calcium channels, which provides another reason that methamphetamine can cause arrhythmias. Together, these interactions lead to prolonged repolarization of the heart cells, another abnormality that is associated with greatly increased risk of sudden death (Figure 20.11).

The World Drug Report 2010, published by the United Nations Office of Drug and Crime Control (UNODC), shows that Saudi Arabian authorities confiscated 12.8 metric tons of amphetamine in 2008. A total of 24.3 metric tons of amphetamine were seized worldwide that year, with 15.3 metric tons seized in the wider Middle East, where abuse of amphetamine-like drugs is becoming an increasing problem. According to the UNODC, Captagon is the brand name for a pharmaceutical drug developed in the 1960s to treat attention-deficit hyperactivity

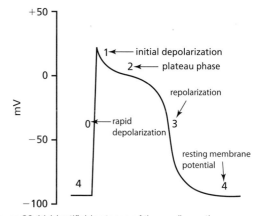

Figure 20.11 Identifiable stages of the cardiac action potential.

disorder (ADHD). Production was discontinued in the 1980s. Pharmaceutical grade Captagon contains a synthetic stimulant called fenethylline. Narcotic manufacturers in south-eastern Europe are taking advantage of Captagon's reputation as a stimulant and producing counterfeit Captagon tablets, stamped with the Captagon logo, but containing amphetamine – a controlled substance – as well as other chemicals, including caffeine. In general, Captagon should produce amphetamine-like effects, but the clinical picture may be clouded by the presence of toxic adulterants.

Opiates and opioids

The term 'opiates' refers to morphine, other contents of the opium poppy (such as codeine) and compounds made by modification of the morphine molecule. Box 20.1 lists commonly abused opioids. Opioids are synthetic molecules. Opiates and opioids both exert their effects by binding to the μ_1 opiate receptor located on neurons throughout the brain. Similar receptors are also found in the intestine, explaining why opiate users are almost always constipated. Stimulation of the μ_1 receptor relieves pain, depresses respiration and reduces gut motility. The only important difference between heroin, morphine and all the other synthetic opioids is their relative affinity for the μ_1 receptor. Some opioids conform to the shape of the μ_1 receptor better than others and, accordingly, produce greater or lesser effect, with some synthetic opioids being more than 1000 times as potent as morphine itself.

Opiate use can be accompanied by numerous medical complications often related to the process of injecting itself. However, there are some complications that are specific to opiates and opioids. Heroin smokers, for example, can develop a specific type of brain degeneration that is not very different from 'mad cow' disease; however, these cases remain very uncommon.

Several features of opiate abuse do merit special consideration. Tolerance is one of these. With chronic use, the user becomes less and less responsive to the drug's effects and must increase the dosage. This phenomenon is just as much a problem for hospital patients as it is for addicts. Tolerance to different opiate effects emerges at different rates. Tolerance to the pain-relieving effects of morphine emerges quickly, but tolerance to morphine-induced respiratory depression emerges very slowly. This differential effect often leads to potentially life-threatening situations. Clinicians need to be aware of the physical effects of intoxication with these drugs, and the symptoms produced by their withdrawal. Perhaps the best-known sign of acute use of opiates is the presence of pinpoint pupils (Figure 20.12). Withdrawal from opiates ('clucking', 'rattling') leads to a number of different symptoms, the severity of which is mostly dependent on how severely addicted the individual is: symptoms may include the presence of gooseflesh, rhinorrhoea, lacrimation, yawning, abdominal pain, muscle pain and diarrhoea and vomiting.

Some opiates are much more potent than others. Fentanyl, for example, is more than 100 times more powerful than morphine, because it is a better fit for the μ_1 receptor than morphine. The molecular structure of the opiate can also have an effect on routine drug screening tests. Routine drug screening tests (including the various test kits used in most casualty wards) are antibody based. The antibodies used

Box 20.1 Common opiates and opioids

- Buprenorphine
- Codeine
- Fentanyl
- Hydrocodone
- Kratom
- Methadone
- Meperidine (pethidine)
- Oxycodone
- Oxymorphone
- Propoxyphene
- Tramadol

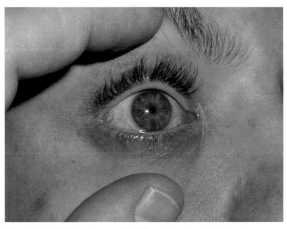

Figure 20.12 Pinpoint pupils following opiate intake.

have usually been designed to attach to morphine and will not react at all in the presence of synthetic opioids such as fentanyl.

The non-narcotic materials used to adulterate heroin by street dealers are called excipients. They are used to increase drug volume in hopes of increasing revenue. The compounds added to enhance drug effects (called adulterants) are relatively insoluble. This lack of solubility causes veins to become sclerotic, explaining the track marks seen in repeated injection users (Figure 20.13). The adulterants used in cocaine production tend to be more soluble and cause far less damage to peripheral veins, even though they can occasionally be quite toxic in their own right. Much of the cocaine sold on the streets in the USA has been adulterated with levamisole, an anti-helminthic piperazine type drug with the ability to cause bone marrow suppression. Similar cases are now occurring in the EU. Occasional clusters of multiple deaths have been reported as a result of the adulteration of street heroin with illicitly produced α-methyl fentanyl (as opposed to the unsubstituted, medicinal fentanyl). This can be problematic for toxicologists because, as indicated above, the presence of fentanyl is not detected by routine screening assays and will not be detected even when routine screening is performed of whole blood using gas chromatography/mass spectrometry.

Finally, there is the problem of genetic polymorphism. The phrase refers to mutations that occur in all opiate receptors and in almost all liver enzymes, including those that metabolize the opiates. Depending on the type of mutation affecting the receptor, drug effects can be minimized, exaggerated or not altered at all. Depending on their ability to metabolize opiates, individuals may be classified as poor, normal, rapid or super-metabolizers, depending on which mutation is present in which gene. Tests are available that can differentiate between different kinds of metabolizers in the living, but they are not generally available for use in autopsy material Undiagnosed polymorphisms often explain why patients fail to respond to what appear to be adequate doses of drug. Genetic polymorphism can also explain the occurrence of unexpected deaths.

Sedative hypnotics

A very long list of prescription medications is available for the treatment of insomnia. The drugs most frequently prescribed for insomnia (which may also have an anxiolytic action) include benzodiazepines (BZs), non-benzodiazepines (nonBZs) and antidepressants. Older drugs, such as long-acting barbiturates and chloral hydrate have fallen into disfavour. Benzodiazepines increase the effect of the neurotransmitter called GABA (γ-amino butyric acid).

In the absence of drugs the GABA$_A$ receptor (GABA$_A$R) binds to GABA, which is the major inhibitory neurotransmitter within the CNS. When it is activated the GABA$_A$ receptor selectively conducts chloride ion through its central pore into the cell. As a consequence, the neuron become hyperpolarized. When a cell is hyperpolarized, action potentials are less likely to occur and neurotransmission is slowed. The active site on the GABA$_A$ receptor is, of course, GABA. However, the receptor also contains a number of other different binding sites, including areas where BZs, nonBZs, barbiturates, ethanol and even inhaled anaesthetics can bind.

Any drug that can bind to the GABA$_A$ receptor is likely to exert sedative, anticonvulsant and anxiolytic effects. Some drugs may produce muscle relaxation while others may produce euphoria. In general, these are very safe drugs. Death from overdose is rare. However, combinations of high doses of BZs with other drugs, such as alcohol, barbiturates, opiates and tricyclic antidepressants may lead to coma and death, mediated primarily by respiratory depression. Flumazenil is an appropriate reversal agent, which should be used with caution because its effects are short-lived and somewhat unpredictable, and re-sedation may occur later. Supportive care in an appropriately monitored setting is usually

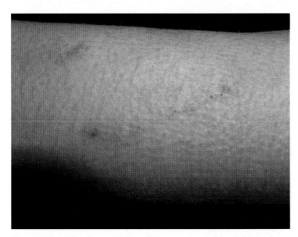

Figure 20.13 Track marks from intravenous drug administration.

sufficient treatment for those who have ingested drugs in this category.

The BZs have long been the drug of choice for the treatment of insomnia, but long-term use leads to dependence and abrupt discontinuation can even lead to the occurrence of seizures. The nonBZ hypnotics are more effective at speeding the onset of sleep than BZs and are thought to have fewer side-effects and drug interactions. Antidepressants are considered third-line drugs for the treatment of insomnia and, in most countries, have not been approved for the treatment of insomnia. Nonetheless, they are widely prescribed, despite the fact that any antidepressant may precipitate serotonin syndrome. A list of the most popular agents is shown in Box 20.2.

Box 20.2 Some common sedative hypnotic drugs

- **Benzodiazepines**
  - Triazolam
  - Estazolam
  - Temazepam
- **Non-diazepines**
  - Eszopiclone
  - Zaleplon
- **Antidepressant**
  - Trazodone
  - Amitryptiline
- **Melatonin receptor agonist**
  - Ramelteon (Rozerem)

Hallucinogens

Criteria for membership in this group are difficult to define. All members are said to share five common properties:

- changes in mood and perception dominate in proportion to any other effects the drug may exert;
- there is minimal impairment of intellect or memory;
- use is not associated with agitation;
- there are minimal side effects;
- craving and addiction do not occur.

Hallucinogens have traditionally been divided into two groups depending on their chemical structure – the phenylalkylamines and indolealkylamines. Mescaline is the best known of the former group while psilocybin (magic mushrooms), bufotenine

(also known as bufotenin or cebilcin) (derived from the skin of certain toads), and LSD (lysergic acid diethylamide; Figure 20.14) are the three best-known indolealkylamines.

In recent years these distinctions have become blurred, as both dissociative anaesthetics (see below) and designer amphetamines such as MDMA (3,4-methylenedioxymethamphetamine, commonly known as ecstasy), share some properties with the hallucinogens. The most important distinction appears to be that, at worst, use of hallucinogens leads only to behavioural toxicity. However, the hallucinatory 'designer' amphetamines have been responsible for many deaths, often a result of hyperthermia and multisystem failure. PMA (paramethoxyamphetamine) appears to be the most dangerous member of this latter group.

The most notorious of the designer amphetamines, by far, is MDMA (Figure 20.15). Shortly after MDMA was introduced into England, reports of MDMA-induced hepatic failure began to appear in major medical journals. MDMA seized by police in the UK is primarily manufactured in clandestine laboratories located in the Netherlands and Belgium. Most reported deaths from MDMA have involved heat-related illness, usually associated with rhabdomyolysis. Substantial experimental evidence also confirms the existence of MDMA-associated neurotoxicity. High doses of MDMA given to rats produce dramatic decreases in brain serotonin concentrations, although animals fully

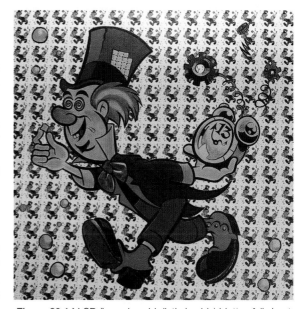

Figure 20.14 LSD (lysergic acid diethylamide) blotter, full sheet.

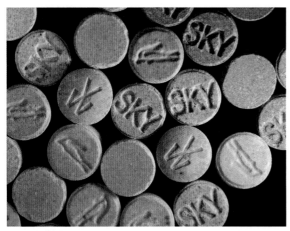

Figure 20.15 MDMA (3,4-methylenedioxymethamphetamine) tablet.

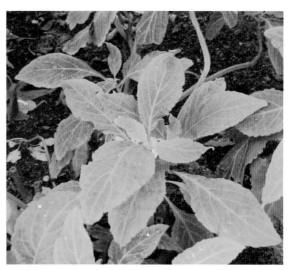

Figure 20.16 *Salvia divinorum*.

recover after 1 week. In controlled human studies, the spinal fluid of MDMA users has been found to contain reduced concentrations of 5-hydroxyindoleacetic acid, the major serotonin metabolite.

Dissociative anaesthetics

Five drugs fall into this category: phencyclidine (PCP), ketamine, γ-hydroxybutyrate (GHB), dextromethorphan and *Salvia divinorum* (Figure 20.16). All are hallucinogens, and the first four share the same mechanism of action: they block the NMDA receptor, the predominant molecular mechanism involved in memory function and learning. *Salvia* has no effect on the NMDA channel. Instead, it specifically blocks the κ receptor. Drugs that bind to the κ receptor produce intense feelings of unhappiness and depression but all have hallucinogenic (psychotomimetic) effects.

Salvinorin A, the active ingredient in *Salvia divinorum*, is the exception. The only reason for taking *Salvia* is to produce hallucinogenic effects, but many potentially useful drugs also stimulate κ-receptors and the psychological side-effects that result from this stimulation can be so strong that the drug cannot be used for its intended clinical purpose (the reason phencyclidine was withdrawn from the human market).

The effects produced by salvinorin A are qualitatively different than those produced by the other hallucinogens such as LSD or mescaline, and the mechanism of action is not understood. It is known that κ-opioid receptors also play a key role in the human stress response. Because κ stimulation tends to neutralize the effects of μ_1 stimulation, and some feel the presence of the κ receptor may diminish the possibility of drug overdose. There is also evidence that stimulation of κ receptors in some way protects the neuron from damage; in particular, damage produced by hypoxia/ischaemia is minimized in the presence of κ receptor agonists but, again, the mechanisms involved remain totally unknown.

Marijuana

Marijuana (Figure 20.17), with multiple street names (e.g. weed, hash, skunk), is a drug that interacts with many different receptors. The body itself produces marijuana-like drugs called endocannabinoids. These are compounds with structures similar to that of THC (tetrahydrocannabinol), the active ingredient in marijuana. Endogenously produced endocannabinoids bind with specific endocannabinoid receptors known as C1 and C2. Surprisingly, there is evidence that, in addition to binding C1 and C2, THC also interacts with the benzodiazepine receptor and opioid receptors. THC increases pulse rate in direct proportion to the dose administered. It may decrease cardiac output, and can sometimes cause syncope, particularly in those with pre-existing heart disease.

Whether or not THC relieves pain is still debated, but there is little doubt that, once within the body, THC remains in the body fat stores for a very long time (> 1 month). It is then slowly released back into the circulation by an assortment of different stimuli, including dieting and stress. Both of

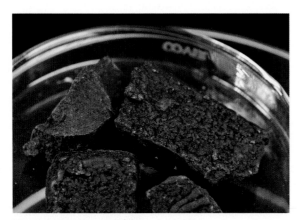

Figure 20.17 Marijuana/hash.

the latter conditions lead to increased secretion of ACTH and cortisol that, in turn, can also cause THC stored in fat to be released. If stress can cause the release of THC stored in fat cells, what is to be made of the driver suspected of driving under the influence who is found to have low concentrations of THC in his blood, even if he had not smoked marijuana for weeks prior to the event? In this case THC stored weeks earlier would have been released. Should he be charged with driving under the influence? It is essential that an appropriate clinical examination be undertaken to determine whether or not there is clear evidence of any drug having been consumed and, if so, whether that drug has an effect on that individual's ability to drive properly. As is also the case with phencyclidine, so much marijuana is stored in fat tissue, the interpretation of post-mortem blood levels is almost impossible. After death, as individuals cells die, they release their drug content and there is no way to differentiate between THC that was ingested just before death from drug that was ingested 1 month earlier.

Multiple new drugs are increasingly becoming available as governments limit the availability and legality of so-called 'legal highs' (see below). For example 'Spice' has recently become popular. It is sold mostly over the Internet and at 'head shops'. Spice is the popular name for a molecule named JWH-018 (1-pentyl-3-[1-napthoyl]indole). It exerts many of the same effects as the cannabinoids but has a completely different structure. Although the structure of Spice is very different from THC, it nonetheless avidly binds at the same C1 and C2 receptor, at exactly the same sites where THC is active. The effects produced are said to be the same as smoking marijuana, but are believed to last much longer. The potential use of this compound as a transdermal pain reliever is under investigation, but if it ever does come to market there will, no doubt, be a thriving black market trade.

Solvents

Solvents such as toluene volatize at room temperature, allowing users to inhale the fumes, a practice referred to as 'huffing'. Use of these agents and others such as glue, or gas fuel for cigarette lighters is much less common now than previously. Glue-sniffing was more frequent in the 1980s but still occurs. Clinical examination may reveal traces of the inhalant, such as glue, around an individual's mouth and face, with the persistent odour of the relevant inhalant. Some individuals may have evidence of singeing of beard or hair, or evidence of old burn injury to the face, as many of the agents used for such practices are highly flammable and do not associate well with lighted cigarettes. Toluene, as opposed to the solvents found in hair spray, dry-cleaning fluid and gasoline, is the agent most often responsible for fatal intoxication. The mechanism seems to be the disruption of normal cardiac electrical activity. Inhalation of any solvent will result in transient euphoria, headache and ataxia. Members of this group selectively destroy brain white matter, and a distinctive pattern can be identified in the MRI scans of chronic abusers. Solvents share some properties with other depressants such as barbiturates, benzodiazepines and even alcohol. However, the solvents, as a group, interact with so many different receptor subtypes that their actual mechanism of action remains unclear.

New synthetic agents and legal highs

These drugs first emerged in New Zealand during the early 2000s, but use has quickly spread to involve Europe and the USA. These drugs are commonly (and sometime incorrectly) known as legal highs. Their legal status is generally an evolving one, and what was legal one day may, by virtue of new legislation, become illegal nearly overnight. Governments are concerned by the proliferation of such substances, many of which may be sold in corner shops or over the Internet, and appear to be taking rapid action to address these problems. All of these newly abused drugs belong to the chemical class known as piperazines, derived from piperazine and benzyl chloride. Piperazines were originally used as worming agents in humans and in veterinary medicine, particularly in the treatment of round worms (especially *Ascaris*); they paralyse the worms so they are flushed out by peristalsis. However, the medicinal use of piperazines is banned in many countries. Ironically, more than half of the cocaine sold in the USA is contaminated with levamisole, a piperazine anti-helminthic, which was initially withdrawn from the US market because it is known to induce bone marrow suppression. Several piperazines derivatives are now in circulation and are discussed below.

1-Benzylpiperazine (BZP) is a stimulant. It is sold as a legal alternative to amphetamine, methamphetamine and MDMA and, on occasion, is misrepresented as MDMA. It interacts with numerous different receptors, but the net effect produced more or less resembles that of an amphetamine type drug. Consequently the adverse effects associated with BZP use are likely to include confusion, agitation, vomiting, anxiety and palpitations. There is strong evidence that higher plasma levels of BZP are associated with an increased incidence of seizures. Co-ingestion of ethanol increases the likelihood of adverse BZP-induced symptoms, but reduces the incidence of BZP seizures.

When taken in small doses the piperazine commonly abbreviated as TFMPP (trifluoromethylphenylpiperazine) is said to produce effects like those of MDMA. However, in large doses, or when combined with BZP, or alcohol or both, it may be toxic. A recent clinical trial employing a fixed dose of TFMPP and BZP had to be discontinued early because so many of the participants experienced agitation, anxiety, hallucinations, vomiting, insomnia and migraine. As with BZP, many of the effects resemble those produced by amphetamines, including increased heart rate and blood pressure and insomnia.

meta-Chlorophenylpiperazine (MCPP) is also a piperazine and a non-selective serotonin receptor agonist. It is sold as legal alternative to illicit stimulants, mostly in New Zealand. Like the other piperazines, MCPP is sometimes sold as faux MDMA. MCPP causes headaches in humans, and has been used as a challenge agent for testing potential anti-migraine medications. Up to 10 per cent of those who take MCPP will develop a migraine headache, and 90 per cent of individuals who commonly suffer from migraines will have an attack if challenged with MCPP. This has tended to limit the use of MCPP as a recreational drug, and may explain why no deaths have been reported after its use. There are also reports that MCPP has been used as a cocaine adulterant.

Harm reduction measures on the club and rave scene have included on-the-spot analysis of drugs to ensure that what has been bought (even though illegal) is what it is purported to be rather than something more dangerous.

An example of the concerns resulting in rapid legal changes is the change of status in England and Wales of all cathinone derivatives, including mephedrone, methylone and methadrone/methedrone (often it appears all these names are used interchangeably by users and scientists), which are Class B drugs under the Misuse of Drugs Act 1971. It is illegal to be in possession of the drugs and to sell them. The substances are controlled under generic legislation (i.e. all cathinone derivatives are covered by the Misuse of Drugs Act).

In 2009, the Advisory Council on the Misuse of Drugs (ACMD) was asked by the government to consider the harms associated with cathinone derivatives and whether they should be brought under the control of the Misuse of Drugs Act. On 29 March 2010, the ACMD recommended that mephedrone and other cathinone derivatives should be brought under the control of the Act as Class B drugs (2). The legislation was passed on 16 April 2010.

As these drugs are relatively new, with little exposure experienced by humans, there are many concerns for possible ill health effects that remain unknown. It should be noted that some amphetamine analogues containing paramethoxy group are known to cause severe hyperthermia and even death owing to concurrent monoamine oxidase inhibitor (MAOI) and monoamine releasing action. The deaths of two young men in Sweden in 2009 were attributed to methadrone overdose.

■ Drug facilitated sexual assault

Drug facilitated sexual assault (DFSA) is a matter of huge public concern. There is now an abundance of data that indicates that alcohol is the most important drug that facilitates sexual assault, and in many cases this has been consumed by the complainant rendering them more compliant and thus vulnerable to assault.

Certain drugs have been identified as having particular potential for use in DFSA and these include, ethanol, chloral hydrate, BZs, nonBZ sedative-hypnotics, GHB, ketamine, opioids, dextromethorphan, barbiturates, anticholinergics and antihistamines. Clinical examination and sampling of blood, urine and hair as soon as possible after an alleged incident may assist in determining the possible drug group involved (if any), and the time at which it was involved. Such information may assist the toxicology laboratory in directing appropriate investigation techniques. Possibly the most important future need is for education to ensure that children and young people understand the implications of drug-induced risky decisions, reduced inhibitions and reduced ability to resist.

One caveat about GHB is that inferences about ingestion cannot be drawn from autopsy material, as might be the case when a fatal sexual assault has occurred. GHB is produced as a post-mortem artefact, both in the urine and the blood, and post-mortem GHB blood measurements are particularly suspect. Different laboratories have different 'cut-offs' for reporting GHB results, and these values may vary from country to country and from laboratory to laboratory.

■ Further information sources

Advisory Council on the Misuse of Drugs. *Consideration of the Cathinones*. http://www.homeoffice.gov.uk/publications/drugs/acmd1/acmd-cathinodes-report-2010?view=Binary (accessed 23 November 2010).

Advisory Council on the Misuse of Drugs. *Consideration of the Naphthylpyrovalerone Analogues and Related Compounds*. http://www.homeoffice.gov.uk/publications/drugs/acmd1/naphyrone-report?view=Binary (accessed 23 November 2010).

Ambre JJ, Connelly TJ, Ruo TI. A kinetic model of benzoylecgonine disposition after cocaine administration in humans. *Journal of Analytical Toxicology* 1991; **15**: 17–20.

Bae SC, Lyoo IK, Sung YH *et al*. Increased white matter hyperintensities in male methamphetamine abusers. *Drug and Alcohol Dependence* 2006; **81**: 83–8.

Brandt SD, Sumnall HR, Measham F, Cole J. (2010) Analyses of second-generation 'legal highs' in the UK: initial findings. Drug Test Anal. Aug;2(8):377–82.

Capasso R, Borrelli F, Capasso F *et al*. The hallucinogenic herb *Salvia divinorum* and its active ingredient salvinorin A inhibit enteric cholinergic transmission in the guinea-pig ileum. *Neurogastroenterology and Motility* 2006; **18**: 69–75.

Chow MJ, Ambre JJ, Ruo TI *et al*., Kinetics of cocaine distribution, elimination, and chronotropic effects. *Clinical Pharmacology and Therapeutics* 1985; **38**: 318–24.

Cone EJ, Holicky BA, Grant TM *et al*., Pharmacokinetics and pharmacodynamics of intranasal 'snorted' heroin. *Journal of Analytical Toxicology* 1993; **17**: 327–337.

Cone EJ, Fant RV, Rohay JM *et al*. Oxycodone involvement in drug abuse deaths. II. Evidence for toxic multiple drug–drug interactions. *Journal of Analytical Toxicology* 2004; **28**: 616–24.

Drummer O. *The Forensic Pharmacology of Drugs of Abuse*. London: Hodder Arnold, 2001.

Du Mont J, Macdonald S, Rotbard N, Bainbridge D, Asllani E, Smith N, Cohen MM. Drug-facilitated sexual assault in Ontario, Canada: toxicological and DNA findings. *Journal of Forensic and Legal Medicine* 2010; **17**: 333–8.

Ferner RE. Post-mortem clinical pharmacology. *British Journal of Clinical Pharmacology* 2008; **66**: 430–43.

Finn SP, Leen E, English L, O'Briain DS. Autopsy findings in an outbreak of severe systemic illness in heroin users following injection site inflammation: an effect of *Clostridium novyi* exotoxin? *Archives of Pathology and Laboratory Medicine* 2003; **127**: 1465–70.

Flanagan RJ, Taylor AA, Watson ID, Whelpton R. *Fundamentals of Analytical Toxicology*. London: Wiley-Interscience, 2008.

Gibbons S, Zloh M. An analysis of the 'legal high' mephedrone. *Bioorganic & Medicinal Chemistry Letters* 2010; **20**: 4135–9.

Goldberger BA, Cone EJ, Grant TM, Caplan YH, Levine BS, Smialek JE. Disposition of heroin and its metabolites in heroin-related deaths. *Journal of Analytical Toxicology* 1994; **18**: 22–8.

Goldberger BA, Cone EJ, Grant TM *et al*. Disposition of heroin and its metabolites in heroin-related deaths. *Journal of Analytical Toxicology* 1994; **18**: 22–8.

Hall J, Goodall EA, Moore T. Alleged drug facilitated sexual assault (DFSA) in Northern Ireland from 1999 to 2005. A study of blood alcohol levels. *Journal of and Legal Medicine* 2008; **15**: 497–504.

Halpern JH. Hallucinogens: an update. *Current Psychiatry Reports* 2003; **5**: 347–54.

Huestis MA, Elsohly M, Nebro W *et al*. Estimating time of last oral ingestion of cannabis from plasma THC and THCCOOH concentrations. *Therapeutic Drug Monitoring* 2006. **28**: 540–4.

Karch S. *A Brief History of Cocaine*, 2nd edn. Boca Raton, FL: CRC Press, 2005.

Karch SB. *Karch's Pathology of Drug Abuse*, 4th edn. Boca Raton, FL: CRC Press, 2008.

20 Licit and illicit drugs

Karch SB, Billingham ME. The pathology and etiology of cocaine-induced heart disease. *Archives of Pathology and Laboratory Medicine* 1988; **112:** 225–30.

Karch SB, Stephens B, Ho CH. Relating cocaine blood concentrations to toxicity – an autopsy study of 99 cases. *Journal of Forensic Science* 1998. **43:** 41–5.

Karch SB, Stephens BG, Ho CH. Methamphetamine-related deaths in San Francisco: demographic, pathologic, and toxicologic profiles. *Journal of Forensic Science* 1999; **44:** 359–68.

Karschner EL, Schwilke EW, Lowe RH et al., Implications of plasma Delta9-tetrahydrocannabinol, 11-hydroxy-THC, and 11-nor-9-carboxy-THC concentrations in chronic cannabis smokers. *Journal of Analytical Toxicology* 2009; **33:** 469–77.

Kugelberg FC, Holmgren A, Eklund A, Jones AW. Forensic toxicology findings in deaths involving gamma-hydroxybutyrate. *International Journal of Legal Medicine* 2010; **124:** 1–6.

Lalovic B, Kharasch E, Hoffer C, Risler L, Liu-Chen LY, Shen DD. Pharmacokinetics and pharmacodynamics of oral oxycodone in healthy human subjects: role of circulating active metabolites. *Clinical Pharmacology and Therapeutics* 2006; **79:** 461–79.

LeBeau MA. Mozayani A (eds). *Drug-Facilitated Sexual Assault: A Forensic Handbook*. London: Academic Press, 2001.

LeBeau MA, Montgomery MA, Morris-Kukoski C, Schaff JE, Deakin A, Levine B. A comprehensive study on the variations in urinary concentrations of endogenous gamma-hydroxybutyrate (GHB). *Journal of Analytical Toxicology* 2006; **30:** 98–105.

Misuse of Drugs Act 1971. http://www.statutelaw.gov.uk/content.aspx?activeTextDocId=1367412 (accessed 23 November 2010).

Poon WT, Lai CF, Lui MC et al. Piperazines: a new class of drug of abuse has landed in Hong Kong. *Hong Kong Medical Journal* 2010; **16:** 76–7.

Ramsay CN, Stirling A, Smith J et al. An outbreak of infection with *Bacillus anthracis* in injecting drug users in Scotland. *Euro Surveillance* 2010; **15:** pii: 19465.

Rosenberg NL, Grigsby J, Dreisbach J et al., Neuropsychologic impairment and MRI abnormalities associated with chronic solvent abuse. *Journal of Toxicology. Clinical Toxicology* 2002; **40:** 21–34.

Stark MM, Payne-James JJ. *Symptoms and Signs of Substance Misuse*. London: Greenwich Medical Media, 2003.

Toennes SW, Harder S, Schramm M et al. Pharmacokinetics of cathinone, cathine and norephedrine after the chewing of khat leaves. *British Journal of Clinical Pharmacology* 2003; **56:** 125–30.

United Nations Office on Drugs and Crime. http://www.unodc.org/ (accessed 23 Novemmber 2010).

Vardakou I, Pistos C, Spiliopoulou C. Spice drugs as a new trend: mode of action, identification and legislation. *Toxicology Letters* 2010; **197:** 157–62.

WHO International Statistical Classification of Diseases and Related Health Problems, 10th Revision. http://apps.who.int/classifications/apps/icd/icd10online/ (accessed 23 November 2010).

Wood DM, Davies S, Puchnarewicz M et al. Recreational use of mephedrone (4-methylmethcathinone, 4-MMC) with associated sympathomimetic toxicity. *Journal of Medical Toxicology* 2010; **6:** 327–30.

Wood DM, Greene SL, Dargan PI. Clinical pattern of toxicity associated with the synthetic cathinone mephedrone. *Emergency Medicine Journal* 2011; **28(4):** 280–81.

Zvosec DL, Smith SW, Porrata T, Strobl AQ, Dyer JE. Case series of 226 γ-hydroxybutyrate-associated deaths: lethal toxicity and trauma. *American Journal of Emergency Medicine* 2011; **29(3):** 319–332.

Chapter

21

- ■ Introduction
- ■ Serotonin syndrome
- ■ QT interval prolongation (long QT syndrome)
- ■ Drugs with unique modes of action
- ■ Further information sources

Medicinal poisons

■ Introduction

Large doses of any medicine may cause cardio-toxicity or neurotoxicity but when toxicity occurs it usually does so as a result of the drug's shared ability to stimulate the same set of brain receptors as are stimulated by abused drugs. Analgesics such as oxycodone and hydrocodone bind to the same set of μ receptors as morphine. Antitussives, such as dextromethorphan, bind the same set of N-methyl-D-aspartate (NMDA) receptors as any other dissociative anaesthetic. Barbiturate drugs are rarely the cause of death except, perhaps, in epileptics, where death is more likely caused by the absence of the drug rather than any excess (sudden unexpected deaths in epileptics – SUDEP). Members of the benzodiazepine family (alprazolam, clonazepam, diazepam, zolpidem) bind the benzodiazepine receptor located on the γ-aminobutyric acid$_A$ (GABA$_A$) receptor acting synergistically with opiates to depress respiration. Second- and third-generation antidepressants cause 'serotonin syndrome', but the underlying mechanism is just the same as that of cocaine – the antidepressants prevent the reuptake of serotonin, leading to the accumulation of excess serotonin in the synaptic cleft

between nerve endings. When prescription medications are considered, two disorders have come to predominate most discussion: serotonin syndrome and QT interval prolongation.

■ Serotonin syndrome

Serotonin syndrome is a potentially life-threatening adverse drug reaction that occurs when excess serotonin accumulates within the synaptic cleft of neurons in the central nervous system. It may be caused by therapeutic drug use, inadvertent interactions between drugs, overdose of prescription drugs or the recreational use of certain other drugs such as cocaine. A spectrum of specific symptoms, somatic, cognitive and autonomic, may occur. In full-blown serotonin syndrome symptoms include: cognitive effects (mental confusion, hypomania, hallucinations, agitation, headache, coma), autonomic effects (shivering, sweating, hyperthermia, hypertension, tachycardia, nausea and diarrhoea) and somatic effects (myoclonus, hyper-reflexia and tremor). A list of drugs known to cause serotonin syndrome is given in Box 21.1.

Box 21.1 Drugs known to cause serotonin syndrome

- Antidepressants
  - Monoamine oxidase inhibitors
  - Selective serotonin reuptake inhibitors
  - Tricyclic antidepressants
  - Bupropion
  - Trazadone
- Opiates
  - Buprenorphine
  - Fentanyl
  - hydrocodone
  - Merperidine
  - Oxycodone
  - Pentazocine
- Stimulant drugs
  - Cocaine
  - All amphetamines
  - Methylphenidate
- Migraine treatments
  - All triptans (agents that bind type 1 serotonin receptors)
- Psychedelics
  - LSD (lysergic acid diethylamide)
  - MDMA (3,4-methylenedioxymethamphetamine, commonly known as ecstasy)
  - MDA (3,4-methylenedioxyamphetamine)
- Miscellaneous agents (many different types of drugs fall into this category)
  - Chlorpheniramine
  - Dextromethorphan
  - Lithium
  - Olanzapine
  - Risperidone
  - Ritonavir

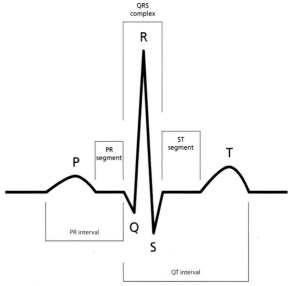

Figure 21.1 Electrocardiogram (ECG) showing QT interval which can be prolonged in the repolarization of cardiomyocytes.

■ QT interval prolongation (long QT syndrome)

Individuals with long QT syndrome (LQTS) experience abnormal prolongation of the QT interval – the portion of the electrocardiogram (ECG) that represents repolarization of cardiomyocytes (Figure 21.1). The QT interval extends from the onset of the Q wave to the end of the T wave. The normal rate–adjusted length for the QT interval is less than 440 milliseconds. A prolonged QT interval favours the occurrence of a lethal form of ventricular tachycardia known as torsades des pointes. The QT prolongation may be caused by genetic aberration or it may be acquired. Even those with the genetic form of the disease may have a perfectly normal-appearing electrocardiogram until some event causes the QT interval to lengthen, become pathologically long and produce an arrhythmia. The diagnosis cannot be made at autopsy except by DNA resequencing. This advanced diagnostic procedure is already being performed at some centres today.

An acquired form of this disorder also exists and is, in fact, much more common than the heritable form of the syndrome. Acquired LQTS is the result of a drug interaction between a drug and one of the channels that controls the orderly sequence of depolarization within the heart's individual cardiomyocytes. This structure in question is called the 'rapid delayed repolarizing channel', abbreviated as hERG. The molecular structure of the hERG channel is shown in Figure 21.2.

Some individuals carry mutations that make them more subject to hERG interactions. The end result is the same as with any hereditary cause of the disease: QT prolongation, arrhythmia and sudden death. Methadone is perhaps the most notorious of the drugs that produce this syndrome but, as indicated in Box 21.2, the list of drugs is a long one and is growing continuously. Routine toxicology screening will not reveal whether this interaction has occurred, and there will be no detectable changes at autopsy, making a thorough review of the medical history mandatory; even then the diagnosis may be impossible to make at autopsy.

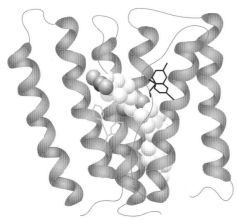

Figure 21.2 Rapid delayed repolarizing (hERG) channel: a computer rendering showing an experimental anti-arrhythmic drug docking in within the central cavity of the hERG potassium channel.

Box 21.2 Drugs causing QT prolongation

All of the drugs listed below have been show to cause ventricular tachycardia (torasades des pointes). Note that many, though far from all, are either drugs intended to treat cardiac arrhythmias or macrolide antibiotics.

- Amiodarone
- Arsenic trioxide
- Astemizole
- Bepridil
- Chloroquine
- Cisapride
- Clarithromycin
- Disopyramide
- Dofetilide
- Droperidol
- Erythromycin
- Halofantrine
- Haloperidol
- Ibutilide
- Levomethadyl
- Mesoridazine
- Methadone
- Pentamidine
- Pimozide
- Procainamide
- Quinidine
- Sotalol
- Sparfloxacin
- Terfenadine
- Thioridazine

■ Drugs with unique modes of action

Some drugs have unique modes of action. Poisoning with phenacetin is now an exceedingly rare event because its proclivity to produce renal disease is well known. However, it is an effective pain reliever by virtue of its actions on the sensory tracts of the spinal cord. Lithium, even though itself devoid of any psychoactive effects, except as a mood stabilizer, has a very complex mode of action. In fact, its mode of action is not known with certainty. There is some evidence that an excitatory neurotransmitter could be involved. It has also been proposed that lithium alters gene expression. Most recently it has been proposed that lithium might restore normal brain function to those with bipolar disorder, and that it somehow does so by deactivating an enzyme called GSK-3B. Chronic lithium poisoning is characteristically associated with greater toxicity than acute ingestion, and is usually manifested by neurotoxicity of rapid onset. Another feature of lithium poisoning is delayed cardiotoxicity, usually manifesting as bradycardia. Diagnosis of poisoning is by measurement of blood lithium concentrations.

No discussion of forensic toxicology would be complete without some mention of insulin poisoning. Insulin poisoning was once a popular means of homicide; now it is rare. Insulin overdose can cause fatal brain damage, but if overdose is suspected it can be confirmed by several different methods. C-Peptide is a peptide that is made when proinsulin is split into insulin and its C-peptide fragment. This event occurs just before release of insulin from the pancreas. If concentrations of the peptide are very low and insulin very high, the disparity would suggest that exogenous insulin had been administered. However, unless the blood specimen is frozen, levels of C-peptide may degrade rapidly. DNA analysis offers another possible approach. Biosynthetic 'human' insulin is now produced by genetic engineering. Some of the bioengineered insulin has a slightly different structure than human insulin and these differences can be detected. A friend, relative or care-giver is almost always the one who carries out homicide by insulin injection.

■ Further information sources

Barile FA (2004). *Clinical Toxicology: Principles and Mechanisms*. Boca Raton, FL: CRC Press.

Boyer EW, Shannon M. The serotonin syndrome. *N Engl J Med* 2005; **352**: 1112–20.

Byard RW. A review of the potential forensic significance of traditional herbal medicines. *Journal of Forensic Science* 2010; **55:** 89–92.

Drummer O. *The Forensic Pharmacology of Drugs of Abuse*. London: Hodder Arnold, 2001.

Ferner RE. *Forensic Pharmacology: Medicines, Mayhem and Malpractice*. New York: Oxford University Press, 1996.

Flanagan RJ, Taylor AA, Watson ID, Whelpton R. *Fundamentals of Analytical Toxicology*. London: Wiley-Interscience, 2008.

Glaister J. *A Text-Book of Medical Jurisprudence, Toxicology and Public Health*. Edinburgh: Livingstone, 1902.

Jones AL, Dargan PI. *Churchill's Pocketbook of Toxicology*. Edinburgh: Churchill Livingstone, 2001.

Luff AP. *Text-Book of Forensic Medicine & Toxicology*, Volumes I and II. London: Longmans, Green and Co, 1895.

Ross IA. *Medicinal Plants of the World*, Volumes 1, 2 and 3. Totowa, NJ: Humana Press, 2005.

Thorpe EL, Pizon AF, Lynch MJ, Boyer J. (2010) Bupropion induced serotonin syndrome: a case report. *Journal of Medical Toxicology* 2010; **6:** 168–71.

Chapter

22

- Arsenic
- Carbon monoxide
- Cyanide
- Lead
- Methanol
- Further information sources

Miscellaneous poisons

Arsenic

When arsenic is detected in a post-mortem tissue sample the significance of its presence is often difficult to determine. The presence of arsenic may indicate acute poisoning or it may indicate nothing at all. This predicament arises because arsenic exists in two forms: organic and inorganic. The term 'organic' indicates that the arsenic is bound to another organic molecule and unable to exert toxicity (the resultant compounds are called arsenosugars and arsenobetaine). In contrast, the term inorganic arsenic indicates that the arsenic atom exists as a salt bound to another cation; this salt may disassociate and then cause poisoning. The arsenic found in oysters from contaminated oyster beds is an example of organic arsenic, whereas the arsenic found in coal deposits is an example of the inorganic form. The standard method used to detect arsenic in post-mortem materials does not differentiate organic from inorganic arsenic, so the mere detection of this compound has little significance, at least not without a very suggestive clinical history.

In its free form, arsenic is highly toxic. This is unfortunate as arsenic is found in the drinking water of millions of people all around the world.

Estimates suggest that more than 13 million Americans, mainly those who use well water, are exposed to toxic levels of free arsenic every day. The entire aquifer of the Indian subcontinent is also contaminated with arsenic, which explains why many Indian herbal remedies are contaminated with arsenic. Mere exposure to arsenic does not guarantee illness because the liver is capable of rapidly detoxifying free arsenic and excreting it from the body. This protective mechanism does have its limits though, and in the presence of massive amounts of arsenic, the liver's ability to detoxify arsenic is overwhelmed.

Arsenic poisoning was once a popular type of homicide, but no longer. Arsenic poisoning is now most likely to be seen in children who have ingested arsenic pigments found in old lead-based paints (the two elements are often commingled). Such paint still exists on the walls of some Victorian era homes and constitutes a health menace.

Three forms of arsenic poisoning are recognized: acute, subacute and chronic. At any stage of the disease the breath may have garlic-like odour (as will a cadaver's tissues at autopsy). In acute poisoning, when 1 g or more of inorganic arsenic has been administered, gastrointestinal symptoms predominate with bloody vomiting and severe diarrhoea. The diarrhoea can be sufficiently copious to cause shock and cardiorespiratory failure.

If the victim dies very quickly, no abnormalities will be evident at autopsy. However, if a few hours pass before death occurs, inspection of the upper gastrointestinal (GI) tract will show that the oesophagus has become red and inflamed. In some instances, the inflammation can be so intense that the bowel is said to have a 'red velvet' appearance. The only other reliable post-mortem change produced by arsenic poisoning is bleeding from the muscle that lines the inner surface of the left side of the heart (an area known as the left ventricular subendocardium). Unfortunately, this is a relatively non-specific abnormality seen in conditions where the blood pressure suddenly collapses; the cardiac changes can be especially prominent when there has been massive blood loss from arsenic-induced bloody diarrhoea.

Chronic arsenic poisoning presents a very different picture and may be difficult or even impossible to prove with certainty. It is sometimes diagnosed as gastroenteritis or, occasionally, neuropathy. Victims may present with vague symptoms of leg and arm pain secondary to arsenic-induced nerve damage. In chronic poisoning the skin may become overly dry and pigmented, especially within the lines of the forehead and neck. Hair loss is common, and there may be swelling of the legs. In the early stages of chronic poisoning, the stomach looks normal, but eventually haemorrhagic gastroenteritis will develop. The liver will contain excessive amounts of fat, but usually only around the edges. The kidney and heart will be damaged, but the damage is only apparent if the tissues are examined with a microscope. The nails may shows 'Mee's lines' – transverse white bands across the fingernails.

■ Carbon monoxide

Intoxication from carbon monoxide (CO) is a phenomenon that occurs in a wide variety of settings worldwide. Carbon monoxide is a major environmental toxin whose effects were described over a century ago by Haldane. It is a colourless, odourless and non-irritant gas produced by the incomplete combustion of hydrocarbons and found whenever organic matter is burned in the presence of insufficient oxygen. The highest concentrations to be found in the modern urban environment are generated by motor vehicles, petrol-powered tools, heaters and barbecues. Ambient air concentrations of more than 100 ppm are considered dangerous to human health. The effects observed include a variety of physical and neurological signs and symptoms ranging from none to death. Exposure occurs in two main ways: (1) acute exposure for varying lengths of time where the effects are generally immediately obvious, and (2) delayed or chronic exposure where the effects may be unrecognized for days, months or years. The diagnosis of CO exposure may be one of exclusion. The problems of recognizing low-grade exposure to CO may result in a considerable underestimation of the problem. It has been estimated that in the USA that there are up to 6000 deaths from CO poisoning per annum, with up to 40 000 emergency department attendances for non-fatal exposure.

Carbon monoxide dissolves in plasma and binds to oxygen-transporting proteins haemoglobin (in plasma) and myoglobin, and the cytochrome system in tissues. The most significant affinity is for haemoglobin. CO is absorbed through the lungs and binds to haemoglobin (Hb) forming carboxyhaemoglobin (COHb). This a reversible reaction that can be described as follows:

$$HbO_2 + CO \rightarrow COHb + O_2$$

The affinity of Hb for CO is up to 250 times greater than that for oxygen and the presence of CO results in a shift of the oxygen–haemoglobin dissociation curve to the left, causing decreased oxygen-carrying capacity and impaired delivery of oxygen to the tissues. Cellular hypoxia results and cardiac function is diminished because of hypoxia. The link between levels of CO and effects is not direct. The amount of uptake is governed by a number of variables, all of which are interrelated and include: relative concentrations of CO and oxygen, alveolar ventilation, duration and intensity of exposure. However, chronic exposure to high levels of CO leads to CO binding to proteins with less affinity than haemoglobin, such as myoglobin and cytochromes of the P450 system, particularly a3. Differential affinity may also account for some of the variations in response to exposure. Hypoxic stress caused by CO exposure alone would not seem to account for some of the longer-term effects and it is believed that CO also initiates a cascade of events culminating in oxidative stress.

The World Health Organization has issued guidelines for the level of CO in the air that will prevent blood COHb levels from rising above 2.5 per cent. Exposure to CO may be difficult to detect. Work, domestic and leisure settings may all account for exposure. If exposure is suspected, it is appropriate to use a system such as the CH^2OPD^2 mnemonic to try to explore the source of environmental exposure (enquiring about Community, Home, Hobbies, Occupation, Personal, Diet and Drug issues). Systematic enquiry is the most efficient way of establishing a cause and a source.

Poisoning by CO is described as a 'disease with a thousand faces' because of its many different clinical presentations. Classic acute CO intoxication is said to cause the triad of cherry-red lips, cyanosis and retinal haemorrhages, but this type is rare. In many cases a more insidious presentation develops and the only indicator may be a general malaise or suspicion of a viral-type illness. Specific symptoms include headache, dizziness, nausea, shortness of breath, altered vision, altered hearing, chest pain, palpitations, poor concentration, muscle aches and cramps and abdominal pain. Sometimes these may occur in clusters and sometimes in isolation. More serious effects include loss of consciousness, myocardial ischaemia, hypotension, congestive cardiac failure, arrhythmias, mental confusion, and mood variation. These symptoms and signs may be present during acute exposure at higher level in non-fatal cases, but also in the more chronic or prolonged exposures.

In addition to the symptoms and signs discussed above there are a variety of neurological, psychiatric and psychological sequelae that may develop days, months and years after initial exposure.

Diagnosis is made by measurement of venous COHb levels; however, there is no absolute level that can confirm the presence or absence of poisoning. A level above 10 per cent is considered to confirm the diagnosis, unless the individual is a heavy smoker (Box 22.1). Concentrations of COHb in arterial blood are not significantly different from venous concentrations and so an arterial sample is not required for diagnosis. Arterial blood gas measurements can show a mixed picture of normal partial pressure of oxygen, variable partial pressure of carbon dioxide, decreased oxygen saturation, all in the presence of a metabolic acidosis. Problems arise, particularly in chronic, lower-dose exposures, because the COHb concentration will revert to 'normal' values once the source of exposure has been removed; however,

the removal process is dependent on the half-life of COHb in the particular setting. Normal COHb levels do not necessarily rule out CO poisoning. See Appendix 3 for more detailed guidelines on diagnosing CO poisoning issued by the Health Protection Agency.

Box 22.1 Haemoglobin concentrations of carbon monoxide (CO) and guideline symptoms

- In non-smokers less than 3% total haemoglobin contains CO
- In smokers 2–10% of haemoglobin contains CO
- 20–30% of haemoglobin causes headache, nausea, vomiting and confusion
- 30–40% of haemoglobin causes dizziness, muscle weakness, confusion, rapid heart beat
- 50–60% of haemoglobin causes loss of consciousness
- Over 60% of haemoglobin causes seizures, coma, death

Table 22.1 shows the symptoms produced by increasing concentrations of carbon monoxide within the body.

Carbon monoxide was once a frequent means of suicide, but changes in technology have led to a marked decrease in the number of deaths. In the 1950s inhaling coal gas accounted for nearly half of all suicides in the UK, but the rate markedly declined after natural gas replaced coal gas in the 1960s. The introduction of catalytic converters for automobiles has reduced, but not quite eliminated, suicides committed by inhaling the exhaust fumes from a car engine operating in an enclosed space. The catalytic converters found in cars today eliminate over 99 per cent of the carbon monoxide produced but, even then, very substantial amounts

Table 22.1 Symptoms produced by carbon monoxide

Concentration (ppm)	Symptom
35	Headache, dizziness
100	Headache, dizziness
200	Headache, loss of judgement
400	Frontal headache
800	Dizziness, nausea, convulsions
1 600	Tachycardia, nausea, death in less than 1 hour
3 200	Tachycardia, nausea, death in less than 20 minutes
6 400	Convulsions, respiratory arrest, death in 1–2 minutes
12 800	Unconsciousness after two breaths, death in 3 minutes

of carbon monoxide may be generated if a car is left with its engine running in a closed garage. The majority of accidental poisonings and suicides by carbon monoxide occur as a result of burning charcoal in a confined space. In the most frequent scenario, a charcoal barbecue is lit in a closed room. If death was solitary and intended, then the windows and doors are likely to have been sealed off. If not, it may be difficult to determine whether or not the cause of death was accident or suicide.

■ Cyanide

Cyanide ions prevent cells from utilizing oxygen; they inhibit the enzyme cytochrome c oxidase. High concentrations of cyanide lead to cardiac arrest within minutes of exposure. Exposure to lower levels of cyanide over a long period (e.g. after use of cassava roots as a primary food source, which is a relatively common occurrence in tropical Africa) results in increased blood cyanide levels, which can cause weakness and a variety of symptoms including permanent paralysis. Cigarette smoking also increases blood cyanide concentrations, although most of the time the increase is asymptomatic and blood concentrations modest. In non-smokers, the average blood cyanide concentration is less than 0.01 μmol/L, rising to 1 mol/L immediately after smoking. In chronic smokers concentrations may be 10 times higher.

Large infusions of sodium nitroprusside, used to treat hypertensive emergencies, can lead to serious cyanide poisoning, but more commonly cyanide poisoning is encountered in fire survivors, as many contemporary fabrics and building materials contain plastics that can liberate cyanide during combustion. Cyanide is said to have the smell of bitter almonds, but approximately 10 per cent of the general population are congenitally unable to perceive this smell. This rarely leads to exposure in the autopsy suite because, in the course of normal circumstance, multiple staff members will be present and at least one is like to perceive the odour.

■ Lead

Routes of lead exposure include contaminated air, water, soil, food and certain lead-containing consumer products, particularly those made in China. In adults the most common cause of lead poisoning is occupational exposure, whereas in children it is the lead paint that exists in older homes. Aged lead paint is likely to peel off walls and may look like an attractive comestible to children. Lead is toxic because it can substitute for calcium in many fundamental cellular processes, although how it does so is not entirely clear: neither the electronic structures nor the ionic radii of the two elements bear any particular resemblance. Nonetheless, lead can cross red blood cell membranes as well as the blood–brain barrier and enter the neuroglia cells which support brain function. This explains why exposed children may develop permanent learning and behavioural disorders.

Symptoms of lead poisoning include abdominal pain, headache, anaemia, irritability and, in severe cases, seizures, coma and death. X-rays will expose dense lines in the long bones of children and red cells undergo a change known as basophilic stippling, where blue-staining remnants of destroyed DNA are seen lining the margins of the red cells. This change is diagnostic for lead poisoning. The main tool for diagnosis is measurement of the blood lead level. Treatment depends on the blood level and is designed to remove the lead from the body (chelation therapy).

■ Methanol

Like ethanol, methanol can cause fatal central nervous system (CNS) depression but, in addition, it is also toxic because it is metabolized to produce formic acid (present as the formate ion) via formaldehyde in a process initiated by the enzyme alcohol dehydrogenase. All of these processes occur in the liver. Formate is toxic because it inhibits mitochondrial cytochrome c oxidase, causing hypoxia at the cellular level. Methanol also causes metabolic acidosis. Methanol poisoning most often occurs after drinking windscreen-washer fluid, but methanol is also used in copy machines and can be found in many other products, even embalming fluid. Methanol poisoning still remains a well-known consequence of 'moonshine' liquor ingestion, although this practice is increasingly uncommon. When paediatric poisoning occurs it is usually the result of having ingested methanol-containing household products. Ingestion of even small amounts of methanol, in addition to causing profound metabolic acidosis, may lead to blindness or even multi-organ system failure and death.

The initial symptoms of methanol intoxication include CNS depression, with headache, dizziness, nausea, lack of coordination and confusion. Large doses quickly lead to unconsciousness and death. Once the initial symptoms have passed, a second set of symptoms can be observed 10–30 hours after the ingestion. These include blindness and worsening acidosis. These secondary symptoms are caused by accumulating levels of formate in the bloodstream. The process may progress to death by respiratory failure.

Methanol poisoning can be treated with the antidotes ethanol or fomepizole, the goal of using either is to compete with alcohol dehydrogenase so that the methanol is excreted by the kidneys instead of being converted into toxic metabolites. Supplemental treatment with sodium bicarbonate for metabolic acidosis and haemodialysis or even haemodiafiltration can be used to remove methanol and formate from the blood.

Because of its toxic properties, methanol is frequently used as a denaturant additive for ethanol manufactured for industrial uses as this addition of methanol exempts industrial ethanol from liquor excise taxation. Methanol is often referred to as 'wood alcohol' because it was once produced chiefly as a by-product of the destructive distillation of wood.

■ Further information sources

Andresen H, Schmoldt H, Matschke J, Flachskampf FA, Turk EE. Fatal methanol intoxication with different survival times – morphological findings and postmortem methanol distribution. *Forensic Science International* 2008; **179:** 206–10.

Balakumar P, Kaur J. Arsenic exposure and cardiovascular disorders: an overview. *Cardiovascular Toxicology* 2009; **9:** 169–76.

Barceloux DG, Bond GR, Krenzelok EP, Cooper H, Vale JA; American Academy of Clinical Toxicology Ad Hoc Committee on the Treatment Guidelines for Methanol Poisoning. American Academy of Clinical Toxicology practice guidelines on the treatment of methanol poisoning. *Journal of Toxicology, Clinical Toxicology* 2002; **40:** 415–46.

Barile FA. *Clinical Toxicology: Principles and Mechanisms*. Boca Raton, FL: CRC Press, 2004.

Bechtel LK, Holstege CP. Criminal poisoning: drug-facilitated sexual assault. *Emergency Medicine Clinics of North America* 2007; **25:** 499–525.

Coentrão L, Moura D. Acute cyanide poisoning among jewelry and textile industry workers. *American Journal of Emergency Medicine* 2011; **29:** 78–81.

Croxford B, Leonardi GS, Kreis I. Self-reported neurological symptoms in relation to CO emissions due to problem gas appliance installations in London: a cross-sectional survey. *Environmental Health* 2008; **7:** 34.

Drummer O. *The Forensic Pharmacology of Drugs of Abuse*. London: Hodder Arnold, 2001.

Ferner RE. *Forensic Pharmacology: Medicines, Mayhem and Malpractice*. New York: Oxford University Press, 1996.

Flanagan RJ, Taylor AA, Watson ID, Whelpton R. *Fundamentals of Analytical Toxicology*. London: Wiley-Interscience, 2008.

Fortin JL, Desmettre T, Manzon C et al. Cyanide poisoning and cardiac disorders: 161 cases. *Journal of Emergency Medicine* 2010; **38:** 467–76.

Gensheimer KF, Rea V, Mills DA, Montagna CP, Simone K. Arsenic poisoning caused by intentional contamination of coffee at a church gathering – an epidemiological approach to a forensic investigation. *Journal of Forensic Science* 2010; **55:** 1116–19. Epub 2010 Apr 8.

Glaister J. *A Text-Book of Medical Jurisprudence, Toxicology and Public Health*. Edinburgh: Livingstone, 1902.

Hall AH, Saiers J, Baud F. Which cyanide antidote? *Critical Reviews in Toxicology* 2009; **39:** 541–52.

Hall JA, Moore CB. Drug facilitated sexual assault – a review. *Journal of Forensic and Legal Medicine* 2008; **15:** 291–7.

Iqbal S, Clower JH, Boehmer TK, Yip FY, Garbe P. Carbon monoxide-related hospitalizations in the U.S.: evaluation of a web-based query system for public health surveillance. *Public Health Reports* 2010; **125:** 423–32.

Ilano AL, Raffin TA. Management of carbon monoxide poisoning. *Chest* 1990; **97:** 165–9.

Jones AL, Dargan PI. *Churchill's Pocketbook of Toxicology*. Edinburgh: Churchill Livingstone, 2001.

Karayel F, Turan AA, Sav A, Pakis I, Akyildiz EU, Ersoy G. Methanol intoxication: pathological changes of central nervous system (17 cases). *American Journal of Forensic Medicine and Pathology* 2010; **31:** 34–6.

Karch S. *Karch's Pathology of Drug Abuse*, 4th edn. Boca Raton, FL: CRC Press, 2008.

Luff AP. *Text-Book of Forensic Medicine & Toxicology*, Volumes I and II. London: Longmans, Green and Co, 1895.

Moffat AC, Osselton, MD, Widdop, B (eds). *Clarke's Analysis of Drugs and Poisons*, 3rd edn. London: Pharmaceutical Press, 2004.

Paasma R, Hovda KE, Jacobsen D. Methanol poisoning and long term sequelae – a six years follow-up after a large methanol outbreak. *BMC Clinical Pharmacology* 2009; **9:** 5.

Payne-James JJ, Robinson S. Carbon monoxide poisoning: clinical aspects. In: Payne-James JJ, Byard RW, Corey TS, Henderson C (eds). *Encyclopedia of Forensic and Legal Medicine*. Oxford: Elsevier Academic Press, 2005.

Piantadosi CA. Diagnosis and treatment of carbon monoxide poisoning. *Respiratory Care Clinics of North America* 1999; **5:** 183–202.

Roychowdhury T Groundwater arsenic contamination in one of the 107 arsenic-affected blocks in West Bengal, India: status, distribution, health effects and factors responsible for arsenic poisoning. *International Journal of Hygiene and Environmental Health* 2010; **213:** 414–27.

Saukko P, Knight B. *Knight's Forensic Pathology*, 3rd edn. London: Hodder Arnold, 2004.

Sheikhazadi A, Saberi Anary SH, Ghadyani MH. Nonfire carbon monoxide-related deaths: a survey in Tehran, Iran (2002–2006). *American Journal of Forensic Medicine and Pathology* 2010; **31:** 359–63.

Singh N, Kumar D, Sahu AP. Arsenic in the environment: effects on human health and possible prevention. *Journal of Environmental Biology* 2007; **28**(Suppl): 359–65.

Sullivan JT, Sykora K, Schneiderman J *et al*. Assessment of alcohol withdrawal: the revised Clinical Institute Withdrawal Assessment for Alcohol scale (CIWA-Ar). *British Journal of Addiction* 1989; **84:** 1353–7.

Tournel G, Houssaye C, Humbert L *et al*. Acute arsenic poisoning: clinical, toxicological, histopathological, and forensic features. *Journal of Forensic Science* 2011; **56**(suppl. 1): S275–9.

Ye X, Wong O. Lead exposure, lead poisoning, and lead regulatory standards in China, 1990–2005. *Regulatory Toxicology and Pharmacology* 2006; **46:** 157–62.

Chapter 23

Principles of forensic science

- Locard's exchange principle
- Scene examination
- Evidence recovery
- Chain of custody
- Sample analysis
- Blood pattern analysis
- Damage
- Fingerprints
- Footwear
- Trace evidence
- Fire investigation
- Firearms
- Further information sources

■ Locard's exchange principle

Much of the work of forensic practitioners is based on the principle described by Edmond Locard (1877–1966) who was director of the crime laboratory in Lyon, France. This principle (also known as Locard's theory) – in simple form 'every contact leaves a trace' – provides a basis for the recovery and interpretation of evidence. When applied to a criminal setting it states that if a perpetrator of a crime comes into contact with a scene (or someone within that scene), then something will be brought into the scene, and something will be taken away. It is for the forensic practitioner to identify what those types of contact were by identifying the contact and putting it into an evidentially sound format.

The principle can be applied in all settings, for example by linking a suspect's DNA to seminal fluid obtained from a complainant's vagina, by identifying paint from a car that has hit an object or by identifying hair from a balaclava used in an armed robbery.

■ Scene examination

The principles of establishing, managing and investigating a crime scene should be similar worldwide. The aim is to secure, identify and preserve evidence that may have value in a subsequent court setting.

A crime scene is an entity which is created when police cordon off an area of interest in relation to an actual or a suspected offence (Figure 23.1). A zone is cordoned off, within which all people accessing or leaving are entered into (and have to sign) a 'scene log'. As such, this provides information as to who has had access to evidence that could have a

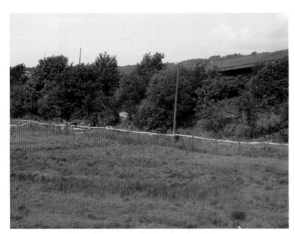

Figure 23.1 Crime scene cordon. Deceased found by motorway, in vegetation. Tape represents police line beyond which entry, exit and activity is controlled and maintained in detail.

bearing on the outcome of a case (Figure 23.1). The scene will be guarded by police or other security personnel. This can be a significant commitment of staff when areas are extensive and the management of personnel is crucial to ensure expeditious and cost-effective progress.

In the UK a Crime Scene Manager (CSM) is in overall charge of the scene and controls the personnel that assist in the examination. The CSM acts as liaison with the Senior Investigating Officer (SIO) as to examination strategy depending on the demands of the enquiry. The CSM and their staff are most often civilian across UK police forces but there are some areas where the Scene of Crime Officers (SOCOs) are still serving police officers. It is usually the CSM who is the point of contact for all those examining the scene as the SIO has overall management responsibility for the case to be taken forward.

At larger incidents, it is likely that a CSM, SOCOs, exhibits officer and photographers would be present. If it is deemed necessary, other specialists such as forensic pathologists or forensic physicians and various other forensic specialists (e.g. a blood pattern expert) may also be in attendance.

Before entering the crime scene a briefing is usually conducted when the facts, as they are known, are presented to parties who will be conducting the initial examinations. Once an examination strategy is decided, the evidence collection can commence. The importance of these briefings cannot be overstated as they ensure an efficient approach with evidence maximized.

Within a crime scene certain precautions need to be taken to ensure that contamination is not introduced (either from investigator to scene or scene to investigator). Wearing overalls, gloves, overshoes and masks ensures that the minimum, if any, cross-contamination will occur. It is best to avoid touching anything if at all possible as all surfaces can harbour evidence. For example, light switches or door handles may be of interest for DNA or fingerprints. Wall or door jambs may be useful for fingerprints so should not be leant on. Staff examining scenes may have to move across the floor on stepping plates as there may be footwear (or other) evidence that still needs to be recovered.

Generally speaking, if there are human remains at crime scenes, examinations are focused on the immediate area around the remains so that they can be removed for a post-mortem examination. The reason for this is simple; remains are prone to rapid changes, especially during the first few weeks of decomposition, making evidence recovery by both scientists and pathologists more challenging.

Once evidence gathering by SOCOs and scientists is complete, other searches can take place. These are the 'fingertip' searches carried out by Police Search Advisory (POLSA) staff. Following this examination, the scene can be closed down. In the case of premises, they may remain in police possession but be made secure and alarmed, or in the case of external areas, the cordon is removed and normal life resumes.

■ Evidence recovery

At a scene, however large or small, once items of forensic interest are found, they are recorded appropriately and assigned an affidavit or exhibit number. They are usually given the initials of the person responsible for the item being 'seized' (very often an exhibits officer) followed by a sequential number, for example 'JDM.1'. The item is usually photographed before being removed carefully, so as not to disturb the relevant evidence, and packaged. There are a number of different types of packaging that can be used for different items. Paper sacks are used for clothing because, if the

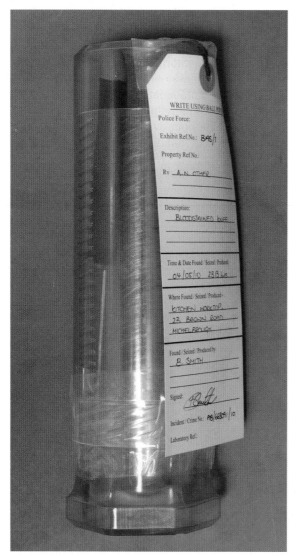

Figure 23.2 Sealed and labelled weapon tube containing a bloodstained knife.

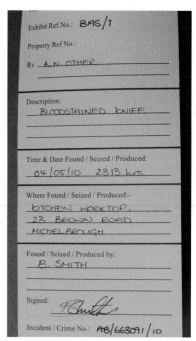

Figure 23.3 A typical exhibit label detailing the unique item number, the item description, the details of where the item was recovered, the time and date on which the item was recovered and the details of the person who recovered the item.

The label is then signed by the person who seized the item (Figure 23.3).

■ Chain of custody

Once an exhibit has been created, each time it is transferred from one place to another, the details need to be recorded. This is the 'chain of custody'. This is achieved by using continuity forms which demonstrate that the exhibit has been passed from one person to another. When an exhibit is placed in a secure store, this fact is logged along with the location of the exhibit so it can easily be relocated when required. Each person who has examined the item as part of their work signs the exhibit label to demonstrate they have seen the item.

Once examinations of an exhibit have been concluded, it is retained for a period of time before it is destroyed or, on occasion, returned. This can be 3 months in more routine cases or at least 30 years in serious cases. Often, items are not destroyed as personnel may realize that advances in technology could reveal evidence that is not at that time apparent.

item is slightly damp, this allows moisture to pass through. Plastic bags can be used for items such as cigarette ends. Plastic tubes that screw together are used for sharp items such as knives or screwdrivers; these are known as weapons tubes (Figure 23.2). Cardboard boxes can also be used for such items with plastic ties to secure the item in place.

If there is no exhibit label integral with the bag, a separate label will need to be filled out and secured to the packaging containing the item. This contains details describing the item, its origin, the person seizing the item and the time and date of seizure.

■ Sample analysis

DNA analysis

What is DNA profiling?

Within most cells in the body there is a nucleus containing 23 pairs of chromosomes. Half of these are inherited maternally and half paternally. The same, or different forms of each complementary area on each paired chromosome (with the exception of the sex chromosomes) may be inherited. DNA is also present in mitochondria within cells; this is inherited through the maternal lineage.

At the time of writing, the most common type of DNA profiling utilizes the fact that there are apparent (comparatively) short regions on chromosomes that repeat themselves a number of times. These are called short tandem repeats (STRs). These are believed to be non-coding and are conserved from generation to generation. The amount of repeats varies between individuals but the range of variation is relatively low and, by themselves, each STR (so-called allele) occurs quite commonly (generally between 5 per cent and 20 per cent of the population). A person can have the same (homozygous) or different STRs (heterozygous) at each region (locus) that is analysed. The power of DNA analysis is realized when one considers that (in the UK) 10 different loci are analyzed, giving a total of 20 alleles in each process.

How is a DNA profile obtained?

A sample that is taken for analysis undergoes a number of steps before a DNA profile can be obtained. The first step is to dissolve the sample in appropriate chemicals to ensure the maximum amount of DNA can be recovered from the source material. This is decided by the analyst but the more information that can be given about the provenance of a sample, the better. For example, a ground tooth would receive very different treatment from that of a cigarette end.

Following this 'extraction' stage, the amount of DNA within the sample is estimated. This is usually minute and measured in terms of nanograms (10^{-9} g). This stage is carried out so that the correct amount of the extracted sample is removed for the next stage (amplification) as the reactions are very sensitive and need to have optimum chemical concentrations.

Amplification is carried out using the polymerase chain reaction (PCR), which uses an enzyme-catalysed reaction over a number of cycles. Each PCR cycle, if it were 100 per cent efficient would double the amount of DNA present within each sample. There are 28 cycles in a standard analysis in the UK using the Second Generation Multiplex Plus (SGM+; Applied Biosystems, Foster City, CA, USA) system. This analyses 10 loci, each on different chromosomes in addition to a sex text. The alleles that are amplified are tagged with a fluorescent dye.

The loci that are amplified vary in the number of repeats that are commonly encountered and so a range in size and thus molecular weight exists. This is exploited by the equipment used to process the amplified sample so a profile can be obtained. The sample is subjected to capillary electrophoresis over a high potential difference. This means that the low molecular weight alleles pass through the capillaries more rapidly than those of a higher weight. This enables an efficient compilation of the profile. As each of the alleles has been tagged with the fluorescent dye, they are detected as they pass through the analytical process. A size standard is also run through each sample set to ensure the sizing of each allele is correct.

As each allele passes through the reader it registers as a peak in intensity of the fluorescent dye. This is translated onto an electropherogram (EPG) which represents a DNA profile as a series of peaks along a graphical line (Figure 23.4).

If a profile has been obtained from a sample such as a blood stain, it can then be compared with a reference sample from an individual believed to be connected to the case. These are most commonly mouth (buccal) swabs but can also be blood samples or tissue samples from a body.

If DNA profiles do not match then they could not have come from the same person. If there are only one or two areas that do not match then, as DNA is inherited and is more similar between family members than unrelated people, one may suspect that the sample under consideration originated from a closely related individual and may current more investigation. If profiles match, then they could be from the same person and the probability is extremely low that there is someone else who has the same profile with the exception of identical twins.

When there is a partial (or incomplete) profile, this can be used to compare with reference samples and a statistic can be provided as to the likelihood of a match with a reference sample. The more incomplete a sample, the more people may be expected to match

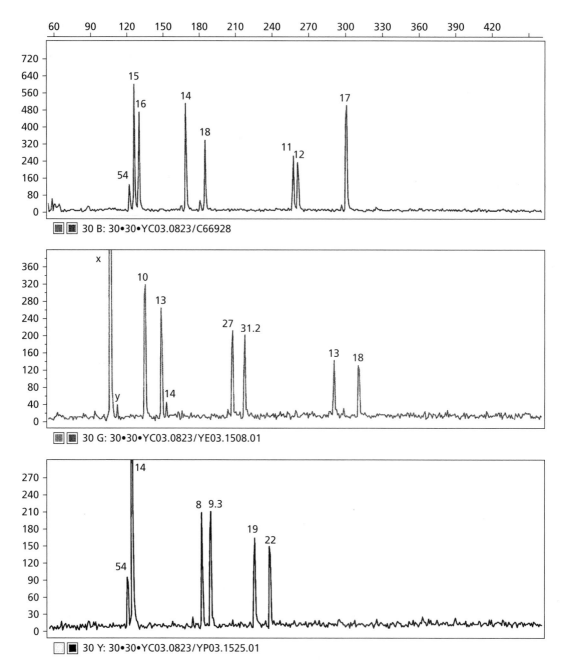

Figure 23.4 Figure showing a DNA profile graphically represented as an electropherogram (EPG).

by chance. Conversely, the more information there is across a profile, the lower will be the probability of a random match. The way in which the statistics are calculated assume a high degree of independence between loci as they are on different chromosomes. Put simply, one multiplies the rarity value of each allele across a profile for the number of alleles that are present. Even if the allele occurs in 50 per cent of the population, one can see how, even with

10 alleles present out of a possible 20, the chance of a random match is low.

DNA Statistics and Bayes Theorem

Discussion of DNA profiling inevitably involves terms such as 'likelihood of a match', or 'probability'. These are used in the expression of the strength of the evidence and the methodology used relies on the use of Bayesian statistics, so-called from the theories developed by Thomas Bayes, an 18th Century clergyman. These differ from other types of statistical analyses that are more commonly encountered in scientific analyses as they use a measure of subjectivity to assist in determining the probability of an outcome. For example, when tossing a coin it would be generally accepted that there is a 50% chance (or the probability is 0.5) that the outcome would be heads. If, however, the coin has a small weight attached to one side, this would affect the outcome and may lend bias to one side. Such considerations bring into play additional information that can be used to condition the calculated probability of a given hypothesis. In summary, there is an uncertain event, to which one wishes to assign a probability as to the outcome. With additional information, Bayesian statistics assist in providing a model to determine that probability.

In relation to DNA evidence, if we consider a single DNA profile from a crime scene that matches a given individual, one can assess the probability of two hypotheses:

A. The DNA originated from that person
B. The DNA originated from another, random, person

The probability of the outcome being true in regards to hypothesis (A) is one.

Looking at the alternative hypothesis (B), one has to consider a number of factors such as the rarity of each allele, any potential knowledge of the ethnicity of the subject, and any other factors. This probability can be extremely small for a full profile but the probability increases with regards to incomplete profile and analysis is complicated when it comes to the interpretation of mixed DNA results.

It is very important when considering DNA evidence (and indeed other forensic evidence), that it is expressed as the probability of the scientific evidence given the hypotheses under consideration, and not the probability of the hypothesis given the evidence. This is termed transposing the conditional and can lead to a complete misrepresentation of the scientific evidence in court.

Mixed DNA Results

A DNA profile can often be a mixture of DNA from more than one person. This is very common, especially in cases of sexual assault and can lead to significant complications in interpretation. If a case involves people who are closely related this can also complicate analysis as they are more likely to share alleles that unrelated people. SGM+ DNA profiling is a very sensitive technique. Typically, it is possible to get a complete DNA profile from less than 300 cells. This ability to get a DNA profile from small amounts of biological material emphasises the need to reduce contamination risks as far as possible.

Other forms of DNA analysis

Low template forms of DNA analysis exist with the purpose of obtaining profiles from very small quantities of DNA. These can be divided into two different methodologies. One method is to take a different form of analysis whereby specialist techniques are used to improve the existing technology within the 28-cycle system. The second is to increase the number of cycles. One such technique using 34 cycles is low copy number (LCN) DNA. Challenges exist in the interpretation of LCN profiles as very small amounts of DNA are amplified. It is thus reported by consensus (more than one result compared) with great care taken over the interpretation. This does not prevent it being an excellent tool to detect DNA left in very small amounts (for example by touch).

The Y-STR DNA technique uses the same STR-based technology as SGM+ but looks at a number of STRs on the Y-chromosome (i.e. only from males). This can be extremely useful in cases of sexual assault when amounts of male DNA are very low compared with female within a sample and it is difficult to separate the two. Results would be expected to be the same with related males.

Mitochondrial DNA analysis can be used where nuclear cellular material is low, for example from hair shafts or in cases where decomposition has meant that much of the DNA that would have been used for SGM+ has degraded. Such analyses look at two main sites on the genome. As mitochondrial DNA is inherited from the mother, female relatives and children from the same mother would be expected to have the same mitochondrial DNA profile.

Single nucleotide polymorphisms (SNPs) are areas where single base-pair variation occurs. As it looks at such small areas, this can be used in cases where DNA is severely degraded (for example by heat). This type of DNA analysis was used to identify individuals from the World Trade Centre in 2001.

National DNA Database

In the UK, the National DNA Database holds the details of people arrested in connection with different offences as well as data relating to crime stains for which no reference profile has been found to match. It is currently the largest such database in the world. Samples can be searched against the database in attempts to identify whether or not there could be a match with a person whose profile has already been loaded for another reason. Whenever a new profile is loaded to the database, it is searched against existing profiles. In this way, many people have been linked to case stains. The database accepts samples profiled using the SGM+ system.

There is considerable concern about the National DNA Database among many, including those with an interest in civil liberties about the appropriateness of retention and the delay or absence of destruction of profiles. This can be with regards to those who never go to trial for the allegation for which they were arrested, those who are acquitted and the vulnerable, such as children.

Body fluid analysis

Forensic scientists will often be requested to conduct searches for a number of body fluids, including blood, semen, saliva, urine, faeces and others in attempts to identify individuals (and in some instances species) who may have left the stains (using DNA analysis) as well as interpreting them in the context of their location.

Blood

Blood is identified by its colour and the chemical reaction it gives when a presumptive test is applied. In the absence of one of these factors, one cannot confirm the presence of blood. Blood does not always appear red/brown in colour and can vary to yellow or even clear depending on the type of stain which has been left. This can make it very challenging to locate stains on a darker surface.

Stains that are to be tested are scraped with the edge of a piece of sterile filter paper that has been folded. The presumptive tests used are Leuco-malachite Green (LMG) or Kastle–Meyer (K-M). Both involve the addition of the reduced form (colourless) of each reagent to the filter paper followed a few seconds later by hydrogen peroxide. If a colour change occurs after the addition of both

chemicals, and the colour of the original stain was typical (to green for LMG, pink for K-M) of a bloodstain, then the presence of blood is confirmed. The colour change occurs as blood has a peroxidise-like activity from haemoglobin, which catalyses the oxidation of each chemical.

False positive reactions can be obtained from vegetation and certain oxidizing chemicals, hence the importance of waiting between adding the K-M or LMG before the hydrogen peroxide.

Blood stains as small as 1 mm in diameter can provide a DNA profile. However, if possible it is best to take a larger sample as the percentage of white blood cells within the sample is not known, as levels may vary between different individuals.

When bloodstains cannot be seen, different methods of detection need to be used. For example wiping filter paper in a systematic manner over areas and sequentially testing these can help localize staining on dark surfaces.

Semen

Human semen is made up of both a liquid and a cellular fraction in unvasectomized post-pubescent males. Semen is detected by forensic scientists using the acid phosphatase (AP) test, as acid phosphatase occurs in high levels in human semen. When testing clothing or other larger items this involves a press-test of filter paper onto a dampened item suspected to bear semen staining. The filter paper is then removed and sprayed with the AP reagent. If a purple colour develops, the presence of semen is indicated (Figure 23.5). This is confirmed by locating the stained area on the garment and extracting some of the stain before making up a microscope slide containing some of the extract. If spermatozoa are seen, the presence of semen is confirmed.

If swabs are to be tested they can also be pressed onto a piece of filter paper before AP is applied or, alternatively, the swab can be extracted, the cellular fraction spun down and a fraction of the liquid supernatant tested instead to conserve cellular material. In a similar manner, a microscope slide is made to search for spermatozoa.

It is important to note how much semen is found on different swabs from different areas of the body as this can have a bearing as to how recently semen was deposited.

It should be noted that in houses where adult male clothing is washed with the rest of the laundry,

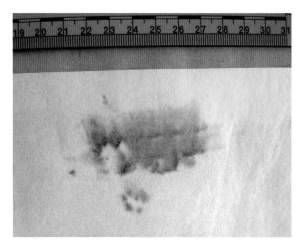

Figure 23.5 A positive reaction result for acid phosphatase (AP), indicating that semen could be present, after application of the AP reagent (photographed at 2 minutes after application).

sperm cells found normally on their underwear may be expected to be transferred to other items within the wash. Washing items will not remove all sperm cells from an area of staining but will remove the chemical that will react with AP reagent. Therefore, if looking for older stains, it can be worthwhile examining exploratory areas to look for sperm cells despite a negative AP reaction. In such instances it is best practice to analyse also a control area to demonstrate the absence of such concentrations elsewhere.

Bacterial infections can give false reactions with AP reagent (a pinkish colour). False positive can also occur from vaginal AP; however, generally only AP from semen produces the quick change to a strong purple colour.

If a male has been vasectomized successfully, no sperm cells should be present within an ejaculate. In these cases, a second chemical test can be used to confirm the presence of semen. This is for prostate specific antigen (PSA) and uses an antibody-based technique to demonstrate the presence of PSA. The Florence Iodine test can also be used, where a small amount of the reagent is introduced to a slide carrying some of the extracted stain. If characteristic brown crystals form then the presence of semen is confirmed. However, this method is not very sensitive and caution should be taken in the interpretation of the results.

Saliva

As saliva stains are usually translucent, a test used to locate and identify such stains is very important.

The locator test detects the presence of amylase, an enzyme found in high levels in human saliva. The most commonly used method for amylase is the Phadebas test (Magle Life Sciences, Lund, Sweden) which can be used in two ways. It can be used in a press-test whereby Phadebas paper is placed against the item under test and wetted. If a uniform blue colour develops, the presence of amylase is confirmed. Depending on the location and strength of the reaction, an opinion can be given as to the presence of saliva. The areas giving positive chemical reactions can then be isolated and submitted for DNA analysis. In cases where allegations of kissing/licking/biting/sucking different parts of the body have been made, this can be a very useful test to employ.

The Phadebas test can also be used as a tube test whereby stains/swabs are extracted and measured quantities of liquid supernatant can be added to a solution of the test reagent. This method can be extremely useful in cases where staining is suspected to be very light as it is highly sensitive and easier to interpret than the press-test method.

Care needs to be taken in the interpretation of Phadebas results as other human body fluids such as vaginal secretions, sweat and faeces can also contain amylase, albeit usually at lower levels. It should also be borne in mind that not all people secrete salivary amylase; therefore, its absence does not mean that saliva was not present.

'Touch' DNA

DNA profiling is often used to identify potential individuals who have handled an item, depositing skin cells, such as on a door handle, for example. It can also be used to assist in the identification of wearers of garments such as gloves or hats and shoes. In some instances, skin cells may be visible microscopically, and sampling appropriately directed. In other instances, a whole area may need to be speculatively swabbed.

Urine and faeces

On occasion, the presence of urine or faeces needs to be confirmed, for example from cases of alleged anal rape or deliberate soiling of items. There is the simple method of dampening and warming items with regard to each body fluid, with the characteristic odour developing, or one can use chemical tests, which are available for both urine and faeces.

In the case of urine, tests such as the dimethylaminocinnamaldehyde (DMAC) test can be employed to detect the presence of urea, a chemical constituent of urine. Other tests can also be employed, for example for the chemical creatinine, another constituent of urine. Both of these tests rely on colour changes to provide positive results.

Stains suspected to be faecal in nature can be tested using Edelman's test, which detects the presence of urobilinogen, a chemical constituent of faeces.

■ Blood pattern analysis

If an individual sustains an injury that bleeds, that blood can be transferred to clothing, footwear and surrounding objects and surfaces. Bloodstain pattern analysis (BPA) can be used to assist the investigator in a variety of ways. It may be possible to determine a sequence of events, the movement of people in the course of an assault, a minimum number of blows and to comment on a possible weapon used to inflict injury. It is also possible to determine the location of an attack site(s) using simple mathematics to determine the point of origin of bloodstains.

The nature and distribution of the staining can vary greatly, depending on several factors among which are:

- the type of blood vessel damaged;
- the location of the damage (exposed or under clothing);
- the mobility and actions of the injured individual after receiving the injury.

Bloodstain patterns are divided into a number of categories from those that result in blood falling with gravity, to contact stains and those distributions that result from forces being applied to the source of the blood (for example impact spatter or cast-off).

Downward drips

Downwards drips are formed when blood falls from a surface (such as the end of a finger) under the force of gravity. If they land on a flat surface, they will make a characteristic circular stain, although if the surface is not smooth (e.g. pavement) the stain can be quite distorted (Figure 23.6).

If blood is dropped onto an absorbent surface such as carpet, the stain can be much smaller while

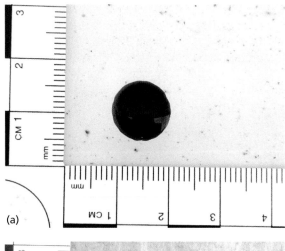

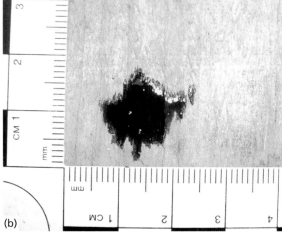

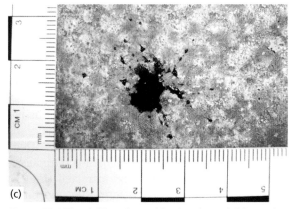

Figure 23.6 Blood dripped onto **(a)** painted metal, **(b)** wood and **(c)** concrete.

still being of the same volume. If a number of drops fall onto the same location, a distribution that could be confused with a more active event is created as the blood makes contact with other wet staining already present. The force of the blood drops falling into wet blood that has already fallen results in a number of smaller, satellite drops being projected away from the area of impact. Such satellite droplets can be projected for quite some distance from the centre of the distribution; this is dependent on the height from which the blood is falling, the texture and absorbance of the surface and the amount of blood already present.

Contact blood staining

Contact bloodstains are formed when a blood-stained item comes into contact with another, non-stained item (Figure 23.7). If a surface is moving when it comes into contact with another surface, and one is bloodstained, a blood smear will result. Contact smears are divided into wipes and swipes. If a surface is contacted, for example, by a bloodstained hand, the resulting stain is a swipe. Conversely, if a clean hand moves through blood staining on a surface, the resulting stain is termed a wipe.

Other types of contact staining commonly encountered are footwear marks and fingerprints left in blood. It can be a matter of great contention as to whether or not a fingerprint was left by a blood-stained finger or whether an impression was made by a finger into an existing wet bloodstain. Scientifically, it can be very difficult to distinguish between the two alternatives.

In cases involving marks, there may be areas of the mark that are so faint that they cannot be resolved by the eye, or indeed the camera lens. Such marks require enhancement and there are a variety of chemicals available that will effectively enhance marks in blood.

Impact spatter

When someone is struck in an area that bears wet blood staining, the stains can be broken up and projected away from the area of impact. The staining that results is termed impact spatter and is characterized by a number of different sized blood stains on surrounding surfaces. The greater the force that is applied the smaller the stains tend to appear. If stains are projected in a perpendicular direction onto a surface they will appear circular. If there is an angle less than 90°, the stains become elliptical in shape and may have a characteristic tail, having the appearance of an exclamation mark (Figure 23.8). By careful measurement and the application of some simple mathematics, it is possible to determine the angle of incidence with the surface and thus the trajectory that the drop of blood would have made. By measuring a number of different stains it can be possible to locate an area where the impact occurred.

The force made by the discharge of a firearm can create bloodstains so small they are termed misting. Such staining will travel forwards as well as backwards towards the weapon if it is in close enough proximity to the wound.

Coughing or sneezing may create patterns similar to impact spatter if an individual has blood within their airways. It may be possible to see some alteration of the staining because of the mucus content of such stains but care needs to be taken in interpretation.

Cast-off

Cast-off is formed when an item bearing blood staining is moved through the air with sufficient

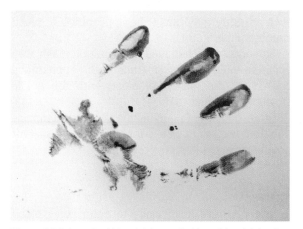

Figure 23.7 A contact bloodstain created by a bloodstained hand touching a wall.

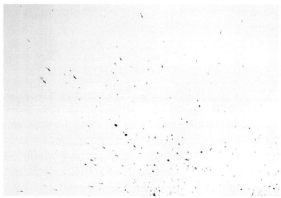

Figure 23.8 A typical impact spatter pattern. The source of wet blood was located at the centre of the bottom edge of the picture.

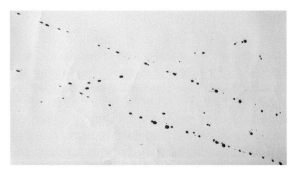

Figure 23.9 Cast-off blood patterns created when a baseball bat wet with blood was swung through the air.

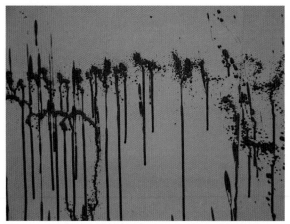

Figure 23.10 Projected blood pattern: arterial spurt/gush.

force to drive blood from its surface. For example, if an individual is repeatedly beaten with a baseball bat, blood may gather on the face of the bat each time it is raised and lowered, and this blood may be driven off by centrifugal forces. Such staining is often in a line, hence the common term 'in-line' cast-off (Figure 23.9). Owing to the movement of the end of such a weapon, the staining can form a figure of eight pattern. Items such as knives and fists can also produce cast-off.

Arterial spurting

When an artery is damaged (e.g. by a knife or blunt impact), blood is projected under high pressure, which does not happen with venous bleeding (the venous system being a low-pressure system). If the injury is exposed, blood can be projected over some distance, landing on adjacent surfaces. As a result of the quantity of blood being expelled from the body, such staining can be very heavy and will form a very characteristic pattern of large stains and runs. There may also be a wave-like pattern to the stains because the pressure with which the blood is forced from the body reflects the pumping action of the heart (Figure 23.10).

Physically altered blood stains

Bloodstains can be physically altered over time or by the addition of other body fluids. This may mean that the blood/admixture does not have the expected appearance, or have the same physical properties as whole blood. On occasion, injuries can be inflicted following a gap in time after an initial assault and blood may have begun to clot. Subsequent blows can result in unusual stains being observed. These may be an admixture of blood and mucus/saliva if

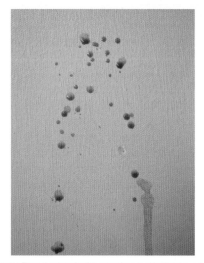

Figure 23.11 Blood mixed with another body fluid projected onto a wall. Note the dilute appearance.

injuries are to the facial area, or other body fluids such as urine may affect the appearance of blood staining (Figure 23.11).

Someone who has bled into their stomach may vomit so-called 'coffee grounds' – the appearance caused by the mixing of blood with the acidic stomach contents.

Other body fluids may mimic blood; decomposition fluid is often mistaken for evidence of a violent assault where none has occurred.

Luminol

If attempts have been made to clean away blood staining, the scientist can use chemical means to visualize staining that may have been present prior

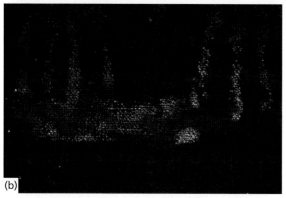

Figure 23.12 (a) A section of carpet with no blood staining visible. (b) The same section treated with luminol, revealing superimposed hand and footwear marks.

to those efforts. The use of luminol, a highly sensitive chemiluminescent compound can help the scientist visualize where blood staining had been present before any such cleaning efforts. It should be noted that the carrier for this chemical is primarily water so its use should be one of the final actions at a scene (Figure 23.12).

■ Damage

When items are broken, it can be possible, by visual and microscopic examination, to tell whether or not two or more items are fragments of one original item; for example, the two broken halves of a plate. This is achieved by comparing both gross features as well as finer details. The more points of comparison that can be made, the stronger the opinion that can be offered.

By examining the edges and fibre damage to clothing items that have been torn or cut, it may be possible to comment on what type of damage

actually occurred as in many cases where allegation of tearing occur, a cut has been used to start a tear. It is also possible to comment on how recently damage may have occurred.

Using controlled tests and reconstructions, it is also possible to comment on whether or not a specific item or action caused an area of damage.

■ Fingerprints

Fingerprints are formed within the womb at approximately 12 weeks of gestation and apart from damage by environmental factors, do not alter during one's lifetime. There is some debate as to the purpose of these ridges with support for the notion that the presence of fingerprints leads to an increase in grip and/or enhances the sensitivity for the perception of texture. The overall nature of a fingerprint can be described as loops, whorls or arches, describing the overall appearance of the ridges when taken together. On a smaller scale the ridges themselves form the next level of detail within the fingerprint; they can terminate or can divide into two. These characteristics enable particular patterns to be formed that are termed ridge ending, bifurcation, short ridge, spur, dot, bridge, lake or delta. Furthermore, the sweat glands on the ridges themselves give an additional area for comparison should this be required.

As there are sweat glands within the ridges, an impression of these secretions can be left as a fingerprint on a surface (latent marks). Such marks usually comprise a mixture of water-soluble and fat-soluble compounds. As the fingerprint is made up of compounds from the body, their chemical composition can reveal, for example, that someone is a smoker or drug user. It is often necessary to use specialized light or chemical enhancement on fingerprints so that all available parts of the mark can be seen. Different wavelengths of light and specialized chemicals are used to enhance the different compounds within the fingerprint (Figure 23.13).

Fingerprints may also be left (patent marks) if there is a contaminant such as ink, blood or paint – for example on the finger before it makes contact with a surface. Another way of leaving a fingerprint is to make an impression into a surface, such as one coated with grease or blood (Figure 23.14).

It is the theory that fingerprints are unique to each person that enabled them to become one of the primary methods by which identifications of

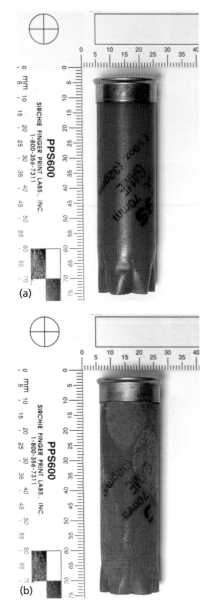

Figure 23.13 A fired shotgun cartridge: **(a)** untreated, and **(b)** treated with cyanoacrylate (superglue) fumes, revealing finger marks.

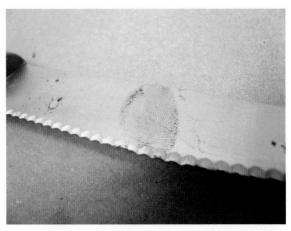

Figure 23.14 A finger mark in blood left on the blade of a knife. The finger was wet with blood prior to touching the blade.

suspected offenders were made. Fingerprints have been used for many years to identify individuals and, for example, have been known to confirm identity by the Chinese in the third century.

Fingerprints were traditionally recorded from an individual by coating their fingers with black ink and rolling them onto a card form. A record of the palm is now also taken. This ensures that all available detail is recorded. While this method is still the main way by which fingerprints are recorded,

scanning machinery is more commonly being used and as technology improves, will supersede the ink-based method.

Databases of fingerprints are held on a card-based system using the 'Tenprint' forms used to take inked fingerprints (Figure 23.15). In recent years each individual's ridge detail characteristics have also been loaded onto computer-based searchable databases. In the UK this was initially NAFIS (the National Automated Fingerprint Identification System) but this only held data from England and Wales. IDENT1 now combines data from England, Scotland and Wales allowing the search of some 6.5 million records against marks (including palm marks).

■ Footwear

Footwear marks

When people wearing footwear come into contact with a surface they often leave an impression. The extent to which this occurs may depend on many factors, such as how dirty the sole of the shoe is or the floor surface itself. The resulting footwear impression can be photographed, lifted using a variety of media or it can be recovered whole (marks on paper for example) and submitted to a laboratory for a suitable method of enhancement.

There are many different methods of enhancing footwear marks, some of which are used in the enhancement of fingerprints. Often photographing under controlled lighting conditions or the addition of specialist light sources can improve the detail

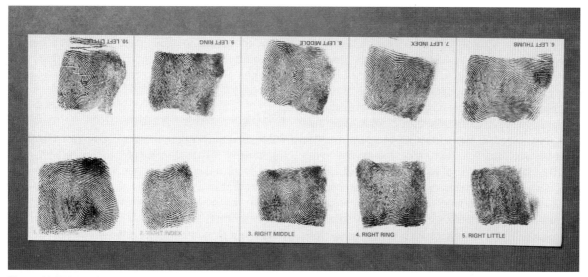

Figure 23.15 Inked fingerprints used as exemplars for comparison.

within a mark. When a mark warrants a more intensive examination (for example in a serious assault) the enhancement may be carried out using chemicals. For soil deposits potassium or ammonium thiocyanate, can be used which reacts with metallic ions in the soil. Marks in blood may be enhanced using Amido Black solution, which reacts with the proteins in the blood. There are many other methods of chemically enhancing marks.

To carry out a comparison of the recovered footwear marks with a suspect shoe, a test impression of the sole pattern is required. This can be prepared by brushing the sole with aluminium or black powder and then placing the shoe, sole side down, onto adhesive plastic. The plastic is then placed onto an acetate sheet and labelled to both identify the shoe but also ensure the correct orientation of the impression. This can then be laid over the photograph of the mark recovered from the crime scene and a comparison carried out.

When shoes are compared various details are considered. As the footwear is worn, general wear characteristics develop in the areas of the sole that come into contact with the ground. Damage detail in the form of cuts and nicks may also be formed in a random fashion on the sole of the footwear (Figure 23.16). Examination of footwear involves comparing the sole pattern, size and degree of wear in the mark found at a scene with a test mark made from an item of footwear. If damage detail is present in the scene mark, and it corresponds to damage in the test mark, it is sometimes possible

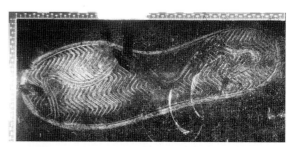

Figure 23.16 Recovered footwear mark showing damage features.

to state conclusively that a mark left at the scene was made by a particular shoe and by no other.

When determining the size of a sole pattern it is not usually possible to establish the exact size because of the many variations in sole patterns of a particular model throughout the population. It is preferable to estimate the size of a shoe from its sole pattern by giving a range of sizes that the shoe could be. This allows for variation in sole pattern between different moulds and manufacturers.

Footwear marks and skin

When contact is made with a person with a degree of force, by kicking or stamping, then skin deposits may be transferred to the inner surface of clothing while next to the skin. For this transfer to occur there must be a sufficient degree of force. Such deposits may require specialist light sources and chemical treatment to increase the contrast of the mark with the background and allow photographic recording.

When forceful contact is made directly to the surface of the skin, it is possible that patterned bruising may be left on the skin forming a mark characteristic of the surface that made the contact. In the instance of shoe marks the surface is often made up from regularly spaced components that may leave an impression matching the components. Alternatively, the pressure exerted during such a forceful contact may force blood in the surface of the skin into the gaps between the sole pattern components, leaving what is often referred to as a negative impression. The comparison of such marks with test impressions taken from the soles of shoes may be possible depending on which part of the body bears the impression. Forceful contact with skin that is close to a bone often carries a greater degree of detail. However as the surfaces are not flat they can often present a distorted impression that is difficult to compare. Photographic overlay techniques can be used to determine comparisons.

■ Trace evidence

This type of evidence can include anything that has been transferred by means such as contact with a surface or a person and this is the practical application of Locard's Exchange Principle. Often the material is very small and requires microscopic examination. Organic material such as pollen can be considered as trace evidence but more often it involves man-made materials such as glass, paint and fibres.

Glass

Glass is manufactured for use in construction by floating it on the surface of molten tin. This produces a glass that is very flat and can be mass produced. A mixture of silicon and various other minerals is added to a furnace and then poured onto the molten tin. Glass can also be moulded into containers or pressed into sheets with patterns. When glass is broken, small fragments are showered into the surrounding area. If a person were near to the breaking glass it would be expected that some of these fragments would transfer to the individual. These fragments will remain on the individual's clothing until such time that they fall off. The length of time that these glass fragments remain on clothing would depend on many factors, such as the type of clothing and the activity of the individual.

Glass fragments recovered in the laboratory or from assault victims and suspects can be compared with another source of glass by various means, including the measurement of their refractive index and their chemical composition.

Paint

There are many different types of paint for many different uses. If damage is caused to a painted surface then small flakes can be transfer red. In the case of road traffic collisions there may be a two-way transfer of material. Once recovered, paint evidence is examined microscopically to identify it and whether it is made up from different layers of paint. Each type of paint may be discriminated by its colour, texture and composition. Various light sources may be used to distinguish different types of paint or the components can be identified using chemical tests and analytical techniques such as chromatography and spectrophotometry.

In cases where there are multiple layers of paint in a sample, it may be possible to state that the evidential sample, came from a suspect car; however, often it is used as corroborative evidence in a case. In the case of graffiti cases it is possible to recover microscopic particles of aerosolized paints in colours that match the colours used in a specific incident of vandalism.

Fibres

Clothing and soft furnishings are made in a wide array of fabrics that come from all manner of sources. Natural fibres, such as wool, cotton and linen have been used for centuries and they are often combined with man-made fibres to improve their versatility. Within the types of fibre used there may be many different dyes and other materials incorporated into them which give different properties to the finished garment. All of these characteristics enable the forensic fibre examiner to identify sources of fibres and compare them with fibres that have been transferred to other garments or furnishings. Identification of the fibres involves microscopic and analytical techniques and it is possible to use the results in tandem with the number and location of the recovered fibres to give an interpretation of the circumstances that caused the transfer to occur. For example, it may be possible to state in which seat of a car a suspect was sitting where their version of events does not fit the incident. It is sometimes possible to find an original source of a fibre that is prevalent in a case by going to manufacturers and obtaining details of the amount and geographic distribution of a particular product.

◼ Fire investigation

Fires are investigated by a wide range of professionals for a diverse range of objectives. An investigator appointed by an insurance company may wish to determine the cause to establish liability. The fire investigator will be concerned with determining the 'defect, act or omission' that led to the fire to improve fire prevention. The forensic scientist may be attempting to determine whether or not a criminal act has taken place and, if so, what evidence can be recovered from the scene to link to an offender or assist in the police inquiry. The forensic pathologist may be attempting to determine whether a body found within the fire scene had been assaulted or had died prior to the fire. On many occasions it may be appropriate for these parties to carry out a joint examination.

Regardless of these objectives, all the investigators will be interested in determining two principal facts: first, the origin (or seat) of the fire must be determined, and second a consideration of what may have started it (i.e. the 'where' and 'how'). It is vital to determine the origin and cause in that order. The more imprecise the area of origin then the more potential causes may have to be considered.

All fires require a combination of oxygen, fuel and heat. Oxygen is normally freely available in air and fuel is provided by almost any material given the right conditions. The heat, initially, is provided by a source of ignition, such as from a lit match, cigarette or heating appliance. Thereafter, the fire provides its own source of heat in a chain reaction.

Once ignited, a fire spreads through a number of mechanisms. These include radiation (or direct flame impingement), convection (the movement of hot air currents) and conduction (the transfer of heat energy through a material). Two types of fire are recognized: smouldering combustion and flaming combustion. Typical examples of smouldering combustion include a lit cigarette or a barbeque; a garden bonfire would be described as an example of flaming combustion.

Smouldering is a form of flameless combustion. Certain materials are prone to this when ignited. These are principally natural materials that produce a rigid char on combustion, such as cotton and cellulose-based materials (e.g. wood). Smouldering combustion can also be produced when the oxygen levels are reduced during burning, such as in a sealed room. Smouldering fires can, however, transform into flaming fires and vice versa. The rate of smouldering will vary depending on the nature of the materials involved. Due to the nature of smouldering fires, they can produce intense but quite localized burning patterns. This assists in distinguishing the burning patterns produced by flaming and smouldering fires.

Smouldering fires spread by direct contact and hence result in severe yet localized damage. In contrast flaming fires spread by a variety of mechanisms including direct flame impingement, radiation and convection. Flames and radiated heat can therefore ignite materials such as paper several feet away from the original fire. Hot gases rise from the flaming fire to ceiling height and then spread throughout a room or rooms. This layer of hot air and gases can reach temperatures of several hundred degrees centigrade. The heat from this layer radiates down from the ceiling and can ignite items well away from the original fire. By this mechanism, light shades and the tops of curtains can be ignited.

An understanding of these fundamental mechanisms is essential to correctly identify the origin of the fire and not be misled by false indications. For example, a fire in a typical domestic lounge will spread across the ceiling and may ignite the tops of the curtains. If these then fall to the floor, the casual observer might mistakenly infer a second seat of fire.

Although a fire may damage or destroy items of interest this is not inevitably the case. It may be possible, by careful observation and the use of excavating and reconstruction techniques, to determine the cause of a fire despite severe damage.

Several complementary methods are used to determine the origin of the fire. As a general rule, fires will tend to spread upwards and outwards. A good place to start, therefore, is by finding the lowest area of severe damage. Heat and flames are quite directional and will leave patterns of charring in some places and protected areas in others. All of these will assist in determining the origin of the fire.

The area of origin can be determined by scorch or char patterns, comparing the relative damage of similar items, the distortion or melting of metals and other heat- and time-related observations. It may sometimes be necessary to determine the cause, or probable cause, by a process of elimination.

Exposed surfaces can become charred during a fire or smoke may be deposited. Other surfaces may be protected from the effects of heat and smoke leaving 'cleaner', less damaged areas. These 'protected' areas enable the investigator to reconstruct items and establish their position and condition at the time of the fire.

Having established, with reasonable accuracy, the origin of the fire, it is then necessary to consider the potential causes. The presence of electrical or heating items needs to be established and may require further laboratory examination and testing for appliance malfunction or misuse. Consideration would also be given to the possible involvement of a discarded lit cigarette or a naked flame, such as from a match, lighter or candle. The presence of a severe, yet localized pattern of damage may be indicative of a smouldering fire, such as initiated by a lit cigarette.

There are some typical indications of a deliberate fire, such as multiple points of ignition, the use of a flammable liquid, a modified fuel load (e.g. the armchairs stacked on top of the sofa!) the presence of an incendiary device or timing mechanism. A deliberate act may also be inferred by indirect forensic evidence. The presence of a broken window at a point of entry, footwear or tool marks, a drop of blood or snagged fibres could all indicate a suspicious event.

In many respects a fire scene should be treated and investigated as a crime scene and the investigator should have a thorough awareness of a wide range of forensic techniques available for analysis and interpretation of findings.

■ Firearms

A firearm (see also Chapter 10) can be defined as 'a lethal barrelled weapon of any description from which any shot, bullet or missile can be discharged'. There are two main types of firearm: those with smooth-bore barrels, which usually fire groups of shot, and those with rifled barrels, which usually fire single bullets. Both of these types of weapon

rely upon the deflagration of a solid propellant to produce the gases that propel the projectile(s).

Air guns and air rifles form a separate group of weapons that rely upon compressed gas, such as air or carbon dioxide, to propel a projectile; however, most of these weapons, even low-power ones directed appropriately have the ability to cause lethal injury and can therefore be classed as firearms.

Shotguns

Shotguns, commonly used as sporting and farming weapons, are long-barrelled, smooth-bore firearms that are used to discharge cartridges that usually contain a number of shot. These guns may have single or double barrels, commonly 26–30 inches (66–76 cm) in length; the double-barrelled weapons are arranged either 'side by side' or 'over and under'. The length of the barrel makes handling and hiding shotguns difficult and so it is not uncommon for the barrels to be shortened for criminal activities. This shortening of the barrel has little impact on the effectiveness of the gun, especially over short to middle distances. A shotgun generally has an effective range of about 33–55 yards 30–50 m and, although it is unlikely to kill an individual at this range, it may well cause serious and painful injuries, and there is no doubt that shotguns can be devastating weapons.

The cartridges for shotguns consist of a metal base, or head, containing a central primer cap, supporting a cardboard or plastic tube containing the propellant charge and the shot, which is closed by a thin disc or a crimp at the end of the tube. The shot may be contained within a plastic wad or there may be discs of felt, cork or cardboard acting as wads above and below the shot. The plastic wads open into a petal-shape in flight and may themselves contribute to an injury, especially at close range (Figure 23.17).

Shotgun cartridges are designated according to the size of the individual shot contained within and can vary significantly in number depending on the shot size (typically 6–850 in number for a 12-bore cartridge). There are also cartridges that contain a single heavy projectile, commonly referred to as a 'slug'. The types of wound produced by a shotgun will be dependent on the calibre, shot size and distance at which the shotgun was discharged from the target.

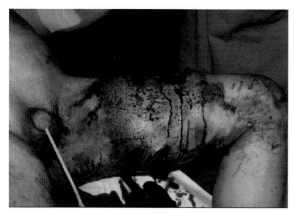

Figure 23.17 Upper thigh injury caused by close range discharge of shotgun to outer leg – bruising, swelling, tissue disruption and lacerations caused by discharge.

Rifled firearms

This group of firearms usually fire one bullet at a time through a barrel that has had a number of spiral grooves cut into the bore. The resultant projections, referred to as 'lands', engage with the bullet and impart gyroscopic spin that produces a more stable and accurate trajectory. Rifled weapons fall into two main groups: hand guns and rifles.

Revolvers and pistols are short-barrelled hand guns. Revolvers contain a rotating cylinder into which cartridges are manually loaded. Pistols, or semi-automatic hand guns, usually contain a magazine enclosing the cartridges located within the grip. The firearm is discharged when the cocked firing pin, or striker impacts on to the primer cup in the base of the cartridge by pulling the trigger. The main difference in the two types of firearm is the method of operation (Figure 23.18).

In the revolver, the cylinder rotates to align a new cartridge with the firing pin and the barrel, which is achieved by either pulling the trigger (double action) or by manually cocking the hammer and subsequently pulling the trigger (single action). The fired cartridge cases remain in the gun until they are manually unloaded.

In a pistol, the forces generated each time a cartridge is discharged are used to recycle the weapon, which involves extracting and ejecting the fired cartridge case, resetting the firing mechanism and loading a new cartridge from the magazine into the chamber. For semi-automatic weapons this occurs each time the trigger is pulled.

Rifles are long-barrelled weapons that are designed to accurately fire projectiles at targets at

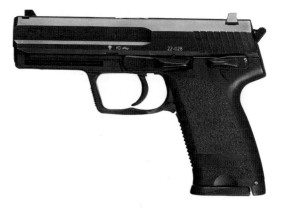

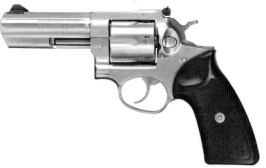

Figure 23.18 Revolvers and pistols. **Top:** Heckler & Koch USP (Universal Service Pistol), Germany, 1993. Calibre 9 mm parabellum. **Bottom:** Ruger GP–100, USA, 1987. Calibre .357 Magnum.

a much greater distance than revolvers or pistols. Rifles have been designed to use many different types of operating mechanism, ranging from single shot bolt-action rifles to fully automatic gas-operated assault rifles, some of which are capable of firing in excess of 700 cartridges per minute.

The cartridges for rifled weapons consist of a metal cartridge case, usually constructed of brass, steel or aluminium, a primer cup located in the base, propellant contained within the cartridge case and a single bullet fitted into the mouth of the case. The size and design of the cartridge is dependent on the weapon in which it is to be used and the desired ballistic performance of the projectile. Rifle cartridges usually have a larger case to bullet ratio, thus a larger propellant load, than hand gun cartridges. This is due to the fact that rifle cartridges are required to be effective over a much greater distance (up to 1.2 miles [2 km]) (Figure 23.19).

Bullet size (or calibre) and design are also very varied and are primarily concerned with ballistic performance and the ability of the projectile to transfer its kinetic energy to the target on impact. The formation of wounds is related to the transfer

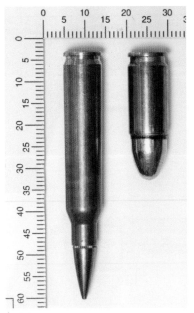

Figure 23.19 A 9 × 19 mm Luger semi-automatic pistol cartridge (top), and a NATO 5.56 × 45 mm automatic rifle cartridge (bottom).

of the energy of the bullet to the body tissues, and many types of ammunition are designed to result in specific wound patterns.

Forensic investigations

Forensic scientists are able to analyse the evidence that is generated at the scene of a crime involving the discharge of a firearm. This includes projectile trajectory and range–of-fire determinations. These aid in the reconstruction of shooting scenes, and the examination of fired bullets and cartridge cases recovered from a crime scene can be used to compare the marks observed with those produced from the discharge of a firearm suspected to have been used in the crime. This information can then be entered into a firearms database that allows the determination of links between scenes at which the same firearm may have been used and to establish gun crime trends, both nationally and internationally.

In addition, forensic scientists can use specialist equipment to determine the velocity and kinetic energy of a projectile in flight, which can be used to establish the ballistic performance of a projectile and the lethality of a weapon/ammunition combination. In the UK this is routinely used to determine if air weapons have lethal potential or are especially dangerous according to current UK firearms legislation.

■ Further information sources

Bär W, Brinkmann B, Budowle B et al. DNA Commission of the International Society for Forensic Genetics: guidelines for mitochondrial DNA typing. International Journal of Legal Medicine 2000; **113:** 193–196.

Gill P, Jeffreys AJ, Werrett DJ. Forensic application of DNA 'fingerprints', Nature 1985; **318:** 577–9.

Hedman J, Dalin E, Rasmusson B, Ansell R. Evaluation of amylase testing as a tool for saliva screening of crime scene trace swabs. Forensic Science International, Genetics 2010; [Epub ahead of print].

Jeffreys AJ, Wilson V, Thein SL. Individual-specific 'fingerprints' of human DNA. Nature 1985; **316:** 76–9.

Montani I, Comment S, Delémont O. The sampling of ignitable liquids on suspects' hands. Forensic Science International 2010; **194:** 115–24.

National DNA Database. http://www.npia.police.uk/en/8934.htm (accessed 24 November 2010).

Nicklas JA and Buel E (2003) Quantification of DNA in forensic samples, Analytical and Bioanalytical Chemistry, **376:** 1160–1167.

Syndercombe Court D. DNA Analysis – current practice, problems and futures. In: Gall J, Payne-James JJ (eds) Current Practice in Forensic Medicine. London: Wiley, 2011.

Virkler K, Lednev IK. Analysis of body fluids for forensic purposes: from laboratory testing to non-destructive rapid confirmatory identification at a crime scene. Forensic Sci Int 2009; **188:** 1–17.

Chapter 24

Allied forensic specialties

- Introduction
- Forensic ecology
- Forensic archaeology
- Forensic anthropology
- Forensic odontology
- Forensic photography
- Further information sources

Introduction

Forensic medicine and science are supported by, and to some extent include other medical, quasi-medical and scientific disciplines each of which may have a significant and often principal role in forensic casework. Investigators should be aware of the range of these disciplines and ensure that the skills and expertise of all appropriately trained practitioners and their specialties are used to their optimum extent. Examples of such specialties, some of which are referred to in earlier chapters are outlined below.

Forensic ecology

Forensic ecology is the use of environmental evidence types to assist in investigating crime, both outdoors and indoors. There are many specialities that may be used and not all are discussed in this text (such as soil and botanical analyses). The following provides an introduction to some of the most commonly encountered areas of forensic ecology: diatomology, palynology and entomology.

Diatomology

Diatoms are algae, microscopic unicellular plants, which can be found in saltwater, freshwater, soils and damp surfaces. They are very diverse with over 100 000 species known. They have a unique silica cell wall called a frustule which makes them very robust and allows them to withstand harsh conditions (Figure 24.1). As they are classed as algae, they rely on the sun for their energy and as such are found in well-lit surface layers of water. When

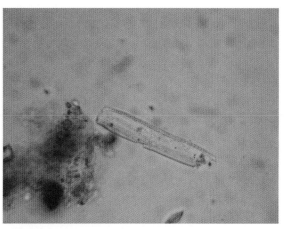

Figure 24.1 Diatom showing silicon frustule.

diatoms die, their skeletons sink to the bottom layers of water.

It is not always possible to determine whether drowning occured at a post-mortem examination when a body has been found in, or near, water. The presence or absence of diatoms within the body can assist in such an investigation. When water has been inhaled into the lungs (and this can be as much as 250 mL), any diatoms present may enter the bloodstream via the lung parenchyma. The heart continues to pump circulating diatoms around the body to all organs. The presence of diatoms within the body suggests that the person was alive when they entered the water and that drowning was the cause of death or played a significant part in the cause of death.

Diatoms cannot pass through the gastrointestinal tract wall and thus diatoms swallowed in food or in the process of drowning will not enter the bloodstream, and this again may provide additional information.

By extracting diatoms from organs that have been collected under the correct conditions to protect against contamination, the scientist can comment on whether or not drowning contributed to death. Caution must be used in the interpretation of diatoms and there remain considerable differences of opinion related to that interpretation (see also Chapter 16).

Forensic palynology

Forensic palynology uses analysis of pollen, spores and other microscopic particles. Pollen grains are produced by seed-bearing plants, flowering plants and cone-bearing non-flowering plants, while spores are produced by ferns, mosses, algae and fungi. Palynology also comprises the study of other microscopic entities such as insect and plant remains, particularly micro-charcoal (microscopic particles of charred plant material). Collectively these are referred to as palynomorphs.

Pollen is seasonally and geographically sensitive and may be dispersed by water, wind and insect activity throughout the year. It settles on surfaces in much the same way as dust and is invisible to the naked eye. In the same way that fibres are trace evidence and can be transferred from one surface to another through contact, pollen may be collected on shoes, clothing and tyres, for example, when in contact with soils and vegetation. In addition, airborne pollen collects in the nasal cavities as one breathes. An experienced palynologist can identify individual pollen grains and spores and reconstruct a habitat from a pollen assemblage of samples collected.

Pollen evidence can be used to:

■ link people, vehicles, and objects to a known scene or deposition site;
■ identify habitats or geographical locations relevant to police investigations;
■ prove or disprove alibis;
■ help determine the fate of an individual prior to death;
■ assist in determining the season and location in which an individual died;
■ help determine possible locations of a missing person by looking at the clothing of a suspected offender;
■ assist in determining the country of origin of illicit drugs.

Forensic entomology

Forensic entomology is the application of knowledge about insects to assist in legal investigations, the vast majority of which are suspicious deaths or murders. The most commonly encountered insects are blowflies, but other flies and beetles are often found. Blowflies are especially useful to the investigator as they are most often the first invaders of decomposing material. In warmer temperatures, blowflies can begin laying eggs on a body within a few hours of death. When temperatures are cooler, or if the body is concealed, such behaviour may be delayed or impeded.

In cases where a body is enclosed, for example within a container or in a grave, blowfly access may be prevented due to the physical size of the flies. Under these circumstances, other, smaller flies may be the first to commence egg–laying. Conversely, an infestation involving particular insects may be present when not expected, indicating a body has been moved since the infestation first occured.

Forensic entomology can also be used in cases of neglect, where fly eggs and larvae will develop in unhygienic settings. For example, if an individual is wearing a soiled nappy and this has not been changed for some time, this will be attractive to certain species of fly, and egg-laying can occur. As such, any stage of the life–cycle encountered provides very strong evidence and immediately indicates that there has been a period of neglect. It is highly important that such evidence is not disposed of simply due to its unpleasant nature but preserved for future examination.

Insect analysis can assist in providing information about:

- an estimated post-mortem interval (PMI);
- whether or not a body has been moved from one location to another;
- whether a body has been moved between a concealed and exposed environment;
- whether there has been abuse and neglect;
- whether there are public health issues.

Forensic archaeology

Forensic archaeology is concerned with the location, recovery and interpretation of buried evidence, mostly human remains, and associated items that may be within the grave, as well as buried items such as stolen goods, firearms and drugs. Forensic archaeologists are commonly involved in searching for the clandestine burials of missing persons, the interpretation of human remains accidentally found during building operations, skeletal fragments discovered on the surface, or alleged grave sites and ground disturbances requiring investigation.

The forensic archaeologist will use their knowledge of land surface characteristics to determine whether or not there could be a burial site. They could be looking for differences in vegetation growth or abundance, factors that are sometimes only apparent at certain times of year.

Once an area has been identified as a possible burial site, other techniques can be deployed to assist the scientist. One common technique is ground penetrating radar (GPR), which looks for areas that differ from the surroundings under the surface. This could be as innocuous as a deposit of sand within a background of gravel or could be buried remains. Resistivity is used to test areas of ground for electrical resistance. If one area differs from another, further investigation may be warranted. Before undertaking excavation, the archaeologist may wish to use a cadaver dog and vent selected areas using probes to enable odours to be detected by the dog, if possible. Only at that point

will excavation commence as, in many cases, very large areas may have to be searched.

In all situations it is important for maximum evidence to be retained, that any 'finds' need to be left *in situ*. Graves are, in effect, miniature crime scenes and anything within the boundary has been left by the offender. Great care needs to be taken not to disturb the integrity of graves as it could affect the meaning of evidential finds. There are clearly cultural, religious, legal and other factors that may affect how such investigations can proceed.

Forensic anthropology

Anthropology is the study of the biological and cultural aspects of humans. A scientific background including the understanding of the morphology of the skeleton and the reconstruction of life histories led to the development of forensic anthropology, initially identifying human remains in the medicolegal setting. This has expanded considerably and now forensic anthropologists are concerned with all aspects of identity, both in the living and the dead. A common question to be addressed is whether or not bones that are found are human or animal. This can have major importance in terms of cost and personnel if a crime can be ruled out at an early stage.

Once bones have been identified as human, the forensic anthropologist will attempt to establish a biological profile of the individual, or individuals. Depending on the completeness of the remains, this may include sex, age at death, height and possible ethnicity. This can be applied to the recently deceased, decomposed remains, skeletal and burnt remains.

Age determination in the living is a need that has expanded in recent years. This is because of an increasing group of individuals who, for a variety of reasons, do not have a known age. This may have major implications as to how that individual is treated in different settings (e.g. asylum applications, criminal cases, care proceedings). The system may be abused by the individual or, to some extent, the authorities may abuse the individual, in both cases because there may be a perception that allotting a person a specific age can benefit whoever is requesting it. Age estimation is a complex area and the anthropologist is well placed to be part of a team that may include physicians, odontologists and radiologists who may all contribute to estimating age as accurately as possible (see Chapter 4, p. 35).

■ Forensic odontology

Forensic odontology is practised by those initially trained as dentists. Forensic odontologists apply their dental skills in the forensic setting and are key players in human identification (of the living and deceased), ageing (of the living and the deceased) and in the identification and interpretation of bite marks (see Chapter 4, p. 35).

Identification by odontological means can be a testing and complex process, as the determination of the anatomy and structure of oral components may be hampered by substantial tissue damage, particularly in the case of mass disaster. Access to teeth (if present) may be hampered by soft tissues damage, rigor mortis or burn damage. Odontologists attempt to identify dental patterns and features and compare these either with known ante-mortem information about the individual or relate such information to known published population data.

Radiological information is widely used to allow comparisons to be made when attempting to identify an unknown body. A dental autopsy follows the method of dental examination in the living so that unique features such as dental restorations can properly be compared with the ante-mortem data. Even with DNA analysis available, identification using odontological techniques remains a cost-effective and expeditious means of establishing identity and remains the key technique considered first in mass disaster identification.

The analysis and interpretation of bite marks remains a contentious and (like many aspects of forensic medicine) an under-researched field. The main questions to be answered with regard to a possible bite mark in the forensic setting are: is it a biting injury and is it human? If the answer to these is yes, the odontologist may be able to identify who has caused the bite. The determination of who has caused the bite is generally a comparative one, frequently using a variety of superimposition techniques. If a suspect is available, then, with consent, a cast is made of impressions of their dentition. A 1:1 image of the impression made (generally using transparent sheeting) is superimposed with a 1:1 overlay of the suspect's dentition for comparison. The transparent overlay remains the most widely used technique of bite mark analysis and comparison, although more sophisticated techniques are being developed.

A forensic odontologist should always be asked to make an assessment where a bite mark is suspected in criminal matters.

■ Forensic photography

Forensic photography is a very specialized area embracing a range of imaging techniques that allow best presentation of visually relevant evidence in an appropriate format. Forensic photographic techniques can include the use of ultraviolet, infrared and polarized light photography, which can be used to enhance or identify items or injuries of interest. A key element of forensic photography is data management of images and how these are stored and reproduced. Forensic practitioners need to work closely with forensic photographers to ensure that the relevance of images taken is best suited to the requirements of the evidential and court process. Poor-quality imaging is now unacceptable and it is appropriate that those most skilled in producing robust evidence are used to provide it for courts and other agencies.

■ Further information sources

Byers ST. *Introduction to Forensic Anthropology: a Textbook*. London: Pearson Education, 2001.

Black S, Aggrawal A, Payne–James JJ. Age Estimation in the Living: a Practitioner's Guide. London: Wiley, 2010.

Cameron, J., Ruddick, R. and Grant, J. (1973) Ultraviolet photography in medicine. *Forensic Photography* (2001), **2:** 9–12.

Clement JG. Odontology (bitemarks, bruising and other injuries to skin). In: Siegal JA, Saukko PJ, Knupfer GC (eds) *Encyclopedia of Forensic Sciences*. London: Academic Press, 2000; 1129–37.

Clement JG. Role of and techniques in forensic odontology. In: Payne-James J, Busuttil A and Smock W, eds. *Forensic Medicine: Clinical and Pathological Aspects*. London: Greenwick Medical Media, 2003; 689–703.

Clement JG and Hill AJ. Odontology: overview. In: Payne-James J, Byard RW, Corey T, Henderson C (eds) *Encyclopedia of Forensic and Legal Medicine*. Oxford: Elsevier Academic Press, 2005; 386–95.

Dirkmaat DC, Cabo LL, Ousley SD, Symes SA. New perspectives in forensic anthropology. *American Journal of Physical Anthropology* 2008; Suppl 47: 33–52.

Faegri K, Ivesen J. *Textbook of Pollen Analysis.* 4ᵗʰ edn (revised) London: Wiley 1992.

Greenberg B. *Entomology and the Law: Flies and Forensic Indicators.* Cambridge, CUP, 2005.

Haglund WD, Sorg MH. *Forensic Taphonomy: the Postmortem Fate of Human Remains.* Boca Raton, FL: CRC Press, 1997.

Lassler AJ, Warnick AJ, Berman GM Three-dimensional comparative analysis of bitemarks. *Journal of Forensic Science* 2009; 54: 658–60.

Martin-de-las-Heras S, Tafur D. Comparison of simulated human dermal bitemarks possessing three-dimensional attributes to suspected biters using a proprietary three-dimensional comparison. *Forensic Science International* 2009; **190:** 33–37.

Marsh N. The photography of injuries. In: Gall J, Payne-James JJ (eds) *Current Practice in Forensic Medicine.* London: Wiley, 2011.

Marshall RJ. Infrared and ultraviolet reflectance measurements as an aid to the diagnosis of pigmented lesions of skin. *Journal of Audiovisual Media in Medicine* 1981; **4:** 11–14

Miller RG, Bush PJ, Dorion RBJ, Bush MA. Uniqueness of the dentition as impresses human skin: a cadaver model. *Journal of Forensic Science* 2009; **54:** 909–14.

Round FE, Crawford RM, Mann DG. *Diatoms: Biology and Morphology of the Genera.* Cambridge, CUP, 1990.

Rowan P, Hill M, Gresham GA, Goodall E, Moore T. The use of infrared aided photography in identification of sites of bruises after evidence of the bruise is absent to the naked eye. *Journal of Forensic and Legal Medicine* 2010; **17:** 293–7.

Scheuer L, Black S. *Developmental Juvenile Osteology.* San Diego, CA: Academic Press, 2000.

West M, Billings J, Frair J. Ultraviolet photography: bite marks on human skin and suggested technique for the exposure and development of reflective ultraviolet photography. *Journal of Forensic Science* 1987; **32:** 1204–13.

West M, Frair J, Seal M. Ultraviolet photography of wounds on human skin. *Journal of Forensic Identification* 1989; **39:** 87–96.

West M, Barsley R, Hayne S. The first conviction using alternative light photography of trace wound patterns. *Journal of Forensic Identification* 1992; **42:** 517–22.

Appendix 1

Guidelines for an autopsy and exhumation

■ Guidelines

1 Where the death is definitely due to crime or if there is a possibility of crime (a suspicious death), the doctor should attend the scene (locus) before the body is moved in order to gain an understanding of the surroundings, blood distribution in relation to the body etc. Notes of attendance, of people present and of the observations should be made. Photographs should be taken of the scene in general, of the body in particular and of any other significant features; these are usually taken by the police.

2 The identity of the body should be confirmed to the doctor by a relative or by a police officer or other legal officer who either knows the deceased personally or who has had the body positively identified to them by a relative or by some other means (e.g. fingerprints).

3 If the remains are mummified, skeletalized, decomposed, burnt or otherwise disfigured to a point at which visual identification is impossible or uncertain, or if the identity is unknown, other methods of establishing the identity of the remains must be used, but the autopsy cannot be delayed while this is done.

4 In a suspicious death, if there can be no direct identification of the body, a police officer must confirm directly to the doctor that the body or the remains presented for autopsy are those that are the focus of the police inquiry.

5 In a suspicious death, the body should be examined with the clothing in place so that defects caused by trauma that may have damaged the body (stab wounds, gunshot injuries, etc.) can be identified. When removed, the clothing must be retained in new, clean bags that are sealed and carefully labelled for later forensic science examination.

6 In suspicious deaths or if there are any unusual features, the body should be photographed clothed and then unclothed and then any injuries or other abnormalities should be photographed in closer detail.

7 X-rays are advisable in victims of gunshot wounds and explosions and where there is a possibility of retained metal fragments, and are mandatory in all suspicious deaths in children.

8 The surface of the body should be examined for the presence of trace evidence: fibres, hair, blood, saliva, semen, etc. This examination may be performed by police officers or by forensic scientists, often with the assistance of the pathologist. Where samples are to be removed from the body itself as opposed to the surface of the body – fingernail clippings, head and pubic hair, anal and genital swabs – these should be taken by the pathologist.

9 Forensic scientists may also wish to examine the body using specialist techniques, and the pathologist must be aware of their needs and allow them access at appropriate times.

10 Careful documentation of the external features of injuries or abnormalities, their position, size,

shape and type, is often the most important aspect of a forensic examination and often has much greater value in understanding and in reconstructing the circumstances of injury than the internal dissection of any wound tracks or of damaged internal organs. Patience is required to perform this examination with care and this part of an examination should not be rushed.

11 The internal examination must fulfil two requirements: to identify and document injuries and to identify and document natural disease. The former may involve the examination of wound tracks caused by knives, bullets or other penetrating objects. It may also involve determining the extent and depth of bruising on the body by reflecting the skin from all of the body surfaces and identifying and describing areas of trauma to the internal organs.

12 A complete internal examination of all three body cavities, with dissection of all of the body organs, must be performed to identify any underlying natural disease.

13 Samples of blood (for blood grouping, DNA analysis, toxicology) and urine (for toxicology) will be routinely requested by the police. Blood should be collected from a large limb vein, preferably the femoral vein, and urine should be collected, preferably using a clean syringe, through the fundus of the bladder. All samples should be collected into clean containers, which are sealed and labelled in the presence of the pathologist. Care must be taken to ensure that the correct preservative is added; if in doubt, ask a forensic scientist for advice.

14 When poisoning is suspected, other samples, including stomach contents, intestinal contents, samples of organs including liver, kidney, lung and brain, may be requested. The storage, preservation and handling of these specimens will depend upon the suspected poison. Specialist advice must be obtained or the samples may be useless.

15 Tissue samples should be retained in formalin for microscopic examination. If there is any doubt, whole organs – brain and heart in particular – should be retained for specialist examination.

16 In all of these aspects of the examination, careful notes must be kept and augmented by drawings and diagrams if necessary. These notes, drawings and diagrams will form the basis for the report.

■ The autopsy

Detailed guidance on the internal examination can be found in textbooks such as 'The Hospital Autopsy' (see 'Further reading' at the end of Chapter 3), but a short summary of the basic techniques is given below.

1 An incision is made from the larynx to the pubis. The upper margin may be extended on each side of the neck to form a 'Y' incision. The extra exposure this brings is useful in cases of neck injury or in children.

2 The skin on the front of the chest and abdomen is reflected laterally and the anterior abdominal wall is opened, with care taken not to damage the intestines. The intestines are removed by cutting through the third part of the duodenum as it emerges from the retroperitoneum and then dissecting the small and large bowel from the mesentery.

3 The ribs are sawn through in a line from the lateral costal margin to the inner clavicle and the front of the chest is removed.

4 The tongue and pharynx are mobilized by passing a knife around the floor of the mouth close to the mandible. These are then removed downward as the neck structures are dissected off the cervical spine.

5 The axillary vessels are divided at the clavicles, and the oesophagus and the aorta are dissected from the thoracic spine as the tongue continues to be pulled forwards and downwards.

6 The lateral and posterior attachments of the diaphragm are cut through close to the chest cavity wall and then the aorta is dissected off the lower thoracic and lumbar spine.

7 Finally, the iliac vessels and the ureters can be bisected at the level of the pelvic rim and the organs will then be free of the body and can be taken to a table for dissection.

8 The pelvic organs are examined in situ or they can be removed from the pelvis for examination.

9 The scalp is incised coronally and the flaps reflected forwards and backwards. The skull-cap is carefully sawn through and removed, leaving the dura intact. This is then incised and the brain removed by gentle traction of the frontal lobes while cutting through the cranial nerves, the tentorium and the upper spinal cord.

10 The organs are dissected in a good light with adequate water to maintain an essentially

blood-free area. Although every pathologist has his or her own order of dissection, a novice would do well to stick to the following order so that nothing is omitted: tongue, carotid arteries, oesophagus, larynx, trachea, thyroid, lungs, great vessels, heart, stomach, intestines, adrenals, kidneys, spleen, pancreas, gall bladder and bile ducts, liver, bladder, uterus and ovaries or testes and finally the brain.

11 Samples should be taken for toxicology and histology as necessary.

12 Make detailed notes at the time of your examination and write your report as soon as possible, even if you cannot complete it because further tests are being performed.

13 All reports should include all of the positive findings and all of the relevant negative findings, because in court the absence of a comment may be taken to mean that it was not examined or specifically looked for and, if a hearing or trial is delayed for many months or years, it would not be credible to state that specific details of this examination can be remembered with clarity.

14 The conclusions should be concise and address all of the relevant issues concerning the death of the individual. A conclusion about the cause of death will be reached in most cases, but in some it is acceptable to give a differential list of causes from which the court may choose.

Appendix 2

Widmark's formula

During the early part of this century, E.M.P. Widmark, a Swedish physician did much of the foundational research regarding alcohol pharmacokinetics in the human body. In addition, he developed an algebraic equation allowing one to estimate any one of six variables given the other five. Typically, we are interested in determining either the amount of alcohol consumed by an individual or the associated blood alcohol concentration (BAC) given the values of the other variables. According to Widmark's equation, the amount of alcohol consumed (A) is a function of these several variables:

From Equation 1
$$N = f(W, r, C_t, \beta, t, z)$$

where:
N = amount consumed
W = body weight
r = the volume of distribution (a constant)
C_t = blood alcohol concentration (BAC)
β = the alcohol elimination rate
t = time since the first drink
z = the fluid ounces of alcohol per drink

Widmark's equation relates these variables according to:

Equation 2
$$N = \frac{Wr(C_t + \beta t)}{0.8z}$$

where:
N = the number of drinks consumed
W = body weight in ounces

r = volume of distribution (a constant relating the distribution of water in the body in L/Kg)
C_t = the blood alcohol concentration (BAC) in Kg/L
β = the alcohol elimination rate in Kg/L/hr
t = time since the first drink in hours
z = the fluid ounces of alcohol per drink
0.8 = the density of ethanol (0.8 oz per fluid ounce)

Worked example

Assume that we are interested in determining the amount of alcohol consumed (number of drinks) given certain information. The information we are given includes: a male weighing 185 lb, r = 0.68 L/kg, Ct = 0.15 g/100 ml, β = 0.015 g/100 ml/h, t = 5 h, and drinking 12 fl oz beers with 4% alcohol by volume. We introduce this information into Equation 2 according to:

$$N = \frac{(180\,\text{lb})(16\,\text{oz/lb})(0.68\,\text{L/kg})(0.0015\,\text{kg/L} + (0.00015\,\text{kg/L/h})(5\,\text{h}))}{(0.8)(0.48\,\text{fl oz/drink})}$$

Note that we had to convert the 0.15 g/100 ml and the 0.015 g/100 ml/h to Kg/L which simply amounts to moving the decimal two places to the left. Solving for A we find:

$$N = \frac{1958.4(0.00225)}{0.384} = 11.5 \text{ drinks}$$

Appendix 3

Diagnosing poisoning – Carbon monoxide. Health Protection Agency guidelines

Patient presenting with:
Headache, nausea/vomiting, drowsiness, dizziness, dyspnoea, chest pain
COULD THIS BE A CASE OF CO POISONING? 1

Ask the patient:
- Do you feel better away from your house or place of work?
- Is anybody else in your family or house experiencing the same symptoms as you?
- Have you recently had a heating or cooking appliance installed?
- Have all gas, coke/coal, wood or oil fired appliances, eg, cookers, fires, boilers at your home been serviced within the last year?
- Do you ever use your oven or gas stove for heating purposes as well as for cooking?
- Has there been any change in ventilation in your home recently, eg, fitting double glazing?
- Have you noticed any sooty stains around appliances or an increase in condensation?
- Does your work involve possible exposure to smoke, fumes or motor vehicle exhaust?
- Is your home detached, semi-detached, terraced, flat, bedsit or hostel? 2

You are suspicious: Could this be a case of CO poisoning?

You are confident: This is **NOT** a case of CO poisoning

Action to take: GP - General Practice ED - Emergency Department
1 **Test for CO**
   GP - breath test for exhaled CO if device is available. (Note: Only indicates recent exposure; interpretation difficult in smokers. For interpretation of results see TOXBASE).
   ED - heparinized venous blood sample for COHb estimation. For interpretation of results see TOXBASE and contact the National Poisons Information Service (NPIS).
2 **Management - Commence oxygen therapy**
   GP - follow advice on TOXBASE; refer to ED if required.
   ED - follow advice on TOXBASE. Contact NPIS for severe poisoning. (See CMO/CNO letter November 2008: www.dh.gov.uk/cmo).
3 **Protect your patient and others** - Contact your local Health Protection Unit (HPU). They will co-ordinate services for your patient and provide further CO guidance. Telephone gas, oil or solid fuel helpline (see Notes).
4 **DO NOT** allow patient home without a warning NOT to use the suspect appliances.
5 **Follow up**
   GP - note that symptoms may persist or develop later.
   ED - advise patient to see GP for follow-up. Note this advice in discharge letter. 3

If patient does not improve
- Contact NPIS for advice.
- Contact local HPU for advice.
- Reconsider diagnosis. 4

Notes

Box 1 Carbon monoxide is a mimic

Carbon monoxide poisoning is notorious for simulating other more common conditions, including flu-like illnesses, migraine, food-poisoning, tension headaches and depression.

Headache is the commonest symptom - think CO!

© Health Protection Agency 2009. Reproduced with permission.

Box 2 Carbon monoxide sources are multiple

The source of CO may be in the home, in the car due to a leaking exhaust system, or in the workplace. Gas, oil, coal, coke and wood heating appliances are the commonest sources in the home.

Malfunctioning heating appliances may be indicated by there being yellow rather than blue flames (if it is not a 'decorative flame' fire) and by the deposition of soot on radiants or on the wall adjacent to the fire. There may be more than one source of carbon monoxide.

Poisoning is not limited to those from lower income groups. Carbon monoxide can leak into a semidetached or terraced house/flat from neighbouring premises. It is unlikely that a patient will know about servicing of appliances at his/her workplace, but it is worth asking about the sort of heating devices in use.

It is also worth asking: "Have you recently started to re-use heating appliances/boilers after the summer break/during an unexpected cold spell?"

Box 3 Stopping further exposure is essential

Preventing further exposure is the most important thing you can do. Breath tests and blood samples may prove inconclusive some hours after exposure has ended: CO levels in the blood decline with a half-life of about 6 hours. Note that a normal concentration of carboxyhaemoglobin (COHb) does not disprove CO poisoning unless the sample has been taken soon after exposure ended. A heparinized venous blood sample should however, always be taken and sent to the local Clinical Chemistry Laboratory for analysis. *For interpretation of results and detailed advice on CO poisoning see TOXBASE and call NPIS.*

If you strongly suspect CO poisoning do not wait for the result of the analysis before taking the other steps listed in Box 3. Contacting the gas (**0800 111999**), oil (**0845 6585080**) or solid fuel (**0845 6014406**) safety services is essential. Contacting your local HPU is essential as they will co-ordinate Environmental Health, Safety, Social and other services to protect your patient and others. Follow-up is important as further consequences of chronic exposure to CO may be delayed, or mild symptoms may persist, multiply or intensify. Recommend the purchase of an audible carbon monoxide alarm for installation in the home.

Index

Index